Principles and Foundations of Health Promotion and Education

Randall R. Cottrell, D.Ed., CHES
University of Cincinnati

James T. Girvan, Ph.D., M.P.H., CHES
Idaho State University

James F. McKenzie, Ph.D., M.P.H.
Ball State University

Allyn and Bacon

Boston ▪ London ▪ Toronto ▪ Sydney ▪ Tokyo ▪ Singapore

Editor-in-Chief: *Paul A. Smith*
Publisher: *Joseph E. Burns*
Series Editorial Assistant: *Sara Sherlock*
Marketing Manager: *Rick Muhr*
Composition and Prepress Buyer: *Linda Cox*
Manufacturing Buyer: *Megan Cochran*
Cover Administrator: *Jenny Hart*
Editorial-Production Service: *Shepherd, Inc.*
Photo Researcher: *Helane Manditch-Prottas*

Copyright © 1999 by Allyn & Bacon
A Viacom Company
Needham Heights, Massachusetts 02494

Internet: www.abacon.com
America Online: keyword:College Online

Library of Congress Cataloging-in-Publication Data

Cottrell, Randall R.
   Principles and foundations of health promotion and education /
Randall R. Cottrell, James T. Girvan, James F. McKenzie.
     p. cm.
   Includes bibliographical references and index.
   ISBN 0-205-27365-3 (alk. paper)
   1. Health education. 2. Health promotion. I. Girvan, James T.,
1946–   . II. McKenzie, James F., 1948–   . III. Title.
RA440.5.C685 1999
613—dc21
                                       98-38235
                                           CIP

Printed in the United States of America

10 9 8 7 6 5 4 3 2 1   03 02 01 00 99 98

CONTENTS

FOREWORD

Health education is an emerging profession, and the authors of this text have made a significant contribution to that emergence. Three audiences should find the text extremely helpful. For students undecided about a major or minor in health education, the text presents an excellent opportunity to make an informed decision. For the undergraduate or graduate health education major, the text is a gold mine of information not only about health education but about the profession of health education. Finally, the text is an invaluable resource for those involved in the professional preparation of health educators. It provides an informative, comprehensive, and insightful perspective for those in the field. It includes the most up-to-date information on health education and health promotion, as well as information on how the field evolved, where it is headed, and what role students can play in shaping its future.

Principles and Foundations of Health Promotion and Education is well organized. From the preface, which provides a clear overview of the text, to the concluding chapter, focusing on future trends, the text integrates theory and practice, knowledge and application, skill development and professional identity, and direction. This is accomplished by clear objectives in each chapter, augmented by excellent "Practitioner's Perspective" boxes throughout, a concise summary, review questions, and a list of activities designed to extend students' knowledge by analyzing and synthesizing the information. This is the case regardless of whether students read the chapter on history or the one on securing the most up-to-date information available on the Internet and World Wide Web.

From a pragmatic perspective, one of the most beneficial aspects of *Principles and Foundations of Health Promotion and Education* is that it introduces students to and describes the different and interesting settings in which health educators practice and the job responsibilities and opportunities within each of those settings. Appropriately noted in the last chapter is the notion of change as a constant and the importance of adapting to change.

The field of health education and promotion is rapidly changing, and all indications are that it will continue to do so at an even accelerated rate as we approach and enter the new millennium. Opportunities have never been greater, and the future has never looked brighter. This text captures this concept and affords readers the opportunity to play an important role in a career which provides personal fulfillment through enhancing the equality of life for all people. Bon voyage.

Thomas W. O'Rourke, Ph.D., M.P.H. CHES
Department of Community Health and College of Medicine
University of Illinois at Urbana—Champaign

PREFACE

Many students enter the field of health promotion and education knowing only that they are interested in health and wish to help others improve their health status. Typically, students' interest in health promotion and education is derived from their own desire to live a healthy lifestyle and not from an in-depth understanding of the historical, theoretical, and philosophical foundations of this emerging profession. Other than perhaps a high school health education teacher, many students do not know any health promotion and education practitioners. In fact, most beginning students are unaware of employment opportunities, the skills needed to practice health education, and what it would be like to work in a given health education setting.

This book is written for such students. The contents will be of value to students who are undecided if health education is the major they want to pursue, as well as for new health education majors who need information about what health education is and where health educators can be employed. The book is designed for use in an entry-level health education course in which the major goal is to introduce students to health promotion and education. In addition, it may have value in introducing new health education graduate students, who have undergraduate degrees in fields other than health education, to the emerging profession of health promotion and education.

Chapter 1, "A Background for the Profession," provides an overview of health promotion and education and sets the stage for the remaining chapters. Chapter 2, "The History of Health and Health Education," examines the history of health and health care, as well as the history of health promotion and education. This chapter was written to help students understand the tremendous advancements that have been made in keeping people healthy, and it provides perspective on the role of health promotion and education in that effort. One cannot appreciate the present without understanding the past. Chapters 3, 4, and 5 provide what might best be called the basic foundations. All professions, such as law, medicine, business, and teacher education, must provide students with information related to the philosophy, theory, and ethics inherent in the field.

Chapter 6, "The Health Educator: Roles, Responsibilities, Certifications, Advanced Study," is designed to acquaint new students with the skills that are needed to practice in the field of health promotion and education. It also explains the certification process to students and encourages them to begin thinking of graduate study very early in their undergraduate programs. Chapter 7, "The Settings for Health Education," introduces students to the job responsibilities inherent in different types of health education positions and provides a discussion of the pros and cons of working in various health education settings. With its "a day in the career of" sections and the "Practitioner's Perspective" boxes, this chapter is unique among introductory texts and will truly provide students with important insights into the various health education settings.

Chapter 8, "Agencies/Associations/Organizations Associated with Health Education," introduces students to the many professional agencies, associations, and organizations that support health promotion and education. This is an extremely important chapter, as all health educators need to know of these resources and allies. We believe that all introductory students should be encouraged to join one or more of the professional associations described in this chapter. For that reason, addresses for most of the professional associations are included in the book. Chapter 9, "The Literature of Health Education," directs students to the information and resources necessary to work in the field. Included in this chapter is basic information related to the Internet and World Wide Web that should be especially helpful to new students. With the explosion of knowledge related to health, being able to locate needed resources is a critical skill for health educators. Finally, health education students need to consider what future changes in health knowledge, policy, and funding may mean to those working in health promotion and education. They must learn to project into the future and prepare themselves to meet these challenges. Chapter 10, "Future Trends in Health Education," is an attempt to provide a window into the future for today's health promotion and education students.

As one reads the book, it will be apparent that certain standard features exist in all chapters. These are designed to help the student identify important information, guide the student's learning, and extend the student's understanding beyond the memorization of content information. Each chapter in the book begins by identifying objectives. Prior to reading a chapter, students should carefully read the objectives, as they will guide the student's learning of the information contained in that chapter. After reading a chapter, it may also be helpful to review the objectives to make certain major points of focus were understood. Following the objectives in each chapter is a list of key terms. Again, it is a good idea to examine these closely prior to reading a chapter and to review them following one's reading. Being able to respond to each objective and define each term is typically of great value in understanding the material and preparing for examinations.

Throughout the book take note of the "Practitioner's Perspective" boxes. These are boxes written by health promotion and education professionals who are currently working in the field. Many of the boxes relate to working in a particular setting, while others focus on such areas as ethics, certification, and philosophy.

At the end of each chapter, the student will find a brief summary of the information contained in that chapter. Following the summary are review questions. Students are encouraged to answer these questions, as they provide an additional method for targeting learning and reviewing the chapter's contents. A short list of activities, designed to extend the reader's knowledge beyond what can be obtained by reading the chapter, is also included. In some cases, students are asked to apply or synthesize the content information. In other activities, students are encouraged to get actively involved with experiences that will help integrate learning from the text with a practical, real-world setting. By completing these activities, students should have a better understanding of health promotion and education.

We readily acknowledge that the information contained in this book represents our bias regarding what material should be taught in an introductory course. There may be important introductory information we have not included, or we may have included information that may not be considered introductory by all users. We welcome and encourage all comments and feedback, both positive and negative, from all users of this text. Only with such feedback can we make improvements and include the most appropriate information in future editions of the text.

Randall R. Cottrell, D.Ed., CHES
James T. Girvan, Ph.D., M.P.H., CHES
James F. McKenzie, Ph.D., M.P.H.

ACKNOWLEDGMENTS

First, we would like to recognize Suzy Spivey, Joe Burns, Sara Sherlock, and Mary Beth Finch of Allyn and Bacon, for their important help in the early conceptualization and development of the book. We would like to thank Barbara Day of Shepherd Inc., and Deb DeBord for their expertise in the editorial and production stages of the book. We would also like to express our appreciation to those health education professionals who reviewed our work: Sherman Sowby, California State University at Fresno; Ernie Randolfi, Montana State University; Marilyn Morrow, Illinois State University; and Kim Stassen, Ball State University. Their thoughtful comments and suggestions greatly helped improve our book.

Finally, we wish to dedicate this book to the people in our lives who mean the most to us: our wives, Karen, Georgia, and Bonnie; our children, Kyle, Kory, Jennifer, Erik, and Anne; and our parents, Russell and Edith Cottrell, Terry and Margaret Girvan, and Gordon and Betty McKenzie. Without their love, encouragement, sacrifice, and support, this book would not have been possible.

1 A Background for the Profession

CHAPTER OBJECTIVES

After reading this chapter and answering the questions at the end, you should be able to

1. Explain why health education should be considered an emerging profession.
2. Describe the current status of health education.
3. Define the following terms—*health, health education, health promotion, health promotion and disease prevention, public health, community health, coordinated school health program,* and *wellness.*
4. Explain the means by which health or health status can be measured.
5. List and explain the goal and objectives of health education.
6. Identify the practice of health education.
7. Explain the following concepts and principles.
   a. Health Field Concept
   b. Levels of prevention
   c. Risk factors
   d. Health risk reduction
      Chain of infection
      Communicable Disease Model
      Multicausation Disease Model
   e. Selected principles of health education—participation, empowerment, and cultural sensitivity
8. Provide a brief overview of epidemiology.

KEY TERMS

adjusted rate
chain of infection
communicable disease
communicable disease model
community health
coordinated school health
   program
crude rate

culturally competent
cultural sensitivity
death rates
disability-adjusted life years
   (DALYs)
discipline
emerging profession
empowerment

endemic
environment
epidemic
epidemiology
health
health behavior
health care organization
health education

health field
Health Field Concept
health promotion
health promotion and disease
   prevention
human biology
life expectancy
lifestyle
mental health
modifiable risk factors
multicausation disease model

noncommunicable disease
nonmodifiable risk factors
ownership
pandemic
participation
physical health
prevention
primary prevention
profession
public health

rate
risk factors
secondary prevention
social health
specific rate
spiritual health
tertiary prevention
wellness
years of potential life lost
   (YPLL)

Health education has come a long way since its early beginnings. As the profession has grown and changed, so have the role and responsibilities of the health educators. The purpose of this book is to provide the readers, those just being introduced to the profession, with a sense of the past—how the profession was born and on what principles it was developed; a complete understanding of the present—what it is that health educators are expected to do, how they should do it, and what theories and models guide their work; and a look at the future— where the profession is headed and how can health educators keep up with the changes in order to be responsive to those whom they serve.

This first chapter has been written to provide the readers with a common background in the terminology, concepts, and principles of the profession. We will briefly discuss why we refer to health education as an emerging profession, look at the current state of the profession, define many of the key words and terms used in the profession, show how health and health status have been measured, outline the goals and objectives of the profession, identify the practice of health education, and discuss some of the basic, underlying concepts and principles of the profession.

An Emerging Profession

"Health education is eclectic in nature. As an applied science, it derives its body of knowledge from a variety of disciplines" (Galli, 1976, p. 158). More specifically, health education's "body of knowledge represents a synthesis of facts, principles, and concepts drawn from biological, behavioral, sociological, and health sciences, but interpreted in terms of human needs, human values, and human potential" (Deeds, Cleary, & Neiger, 1996, p. 11). As the applied science of health education has developed over the years, it has been "labeled" in a variety of ways, including as a process, field, discipline, and/or profession. Most would agree that there is a process or several processes embedded in health education, but to label health education as only a "process" would not be accurate. The words *field* and *discipline* seem much alike and have been used interchangeably, so for the purposes of this discussion we will use the term *discipline.* Thus, the real question comes down to, Is health education a discipline or a profession? We see health education as neither. We see it as somewhere between the two: an **emerging profession.** Though the debate may seem a bit trivial, more technical than significant, or just a question of semantics to the reader, it is important that those studying to be health educators have an understanding of this discussion and be able to see how health education fits into the bigger picture.

One of the reasons a variety of labels have been used to describe health education over the years is the fact that health educators themselves have not been consistent in their use of labels. The labels have varied because those using the labels either do not think it is important to make a distinction or have not given much thought to what the labels mean.

A **discipline** has been defined as "a branch of knowledge or instruction" (Landau, 1979, p. 182). Health education fits this definition, and then some. We see a discipline as something that is smaller than a profession, which has been defined as "an occupation that properly involves a liberal, scientific, or artistic education" (Landau, 1979, p. 528). Or, as Livingood (1996, p. 421) has stated, a **profession** is "the sociological construct for an occupation that has special status." Using these definitions, we see health education as fitting somewhere between a discipline and a profession, thus the term *emerging profession.*

To further support our claim that health education is an emerging profession, it might be helpful to present a list of characteristics of a profession. Upton (1970) felt that the following functions distinguish a profession. The words in the brackets are our opinions on how health education stacks up with each of these characteristics.

1. Provide a unique and essential social service. [Health educators do this.]
2. Require of its members an extensive period of preparation. [Health educators are not in agreement over what constitutes an extensive period of preparation. Some say a bachelor's degree is necessary; others say a master's degree.]
3. Have underlying its practice a theoretical base. [Health educators use a number of theories. See Chapter 4.]
4. Have a system of internal controls that tends to regulate the behavior of its members. [This is emerging with the certification of health education specialist (see Chapter 6), academic program review, and the codes of ethics (see Chapter 8), but as of yet it is not clearly defined for health education.]
5. Have a culture peculiar to the profession. [This is still evolving.]
6. Be sanctioned by the community. [As we state in the next section of this chapter, health education is moving slowly in the right direction, but there are still many who do not recognize the work of health educators.]
7. Have an occupation association that is representative of all and can speak on behalf of all the members of the occupation. [Health education has many associations (see Chapter 8), but none speaks for all.]

Though many of the characteristics on Upton's list can be met by health education, not all can be.

Further, Barber (1988) states that an emerging profession is an occupation which does not rank so clearly high or so clearly low on those attributes that distinguish an occupation from a profession. In other words, Barber indicates that an emerging profession has not been clearly defined by itself or others. We feel Upton's (1970) list and our comments on his list show that health education is an emerging profession.

Stating that health education is not at full profession status is not to say that those who engage in the work—health educators—are not professionals. A professional is "one who pursues as a business some vocation or occupation" (Landau, 1979, p. 528). All health educators, just like all physicians and lawyers, are professionals, regardless of the setting in which they work. Greene and Simons-Morton (1984, p. 388) have described professionals with the following descriptors.

1. They believe in what they are doing.
2. They want to see the job done properly.
3. They do their best.
4. They feel a sense of responsibility for the quality of work done by others in the field.

It is our belief that health educators meet all of these descriptors.

Have we convinced you that health education is an emerging profession? Maybe we have and maybe we have not; however, throughout the remainder of this book we use the term *profession* to represent *emerging profession*. We are also sure the debate (discipline vs. emerging profession vs. profession) will continue.

Current Status of Health Education

In looking back through history, there have been a number of occasions that can be pointed to as "critical" to the development of health education. (See Chapter 2 for an in-depth presentation of the history.) But there has been no time in history in which the status of the profession has been more visible to the average person or as widely accepted by other health professionals as it is today. Much of this notoriety can be attributed to the health promotion period of public health history that began about 1975 in the United States.

The United States' first public health revolution spanned the time period from the late nineteenth century through the mid-twentieth century and was aimed at controlling the harm (morbidity and mortality) that came from infectious diseases. By the mid-1950s, many of the infectious diseases in the United States were pretty much under control (see Figure 1.1). This was evidenced by the improved infant mortality rates, the reduction in the number of children who

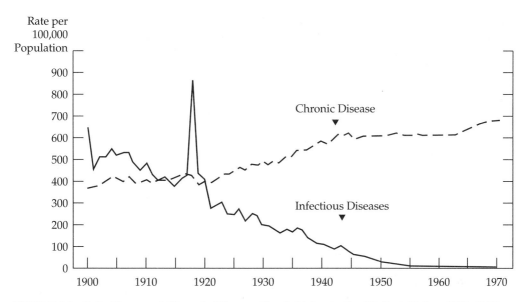

FIGURE 1.1 Infectious and Chronic Disease Death Rates in the United States, 1900–1970.

were contracting childhood diseases, the reduction in the overall death rates in the country, and the increase in life expectancy (see Table 1.1). With the control of many communicable diseases, the country's health focus moved to the major chronic diseases such as heart disease, cancer, and strokes (USDHEW, 1979): diseases that were, in large part, the result of the way people lived.

By the mid-1970s, it had become apparent that the greatest potential for reducing morbidity, saving lives, and reducing health care costs in America was to be achieved through health promotion and disease prevention. At the core of this approach was health education. In 1980, the federal government presented a blueprint of the health promotion and disease prevention strategy in its first set of health objectives in the document called *Promoting Health/Preventing Disease: Objectives for a Nation* (USDHEW, 1980). This document proposed a total of 226 objectives divided into three main areas—preventive services, health protection, and health promotion. This was the first time a comprehensive national agenda for prevention had been developed, with specific goals and objectives for anticipated gains (McGinnis, 1985). In 1985, it was apparent that only about one-half of the objectives established in 1979 would be reached by 1990, another one-fourth would not be reached, and progress on the others could not be judged because of the lack of data (Mason & McGinnis, 1990). Even though not all objectives were reached, "the 1980 planning process demonstrated the value of setting goals and listing specific objectives as a means of measuring progress in the nation's health

TABLE 1.1   Life Expectancy at Birth, at Sixty-Five Years of Age, and at Seventy-Five Years of Age, According to Sex: United States, Selected Years 1900–1995

Year	At Birth Both Sexes	Male	Female	At 65 Years Both Sexes	Male	Female	At 75 Years Both Sexes	Male	Female
1900	47.3	46.3	48.3	11.9	11.5	12.2	*	*	*
1950	68.2	65.6	71.1	13.9	12.8	15.0	*	*	*
1960	69.7	66.6	73.1	14.3	12.8	15.8	*	*	*
1970	70.8	67.1	74.7	15.2	13.1	17.0	*	*	*
1980	73.7	70.7	77.4	16.4	14.1	18.3	10.4	8.8	11.5
1990	75.4	71.8	78.8	17.2	15.1	18.9	10.9	9.4	12.0
1995	75.8	72.5	78.9	17.4	15.6	18.9	11.0	9.7	11.9

Source: Data from National Center for Health Statistics, *Health, United States 1996–97 and Injury Chartbook.* DHHS Publication No. PHS 97-1232, 1997, Public Health Service, Hyattsville, MD.

*Data not available

and health care services" (McKenzie & Pinger, 1997, p. 22). Therefore, the process was repeated in the late 1980s, with the resulting document called *Healthy People 2000: National Health Promotion and Disease Prevention Objectives* (DHHS, 1990a). The planning for a similar document for the year 2010 has been in place for several years, and a tentative framework is in place for its development (DHHS, 1997) (refer to the web site noted with this reference for an update of this document). Such a document, along with the move of the health care industry toward managed health care, should enhance the position of health education in years to come.

Key Words, Terms, and Definitions

In each chapter of this book, you will be introduced to a number of new words and terms that will be important to your understanding the specific content presented in the chapters and that you will use often as you work in the profession. Listing all of these words and terms in this chapter would be overwhelming; however, it is important that all readers have an understanding of some of the more common terms that will be used throughout the book. Like the profession, these words and definitions have evolved over the years. Throughout the past sixty plus years there have been several efforts to try to standardize many of the terms used in the profession. The most recent effort occurred in 1990 (Joint Committee on Health Education Terminology, 1991a, 1991b). During that year, representatives from several professional health education organizations (those represented in the Coalition of National Health Education Organizations—see Chapter 8 for information on the coalition) and the American Academy of Pediatrics convened at a special meeting in Reston, Virginia, for the purpose of updating the terminology of the discipline. Prior to this meeting, the most recent meeting for doing this work was held in 1973 (Johns, 1973). Other presentations of terms and definitions occurred in 1927 (Rugen, 1972), 1934 (Williams, 1934), 1950 (Moss, 1950), and 1962 (Yoho, 1962).

Prior to presenting some of the key terms used in the profession, we think it would be helpful to provide a little more in-depth discussion of the word *health*. Health is a difficult concept to put into words, but it is one that most people intuitively understand. The World Health Organization (WHO, 1947) has defined **health** as "the state of complete mental, physical and social well being not merely the absence of disease or infirmity." This classic definition is important, as it identifies the vital components of health. It further implies that health is a holistic concept involving an interaction and interdependence among these various components. The WHO views health as being only a positive concept, as evidenced by the phrase "the state of complete." In other words, health is a goal to strive for but is not obtainable, because no one ever achieves a "state of complete mental, physical and social well being." It is at this point where we differ with the WHO's definition. We believe health should still be conceptualized as a holistic concept involving mental, physical, and social components, but simply viewed as one's state of being. There are different levels of health, ranging from good to poor; therefore, one can be in a state of good health, a state of poor health, or anywhere in between.

To more fully understand the meaning of health, it is important to understand each of the individual components of health. Utilizing an extensive literature review, Goodstadt, Simpson, and Loranger (1987, p. 59) have aptly described each component of health:

> **physical health**—the absence of disease and disability; functioning adequately from the perspective of physical and physiological abilities; the biological integrity of the individual
>
> **mental health**—(termed *psychological health* by Goodstadt, Simpson, & Loranger, 1987)—may include emotional health; may make explicit reference to intellectual capabilities; the subjective sense of well-being
>
> **social health**—the ability to interact effectively with other people and the social environment; satisfying interpersonal relationships; role fulfillment

The actual number of components to health has been another point of contention. While WHO used three components, others have separated emotional from psychological health and added spiritual to arrive at as many as five components of health. In our discussions, we will maintain emotional and psychological as one domain but will add a spiritual domain. To describe what is meant by spiritual, however, will be left to the individual reader. Goodstadt, Simpson, & Loranger (1987, p. 59) have noted the following description in the literature:

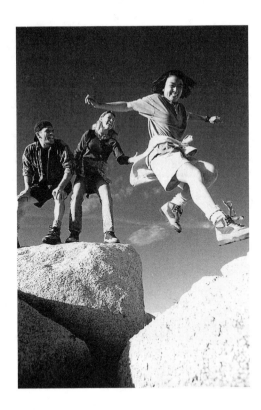

When studying the health of people, all dimensions need to be considered. (Brian Bailey/Tony Stone Images)

Spiritual health—In addition to spiritual health, it has been labeled "personal health"; it has been associated with the concept of self-actualization; it sometimes reflects a concern for issues related to one's value system; alternatively, it may be concerned with a belief in a transcending, unifying force (whether its basis is in nature, scientific law, or a godlike source).

In addition to the word *health* and its various components, it is also important that you have an understanding of the following key terms and definitions:

community health—"includes both private and public efforts of individuals, groups, and organizations to promote, protect, and preserve the health of those in the community" (McKenzie & Pinger, 1997, p. 4)

health education—"any combination of learning experiences designed to facilitate voluntary adaptations of behavior conducive to health" (Green et al., 1980, p. 7)

health promotion—"the combination of educational and environmental supports for actions and conditions of living conducive to health" (Green & Kreuter, 1991, p. 4). (See Figure 1.2 for the relationship between health education and health promotion.)

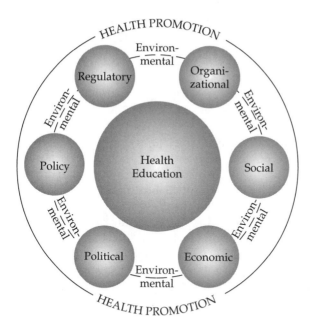

FIGURE 1.2 **Relationship between Health Education and Health Promotion.**

Source: From J. F. McKenzie, & J. L. Smeltzer, *Planning, Implementing, and Evaluating Health Promotion Programs: A Primer.* 1997. Copyright © 1997 by Allyn & Bacon. Reprinted by permission.

health promotion and disease prevention—"the aggregate of all purposeful activities designed to improve personal and public health through a combination of strategies, including the competent implementation of behavioral change strategies, health education, health protection measures, risk factor detection, health enhancement and health maintenance" (Joint Committee on Health Education Terminology, 1991a, p. 102)

public health—"the sum of all official (governmental) efforts to promote, protect, and preserve the people's health" (McKenzie & Pinger, 1997, p. 4)

coordinated school health program—"an organized set of policies, procedures, and activities designed to protect and promote the health and well-being of students and staff which has traditionally included health services, healthful school environment, and health education. It should also include, but not be limited to, guidance and counseling, physical education, food service, social work, psychological services, and employee health promotion" (Joint Committee on Health Education Terminology, 1991b, p. 253; Marx, Wooley, & Northrop, 1998) (Note: In 1998, the term *coordinated school health program* replaced *comprehensive school health program* to distinguish it from comprehensive health education.)

wellness—"an integrated method of functioning which is oriented toward maximizing the potential of which the individual is capable, within the environment where he [sic] is functioning" (Dunn, 1977, p. 9)

Before we leave our discussion about key words and terms of the profession, it should be noted that there is not a 100 percent agreement on terminology. For more on this topic, readers are referred to two articles (Livingood, 1996; Ubbes & Watts, 1995).

Measuring Health or Health Status

Though the definition of *health* is easy to state, trying to quantify the amount of health an individual or a population possesses is not easy. Because of this difficulty, most measures of health are expressed using health statistics based on the traditional medical model of describing ill health (injury, disease, and death) instead of well health. Thus, the higher the presence of injury, disease, and death indicators, the lower the level of health; the lower the presence of injury, disease, and death indicators, the higher the level of health. Out of necessity we have defined the level of health with just the opposite—ill health (Cohen, 1991; McKenzie & Pinger, 1997). In the following sections, we present several of the more common means that are used to quantify health or lack thereof.

Rates

A **rate** "is a measure of some event, disease, or condition in relation to a unit of population, along with some specification of time" (NCHS, 1995, p. 292). Rates are important because they provide an opportunity for comparison of events, diseases, or conditions that occur at different times or places. Some of the more commonly used rates are death rates, birth rates, and morbidity rates. **Death rates** (the number of deaths per 100,000 resident population), sometimes referred to as mortality or fatality rates, are probably the most frequently used means of quantifying the seriousness of injury or disease. (See Table 1.2 for death rates and Table 1.3 formulas to tabulate rates). "The transition from wellness to ill health is often gradual and poorly defined. Because death, in contrast, is a clearly defined event, it has continued to be the most reliable single indicator of health status of a population. Mortality statistics, however, describe only a part of the health status of a population, and often only the endpoint of an illness process" (DHHS, 1991, p. 15). Rates can be expressed in three forms—crude, adjusted, and specific. A **crude rate** is the rate expressed for a total population. An **adjusted rate** is also expressed for a total population but is statistically adjusted for a certain characteristic such as age. A **specific rate** is a rate for a particular population subgroup such as for a particular disease (i.e., disease-specific) or for a particular age of people (i.e., age-specific) (Mausner & Kramer, 1985). Examples include calculating the death rate for heart disease in the United States, or the age-specific death rate for forty-five- to fifty-four-year-olds.

Life Expectancy

Life expectancy is another means by which health or health status has been measured. It, too, however, is based on mortality. Even with this limitation, though,

TABLE 1.2   Death Rates for the Ten Leading Causes of Death: United States, 1995

Cause	Deaths per 100,000 Population
Diseases of the heart	280.7
Malignant neoplasms (cancer)	204.9
Cerebrovascular diseases (stroke)	60.1
Chronic obstructive pulmonary diseases	39.2
Unintentional injuries	35.5
Pneumonia and influenza	31.6
Diabetes mellitus	22.6
Human immunodeficiency virus infection	16.4
Suicide	11.9
Chronic liver disease and cirrhosis	9.6

Source: Data from R. N. Anderson, et al., "Report on final mortality statistics, 1995." in *Monthly vital statistics report;* Vol. 45, No. 11, Supp. 2, 1997, National Center for Health Statistics, Hyattsville, MD.

TABLE 1.3   Selected Mortality Rates and Their Formulas

Rate	Definition	Example (U.S. 1995)*
Age-specific death rate =	$\dfrac{\text{Number of deaths, 45–54}}{\text{Estimated midyear population, 45–54}}$	$\times 100{,}000$ $460.1/100{,}000$
Cause-specific mortality rate =	$\dfrac{\text{Number of deaths (HIV)}}{\text{Estimated midyear population}}$	$\times 100{,}000$ $16.4/100{,}000$
Crude death rate =	$\dfrac{\text{Number of deaths (all causes)}}{\text{Estimated midyear population}}$	$\times 100{,}000$ $880/100{,}000$

Source: Data from National Center for Health Statistics, *Health, United States 1996–97 and Injury Chartbook.* DHHS Publication No. PHS 97-1232, 1997, Public Health Service, Hyattsville, MD.

life expectancy has been described as "the most comprehensive indicator of patterns of health and disease, as well as living standards and social development" (CDC, 1994, pp. 2–8). **Life expectancy** "is the average number of years of life remaining to a person at a particular age and is based on a given set of age-specific death rates, generally the mortality conditions existing in the period mentioned. Life expectancy may be determined by race, sex, or other characteristics using age-specific death rates for the population with that characteristic" (NCHS, 1995, p. 287). The two most frequently used times to state life expectancy are at birth and at age sixty-five. These two times are used because they are means of quantifying the length of life and length of retirement, assuming most people retire at age sixty-five (see Table 1.1). In terms of evaluating the effect of chronic disease on a population, life expectancies calculated *after* birth have been found to be more useful measures than life expectancy *at* birth, because life expectancy at birth reflects infant mortality rates (CDC, 1994).

Years of Potential Life Lost

A third means by which health or health status has been measured is **years of potential life lost (YPLL).** YPLL is a measure of premature mortality (NCHS, 1995) (see Table 1.4). It is calculated by subtracting a person's age at death from seventy-five years. For example, for a person who dies at age thirty, the YPLL are forty-five. Obviously, the earlier someone dies, the greater the YPLL. Some ask why age seventy-five is used instead of a person's projected life expectancy when calculating YPLL. Until 1996, the U.S. government regularly used sixty-five for calculating YPLL because sixty-five was the standard age of retirement (McKenzie & Pinger, 1997). However, today people are living and working longer, thus the switch to age seventy-five.

Disability-Adjusted Life Years

The three measures of health and health status noted previously are commonly used in the United States and other developed countries. However, because mortality does not express the burden of living with disability (for example, the resulting paralysis from an automobile crash or the depression that often follows a stroke), the World Health Organization and the World Bank developed a measure called **disability-adjusted life years (DALYs)** (*World Development Report*, 1993). One DALY is equal to one lost year of healthy life (Murray & Lopez, 1996a). "To

TABLE 1.4   **Years of Potential Life Lost (YPLL) (per 100,000 Population) before Seventy-Five for the Ten Leading Causes of Death: United States, 1995**

Cause	Crude	Adjusted
Diseases of the heart	1,430.2	1,259.2
Malignant neoplasms (cancer)	1,779.4	1,587.7
Cerebrovascular diseases (stroke)	241.1	211.5
Chronic obstructive pulmonary diseases	188.0	161.4
Unintentional injuries	1,098.1	1,155.5
Pneumonia and influenza	126.5	115.3
Diabetes mellitus	169.6	149.9
Human immunodeficiency virus infection	615.0	570.3
Suicide	395.0	405.6
Homicide and legal intervention	399.1	436.4

Source: Data from National Center for Health Statistics, *Health, United States 1996–97 and Injury Chartbook,* DHHS Publication No. PHS 97-1232, 1997, Public Health Service, Hyattsville, MD.

calculate total DALYs for a given condition in a population, years of life lost (YLL) and years lived with disability of known severity and duration (YLDs) for that condition must each be estimated, then the total summed. For example, to calculate DALYs incurred through road accidents in India in 1990, add the total years of life lost in fatal road accidents and the total years of life lived with disabilities by survivors of such accidents" (Murray & Lopez, 1996a, p. 7). For a more thorough explanation of DALYs, the reader is referred to the *World Development Report 1993: Investing in Health* (1993) and *The Global Burden of Disease* (Murray & Lopez, 1996b).

Health Surveys

Data collected through surveys conducted by the National Center for Health Statistics are other means by which health or health status has been measured in the United States. Three examples of such surveys are presented here. The first two, the National Health Interview Survey and the National Health and Nutrition Examination Survey (NHANES) are conducted by the National Center for Health Statistics. The National Health Interview Survey is a telephone interview in which respondents are asked a number of questions about their health and health behavior. One of the questions, for example, asks the respondents to describe their health status using one of five categories: excellent, very good, good, fair, or poor. The NHANES data are collected using a mobile examination center. Through direct physical examinations, clinical and laboratory testing, and related procedures, data are collected on a representative group of Americans. "The examinations result in the most authoritative source of standardized clinical, physical, and physiological data on the American people. Included in the data are the prevalence of specific conditions and diseases and data on blood pressure, serum cholesterol, body measurements, nutritional status and deficiencies, and exposure to environmental toxicants" (McKenzie & Pinger, 1997, p. 175).

The third example of data collected through a survey is the data collected through the Behavioral Risk Factor Surveillance System (BRFSS). These data are collected by individual states through cooperative agreements with the Centers for Disease Control and Prevention (CDC). Through the use of random-digit-dialing telephone survey techniques, each state selects a probability sample from the noninstitutionalized adult population (over eighteen years of age) with telephones. Those selected are asked questions on risk factors, preventive health practices, access to preventive services and health insurance, and a few demographic questions (CDC, 1994).

The Goal and Objectives of the Profession

The ultimate goal of all helping professions, including the profession of health education, is to improve the quality of life, yet quality of life is difficult to quantify (Raphael et al., 1997). However, most feel that there is a direct relationship between quality of life and health status. Quality of life is usually improved when health status is improved, or, as Ashley Montagu (1968, p. 206) has stated, "The highest goal in life is to die young, at as old an age as possible." To that end, "the goal of health education is to promote, maintain, and improve individual and community health. The teaching-learning process is the hallmark and social agenda that differentiates the practice of health education from that of other helping professions in achieving this goal" (NCHEC, 1996, pp. 2–3).

Because quality of life and health status are complex variables, they are not usually changed in a short period of time. In order for people to reach these goals, they usually, over a period of time, work their way through a number of small steps that equip them with all that is necessary to impact both their health status and, in turn, their quality of life. In order to assist people with these steps, health educators have identified a hierarchy of objectives that they have found useful in developing health education/promotion programs. This hierarchy is presented in Table 1.5. Please note that these objectives are presented from easiest to most difficult to achieve. For clarification, we define *easiest* as those that take the least time and resources to accomplish.

The Practice of Health Education

The practice of health education is based on the assumption "that beneficial health behavior in both children and adults will result from a combination of planned, consistent, integrated learning opportunities. This assumption rests on direct evidence from the evaluation of health education programs in schools, at worksites, in medical settings, and through the mass media" (Green & Ottoson, 1994, p. 94). It also rests on evidence from experiences outside the fields of health and education such as community development, social work, agricultural extension, and marketing (Green & Ottoson, 1994). Though the specific work of health educators is outlined in the responsibilities and competencies presented in Chapter 6, the primary role of health educators is to develop—plan, implement, and evaluate—appropriate health education/promotion programs for the people they serve. Though easily stated, this is by no means an easy task. Good health education/promotion programs do not just happen. Much time, effort, practice, and on-the-job training are required to be successful. Even the most experienced health educators find program development challenging because of the constant changes in settings, resources, and target populations (McKenzie & Smeltzer, 1997).

Though the specific steps taken to develop a health education/promotion program vary based on the planning model used (see Chapter 4), most models include the following steps (McKenzie & Smeltzer, 1997, p. 8) (see Figure 4.3):

1. Assessing the needs of the target population
2. Developing appropriate goals and objectives
3. Creating an intervention that considers the peculiarities of the setting

TABLE 1.5 Hierarchy of Objectives and Their Relation to Evaluation

Type of Objective	Program Outcomes	Possible Evaluation Measures	Type of Evaluation
Administrative objectives	Activities presented, and tasks completed	Number of sessions held, exposure, attendance, participation, staff performance, appropriate materials, adequacy of resources	Process (form of formative)
Learning objectives	Change in awareness, knowledge, attitudes, and skills	Increase in awareness, knowledge, attitudes, and skill development/ acquisition	Impact (form of summative)
Behavioral and environmental objectives	Behavior adoption, change in environment	Change in behavior, hazards or barriers removed from the environment	Impact (form of summative)
Program objectives	Change in quality of life (QOL), health status, or risk and social benefits	QOL measures, morbidity data, mortality data, measures of risk (i.e., Health Risk Appraisal)	Outcome (form of summative)

From J. F. McKenzie, & J. L. Smeltzer, *Planning, implementing, and evaluating health promotion programs: A primer.* 1997. Copyright © 1997 by Allyn & Bacon. Reprinted by permission.

4. Implementing the intervention
5. Evaluating the results

Therefore, it becomes the practice of health educators to be able to carry out all that is associated with these tasks.

Basic Underlying Concepts of the Profession

As was noted earlier in this chapter and will be discussed in greater detail in Chapter 2, the profession of health education is one that has been built on the principles and concepts of a number of disciplines and professions. Within health education can be found pieces of community development and organization, education, epidemiology, medicine, psychology, and sociology. In the sections that follow, we present some of the basic underlying concepts of the profession. Please note that we have not exhausted the discussion of each of these topics but, rather, present sufficient information to allow a basic understanding of each.

The Health Field Concept

Shortly after the Canadian government implemented its national health plan that insured health care for all Canadians in 1973, it began to look more closely at the health field as a way of improving the health of Canadians. The **health field** is a term the government described as being far more encompassing than the "health care system." It was a term that was much broader and included all matters that affected health (Lalonde, 1974). Since the health field was such a broad concept, it was felt that there was a need to develop a framework that would subdivide the concept into principal elements so that the elements could be studied. Such a framework was developed and called the **Health Field Concept** (Laframboise, 1973).

The Health Field Concept divided the health field into four elements: human biology, environment, lifestyle, and health care organization. "These four elements were identified through an examination of the causes and underlying factors of sickness and death in Canada, and from an assessment of the parts the elements play in affecting the level of health in Canada" (Lalonde, 1974, p. 31). **Human biology** "includes all those aspects of health, both physical and mental, which are developed within the human body as a consequence of the basic biology of man [sic] and the organic make-up of an individual" (Lalonde, 1974, p. 31). This includes not only the genetic inheritance of an individual but also the processes of maturation and aging and the complex interaction of the various systems of the human body (Lalonde, 1974). The element of **environment** "includes all those matters related to health which are external to the human body and over which the individual has little or no control" (Lalonde, 1974, p. 32). Some examples of things often included in the element of environment are geography, climate, community size, industrial development, economy, and social norms.

The element of **lifestyle** is comprised of the "aggregation of decisions by individuals which affect their health and over which they more or less have control" (Lalonde, 1974, p. 32). In more recent times, lifestyle has been more commonly referred to as **health behavior.** The fourth element in the Health Field Concept is health care organization. **Health care organization** "consists of the quantity, quality, arrangement, nature and relationships of people and resources in the provision of health care" (Lalonde, 1974, p. 32). This fourth element of the Health Field Concept is often referred to as the health care system.

The utility of the Health Field Concept has proved to be very helpful over the years, both in Canada and the United States. Its greatest importance may have been to bring attention to the concept of health promotion and disease prevention. Prior to this point in history, the primary focus of health care had been on the cure of disease, not the prevention of disease. In fact, it was stated that the Health Field Concept put human biology, environment, and lifestyle on equal footing with health care organization (Lalonde, 1974). Since its development, studies using this concept, in both Canada and the United States, have provided a greater understanding of what contributes to morbidity and mortality and what health professionals can do to help improve the health of those whom they serve. One such study was conducted by the Centers for Disease Control and Prevention in the late 1970s. That study examined the premature deaths (deaths prior to age sixty-five) recorded in the United States in 1975. "That study revealed that approximately 48% of all premature deaths could be traced to one's life-style or health behavior. Life-styles characterized by lack of exercise, high-fat diets, smoking, uncontrolled hypertension, and inability to control stress were found to be contributing factors to premature mortality" (McKenzie & Pinger, 1997, p. 21). Studies similar to this one have been conducted in the years since; see Table 1.6 for the results of one such study.

The Levels and Limitations of Prevention

The word *prevention* has already been used several times in this chapter. We now want to formally define the term, present the different levels of prevention, and briefly discuss the limitations of prevention. **Prevention,** as it relates to health, has been defined as the planning for and the measures taken to forestall the onset of, a disease or other health problem before the occurrence of undesirable health

TABLE 1.6   Estimated Contribution of Four Factors to the Ten Leading Causes of Death before Age Seventy-Five

Cause of Death	Lifestyle (%)	Environment (%)	Biology/ Heredity (%)	Inadequate Health Care (%)
Heart disease	54.0	9.0	25.0	12.0
Cancer	37.0	24.0	29.0	10.0
Motor vehicle accidents	69.0	18.0	1.0	12.0
Other accidents	51.0	31.0	4.0	13.0
Stroke	50.0	22.0	21.0	7.0
Homicide	63.0	35.0	2.0	0.0
Suicide	60.0	35.0	2.0	3.0
Cirrhosis	70.0	9.0	18.0	3.0
Influenza/pneumonia	23.0	20.0	39.0	18.0
Diabetes	34.0	0.0	60.0	6.0
All ten causes together	51.5	20.1	19.8	10.0

Source: From J. R. Terborg, "Health promotion at the worksite" in K. H. Rowland & G. R. Ferris (eds.), *Research in Personnel and Human Resource Management, Volume 4,* 1986. Copyright © 1986. JAI Press, Greenwich, CT. Reprinted by permission.

Note: Terborg adapted this from Harris, P. R. (1981). *Health United States 1980: With Prevention Profile.* Washington, DC: U.S. Government Printing Office.

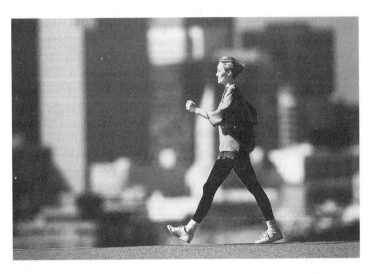

Exercise is an example of primary prevention. (David Madison/Tony Stone Images)

events. This definition presents three distinct levels of prevention: primary, secondary, and tertiary prevention. **Primary prevention** is comprised of those preventive measures that forestall the onset of illness or injury during the prepathogenesis period (McKenzie & Pinger, 1997). Examples of primary prevention measures include wearing a safety belt, using rubber gloves when there is potential for the spread of disease, immunizing against specific diseases, exercising, and brushing one's teeth. And any health education/promotion program aimed specifically at forestalling the onset of illness or injury is also an example of primary prevention.

Illness and injury cannot always be prevented. In fact, many diseases, such as cancer and heart disease, can establish themselves in humans and cause considerable damage before they are detected and treated. In such cases, the sooner a condition can be detected and medical personnel can intervene, the greater the chances of limiting disability and preventing death. Such identification and intervention are known as secondary prevention. More specifically, **secondary prevention** includes the "preventive measures that lead to an early diagnosis and prompt treatment of a disease or an injury to limit disability and prevent more serious pathogenesis" (McKenzie & Pinger, 1997, p. 95). Good examples of secondary prevention include personal and clinical screenings and exams such as blood pressure, cholesterol, and hemocult (hidden blood) screenings; breast self-exams (BSE); and testicle self-exams (TSE).

The final level of prevention is **tertiary prevention.** It is at this level that health educators work to retrain, reeducate, and rehabilitate the individual who has already incurred disability, impairment, or dependency. Examples of some tertiary measures include educating a patient after lung cancer surgery or work-

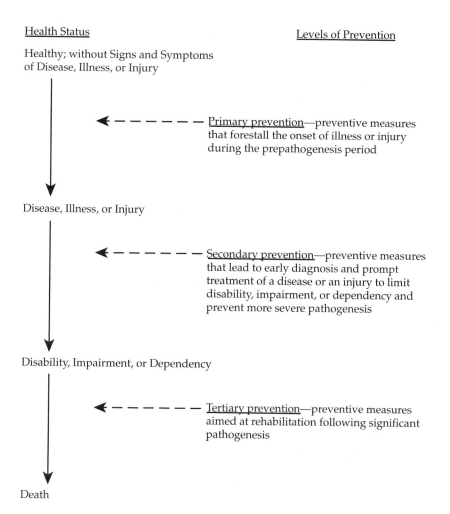

Health Status   Levels of Prevention

Healthy; without Signs and Symptoms
of Disease, Illness, or Injury

◄ — — — — — — Primary prevention—preventive measures
that forestall the onset of illness or injury
during the prepathogenesis period

Disease, Illness, or Injury

◄ — — — — — — Secondary prevention—preventive measures
that lead to early diagnosis and prompt
treatment of a disease or an injury to limit
disability, impairment, or dependency and
prevent more severe pathogenesis

Disability, Impairment, or Dependency

◄ — — — — — — Tertiary prevention—preventive measures
aimed at rehabilitation following significant
pathogenesis

Death

FIGURE 1.3   Levels of Prevention.

From J. F. McKenzie & J. L. Smeltzer, *Planning, implementing, and evaluating health promotion programs: A primer.* Copyright © 1997 by Allyn & Bacon. Reprinted by permission.

ing with an individual who has diabetes to ensure that the daily insulin injections are taken. Figure 1.3 provides a visual representation of the levels of prevention in relation to health status.

Though health educators can intervene at any of the three levels of prevention, and can have a great deal of success in halting or reversing the disease process, it should be obvious from the earlier discussion of the Health Field Concept that prevention is not the "magic bullet" for an endless life. Prevention does have its limits. McGinnis (1985) has noted four major categories of limitations: biological, technological, ethical, and economic. Biological limitations center around life span. How long should individuals expect to live healthy lives or, for that matter, how long should they expect to live at all? Even with the very best inputs and a bit of luck, one should not expect to live longer than 80 to 110 years. Body parts will eventually wear out from use.

Technological advances also have their limitations. Today health care workers have a vast array of highly technical equipment available to help them care for their patients, but technology still has not been able to help the health workers eradicate AIDS or malaria, or to explain the causes of arthritis or Alzheimer's disease.

Prevention is also limited by ethical concerns (see Chapter 5). Even though helmets would increase the chances of survival in automobile crashes, is it ethical to have a law that says all drivers and passengers in automobiles must wear them? Or is it ethical to penalize people via fines, taxes, or surcharges for acting in unhealthy ways such as driving an automobile without a safety belt on, buying and using tobacco products, or for not having a smoke detector and fire extinguisher in the home?

Finally, prevention has economic limitations. Prevention is limited by the amount of money that is put into it. Though the exact figures are difficult to determine, it is commonly understood that less than 5 percent of all dollars spent on health in the United States each year are spent on prevention. Stated another way, over 95 percent of all health dollars in the United States are spent on curing ill health, not on preventing it.

Risk Factors

The Health Field Concept has provided those interested in health with a framework from which the health field can be studied. The levels of prevention and their limitations have provided this same group of people with a time frame from which to plan to help forestall the onset of, limit the spread of, and rehabilitate after pathogenesis or another health problem. What neither of these concepts fully discloses is the focus at which health promotion and disease prevention programming should be aimed. The targets of such programming are **risk factors,** those inherited, environmental, and behavioral influences "capable of provoking ill health with or without previous disposition" (USDHEW, 1979, p. 13). Risk factors increase the probability of morbidity and premature mortality but do not guarantee that people with a risk factor will suffer the consequences.

Risk factors can be divided into two categories: **modifiable** (changeable or controllable) and **nonmodifiable** (nonchangeable or noncontrollable) **risk factors.** The former include such factors as sedentary lifestyle, smoking, and poor dietary habits, things that individuals can change or have control over, while the latter group includes factors such as age, sex, and inherited genes, things that individuals cannot change or do not have control over. It should be noted that these two categories of risk factors are often interrelated. In fact, the combined potential for harm from a number of risk factors is greater than the sum of their individual potentials. For example, it is known that asbestos workers have an increased risk

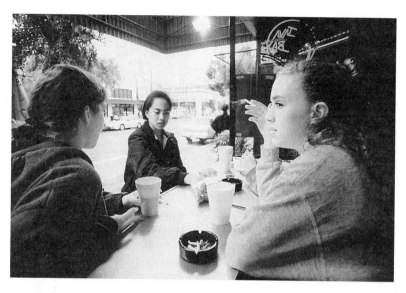

Smoking is a modifiable risk factor. (Martin Rogers/Tony Stone Images)

for cancer because of their exposure to this carcinogen. Further, if they smoke, they have a thirty times greater chance of developing lung cancer than do their nonsmoking co-workers and a ninety times greater chance of getting lung cancer than do people who neither work with asbestos nor smoke (USDHEW, 1979). The rates could go even higher if they have an inherited respiratory disease.

Over the years the knowledge about the impact of risk behaviors has continued to grow. It is now known that better control of many of the modifiable risk factors alone—such as lack of exercise, poor diet, use of tobacco and drugs, and alcohol abuse—could prevent between 40 and 70 percent of all premature deaths, one-third of all acute disabilities, and two-thirds of chronic disabilities (DHHS, 1990b). Because of this knowledge, much of the focus of the work of health educators has been to help individuals identify and control their modifiable risk factors.

Health Risk Reduction

In order to be able to take aim at specific risk factors, it is important that health educators have a basic understanding of both communicable (infectious) and noncommunicable (noninfectious) diseases. A **communicable disease** is "an illness caused by some specific biological agent or its toxic products that can be transmitted from an infected person, animal, or inanimate reservoir to a susceptible host" (McKenzie & Pinger, 1997, p. 84), while a **noncommunicable disease** is one "that cannot be transmitted from infected host to susceptible host" (McKenzie & Pinger, 1997, p. 84). Our intent in this section and the ones that follow is not to present information on all possible diseases and their related risk factors that a health educator may have to develop programs for but, rather, to provide a general understanding of the spread and cause of disease. (See Table 1.7 for leading causes of death and their risk factors.)

Before moving on, we would like to make a special note about one of the terms presented in Table 1.7. The term *leading causes of death* is used in this table. That term refers to "the primary pathophysiological conditions identified at the time of death, as opposed to the root causes" (McGinnis & Foege, 1993, p. 2207). In 1993 McGinnis and Foege conducted a review of literature published between 1978 and 1993 to see if they could identify the root causes of death. Table 1.8 provides a summary of their findings. Such information helps support the program development efforts of health educators.

The Chain of Infection.   The **chain of infection** (see Figure 1.4) is a model that is used to help explain the spread of a communicable disease from one host to another. The basic premise represented in the chain of infection is that individuals can work to break the chain (reduce the risk) at any point; thus, the spread of disease can be stopped. For example, some waterborne diseases are stopped from spreading when the first link of the chain is broken with the chlorination of the water supply, thus killing the pathogens that cause a disease. The risk is reduced by killing the pathogen before it is consumed. The chain can also be broken by placing a barrier between the means of transmission and the portal of entry, as when health care providers protect themselves with surgical masks and rubber gloves. In this case, the risk is reduced by not allowing individuals to expose themselves to the pathogen. With such information, health educators can help create programs that are aimed at "breaking" the chain and reducing the risks.

Communicable Disease Model.   A second model used to describe the spread of a communicable disease is the **communicable disease model.** The elements of this model—agent, host, and environment—are presented in Figure 1.5. These three elements summarize the minimal requirements necessary for the presence and spread of a communicable disease in a population. The agent is the element (or, using the chain of infection labels, the pathogen) that must be present for a disease to spread—for example, bacteria or a virus. The host is any susceptible organism that can be invaded by the agent. Examples include plants, animals, and humans. The environment includes all other factors that either prohibit or promote disease transmission. Thus, "communicable disease transmission occurs when a susceptible host and a pathogenic agent exist in an environment conducive to disease transmission" (McKenzie & Pinger, 1997, p. 85).

Multicausation Disease Model.   Obviously, the chain of infection and communicable disease models are most helpful in trying to prevent disease caused by a pathogen. However, they are not applicable to noncommunicable diseases, which include many of the chronic diseases such as heart disease and cancer. Most of

TABLE 1.7 **Leading Causes of Death, Number of Deaths, and Associated Risk Factors for All Ages: United States, 1995**

Rank	Cause	Number	Risk Factors
1	Diseases of the heart	737,563	Tobacco use, high blood pressure, elevated serum cholesterol, diet, diabetes, obesity, lack of exercise, alcohol abuse, biological factors
2	Malignant neoplasms (cancer)	538,455	Tobacco use, alcohol misuse, diet, solar radiation, ionizing radiation, worksite hazards, environmental pollution, biological factors
3	Cerebrovascular diseases (stroke)	157,991	Tobacco use, high blood pressure, elevated serum cholesterol, diabetes, obesity, biological factors
4	Chronic obstructive pulmonary diseases	102,899	Tobacco use
5	Unintentional injuries	93,320	Alcohol misuse, tobacco use (fires), product design, home hazards, handgun availability, lack of safety restraints, excessive speed, automobile design, roadway design
6	Pneumonia and influenza	82,923	Tobacco use, infectious agents, biological factors
7	Diabetes mellitus	59,254	Obesity (for adult onset), diet, lack of exercise, biological factors
8	Human immunodeficiency virus infection	43,115	Sexual practices, drug misuse, exposure to blood products
9	Suicide	31,284	Handgun availability, alcohol or drug misuse, stress, biological factors
10	Chronic liver disease and cirrhosis	25,222	Alcohol misuse, infectious agents

Source: Data from R. N. Anderson, et al., "Report on final mortality statistics, 1995" in *Monthly vital statistics report;* Vol. 45, No. 11, Supp. 2, 1997, National Center for Health Statistics, Hyattsville, MD.

TABLE 1.8   Actual Causes of Death in the United States, 1990

Cause	Estimated Number of Deaths	Percentage of Total Deaths
Tobacco	400,000	19
Diet/activity patterns	300,000	14
Alcohol	100,000	5
Microbial	90,000	4
Toxic agents	60,000	3
Firearms	35,000	2
Sexual behavior	30,000	1
Motor vehicles	25,000	1
Illicit use of drugs	20,000	< 1
TOTAL	1,060,000	50

Source: Data from J. M. McGinnis & W. H. Foege, "Actual causes of death in the United States" in *Journal of the American Medical Association, 270*(18), p. 2208.

Note: Composite approximation drawn from studies that use different approaches to derive estimates, ranging from actual counts (e.g., firearms) to population attributable risk calculations (e.g., tobacco). Numbers over 100,000 rounded to nearest 100,000; over 50,000, rounded to nearest 10,000; below 50,000, rounded to nearest 5,000.

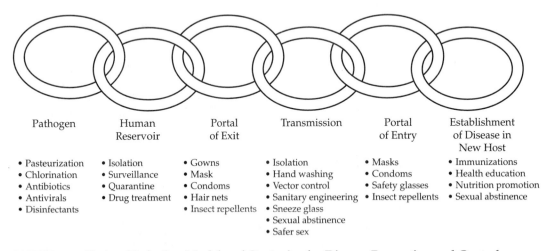

Pathogen	Human Reservoir	Portal of Exit	Transmission	Portal of Entry	Establishment of Disease in New Host
• Pasteurization	• Isolation	• Gowns	• Isolation	• Masks	• Immunizations
• Chlorination	• Surveillance	• Mask	• Hand washing	• Condoms	• Health education
• Antibiotics	• Quarantine	• Condoms	• Vector control	• Safety glasses	• Nutrition promotion
• Antivirals	• Drug treatment	• Hair nets	• Sanitary engineering	• Insect repellents	• Sexual abstinence
• Disinfectants		• Insect repellents	• Sneeze glass		
			• Sexual abstinence		
			• Safer sex		

FIGURE 1.4   Chain of Infection Model and Strategies for Disease Prevention and Control.

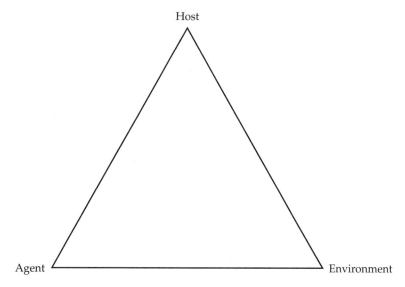

FIGURE 1.5   Communicable Disease Model.

these diseases manifest themselves in people over a period of time and are not caused by a single factor but by many factors. The concept of "caused by many factors" is referred to as the **multicausation disease model.** For example, it is known that heart disease is more likely to manifest itself in individuals who are older, who smoke, who do not exercise, who are overweight, who have high blood pressure, who have high cholesterol, and who have immediate family members who have had heart disease. Note that within this list of factors there are both modifiable and nonmodifiable risk factors. As when using the chain of infection model, the work of health educators is to create programs to help people reduce the risk of disease and injury by helping those in the target population identify and control as many of the multicausative factors as possible.

Other Selected Principles

Several other principles of health education have been noted by Deeds, Cleary, and Neiger (1996). These individuals have identified via the work of others that the principles of participation, empowerment, and cultural sensitivity must be addressed by health educators if health education is to be successful. **Participation** refers to the active involvement of those in the target population in helping identify, plan, and implement programs to address the health problems they face. Without such participation, ethical issues associated with program development come into play, and the target population probably will not support and feel **ownership** of (responsibility for) the program. For example, if the health educators for a large corporation are creating a health promotion program for all employees, they should not begin to plan without the participation of (or at least representation by) each of the segments (clerical, labor, and management) of the employee population.

If health education is going to help people create lasting change, then those in the target population must be empowered as a result of the health education/promotion programming. **Empowerment** is "a social action process that promotes participation of people, organizations and communities in gaining control over their lives in their community and larger society. With this perspective, empowerment is not characterized as achieving power to dominate others, but rather power to act with others to affect change" (Wallerstein & Bernstein, 1988, p. 380). Making a community more safe via a neighborhood watch provides a good example of empowerment. Obviously, police can make a neighborhood safer by regularly patrolling the area. However, because of limited resources in most communities, the police cannot be constantly present in every neighborhood. But the people who live in the area, and are present many more hours than the police could be, can take on the "patrolling" responsibilities. Neighborhood residents can be provided with the knowledge and skills (empowered) to provide an effective "watch" (be the eyes and ears of the police) over the neighborhood. Such empowerment can decrease crime and improve safety.

Health education/promotion programming cannot be effective if it is not sensitive to the culture, beliefs, and concerns of those for whom the program is intended. **Cultural sensitivity** is having and showing respect for cultures other than one's own. Cultural sensitivity is an important principle of health education because of the close relationship that often exists between health and culture.

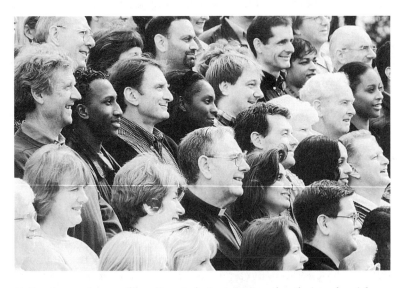

Cultural competency will continue to be important as the ethnic and racial make-up of the U.S. becomes more diverse. (Bob Thomas/Tony Stone Images)

Cultural factors arise from guidelines (both explicit and implicit) that individuals "inherit" from being a part of a particular society, ethnic group, race, or other group (Helman, 1984). Examples include the various beliefs, traditions, and prejudices held by individuals. In order for health educators to be effective in a variety of communities, they need to be **culturally competent.** This means having the knowledge and interpersonal skills to understand, appreciate, and work with individuals from cultures other than their own. It involves an awareness and acceptance of cultural differences; self-awareness; knowledge of the culture of those in the target population; and the adaptation of professional skills to respond to the target population's cultural differences (McManus, 1988). Even services that are provided to all in an equal and nondiscriminatory manner may not take into account the needs of those in the target population and therefore be culturally inappropriate (Davis & Voegtle, 1994).

The Discipline of Epidemiology

As already noted in this chapter, the profession of health education is built on a number of other disciplines and professions. However, one discipline has proven to be extremely important to health education. That discipline is epidemiology. **Epidemiology** is defined as "the study of the distribution and determinants of diseases and injuries in human populations" (Mausner & Kramer, 1985, p. 1). Epidemiology is important to health education because health educators often use epidemiological data to identify the needs of a given population and to evaluate the success of the programs they have planned. Our discussion earlier in this chapter about "measuring health and health status" included a basic component of epidemiology "rates." The terms **endemic** (occurs regularly in a population as a matter of course), **epidemic** (an unexpectedly large number of cases of disease in a population), and **pandemic** (an outbreak of a disease over a wide geographical area, such as a continent) all come from the field of epidemiology. As you continue your preparation to become a health educator, you will find that you will be introduced to more and more epidemiological principles.

Summary

In this introductory chapter, many of the basic principles of the profession of health education were presented. The readers were presented with a brief discussion of why we refer to health education as an emerging profession; a look at the current status of health education; definitions of many of the key words and terms used in the profession, including *health, health education, health promotion,* and *wellness;* an explanation of how health or health status has been measured, including mortality rates, life expectancy, YPLL, DALYs, and health surveys; an outline of the goal and objectives of the profession; the practice of health education, including planning, implementing, and evaluating programs; some of the basic underlying concepts and principles of the profession, including the health field concept, levels of prevention, risk factors, health risk reduction via understanding disease; and the principles of participation, empowerment, and cultural sensitivity. Finally, the chapter ended with a brief discussion about the importance of epidemiology to health education.

REVIEW QUESTIONS

1. Why have the authors chosen to describe health education as an emerging profession?

2. What is the current status of health education?

3. Please define the following terms—*health, health education, health promotion, health promotion and disease prevention, public health, community health, coordinated school health program,* and *wellness.*

4. Explain each of the following means of measuring health or health status.
   - Mortality rates. What is the difference among crude, adjusted, and specific rates?
   - Life expectancy
   - Years of potential life lost (YPLL)
   - Disability-adjusted life years (DALYs)
   - Health surveys

5. Of all the different measures of health presented in this chapter, which one do you think is the best indicator of health? Why?

6. In a given community with a midyear population estimate of 50,000, there were twenty-one deaths due to strokes in the year. What is the rate of stroke deaths per 100,000 population?

7. What is the goal of health education?

8. Name the different levels of objectives of health education.

9. What constitutes the basic practice of health education?

10. Briefly explain the following concepts and principles of health education.
    - Health Field Concept
    - Levels of prevention
    - Risk factors
    - Health risk reduction
    - Chain of infection
    - Communicable disease model
    - Multicausation disease model
    - Selected principles of health education—participation, empowerment, and cultural sensitivity

11. Why is epidemiology such an important discipline for health education?

ACTIVITIES

1. If you have not already done so, locate and read a copy of the government document *Healthy People: The Surgeon General's Report on Health Promotion and Disease Prevention* (USDHEW, 1979). It provides a good background on the health promotion era in the United States.

2. Do you agree with the authors that health education is an emerging profession? Defend your response in a one- to two-page paper.

3. Write your own definitions for *health, health education,* and *health promotion* using the concepts presented in the chapter.

4. Write one paragraph for each of the following:
   - Why do you think the health field concept was so important in getting people to think about health promotion?
   - At what level of prevention do you think it would be most difficult to change health behavior? Why?

5. In a one-page paper, use the chain of infection to outline three different means for preventing the spread of the HIV.

6. In a one-page paper, use the multicausation disease model to explain how a person develops heart disease.

REFERENCES

Barber, B. (1988). Professions and emerging professions. In J. C. Callahan (Ed.), *Ethical issues in professional life* (pp. 35–39). New York: Oxford University Press.

Centers for Disease Control and Prevention (CDC). (1994). *Chronic disease in minority populations.* Atlanta, GA: Author.

Cohen, H. J. (1991). My grandmother said, "If you had your health, you have everything." What did she mean? In M. Feinleib (Ed.), *Vital and health statistics: Proceedings of 1988 International symposium on data on aging* (DHHS pub. no. PHS-91-1482). (pp. 5–9). Washington, DC: U.S. Government Printing Office.

Davis, B. J., & Voegtle, K. H. (1994). *Culturally competent health care for adolescents.* Chicago, IL: American Medical Association.

Deeds, S. G., Cleary, M. J., & Neiger, B. L. (Eds.). (1996). *The certified health education specialist: A self-study guide for professional competency* (2nd ed.). Allentown, PA: The National Commission for Health Education Credentialing, Inc.

Dunn, H. L. (1977). What high-level wellness means. *Health Values: Achieving High-Level Wellness, 1*(1), 9–16.

Galli, N. (1976). Foundations of health education. *The Journal of School Health, 46*(3), 158–165.

Goodstadt, M. S., Simpson, R. I., & Loranger, P. O. (1987). Health promotion: A conceptual integration. *American Journal of Health Promotion, 1*(3), 58–63.

Green, L. W., & Kreuter, M. W. (1991). *Health promotion planning: An educational and environmental approach* (2nd ed.). Mountain View, CA: Mayfield.

Green, L. W., Kreuter, M. W., Deeds, S. G., & Partridge, K. B. (1980). *Health promotion planning: A diagnostic approach.* Palo Alto, CA: Mayfield.

Green, L. W., & Ottoson, J. M. (1994). *Community health* (7th ed.) St. Louis, MO: Mosby.

Greene, W. H., & Simons-Morton, B. G. (1984). *Introduction to health education.* New York: Macmillan.

Helman, C. (1984). *Culture, health and illness: An introduction for health professions.* Bristol, England: John Wright & Son, Stonebridge Press.

Johns, E. B. (1973). Joint Committee on Health Education Terminology: Report of the joint committee on health education terminology. *Health Education, 4*(6), 25.

Joint Committee on Health Education Terminology. (1991a). Report of the 1990 Joint Committee on Health Education Terminology. *Journal of Health Education, 22*(2), 105–106.

Joint Committee on Health Education Terminology. (1991b). Report of the 1990 Joint Committee on Health Education Terminology. *Journal of School Health, 61*(6), 251–254.

Laframboise, H. L. (1973). Health policy: Breaking it down into more manageable segments. *Journal of the Canadian Medical Association, 108*(Feb. 3), 388–393.

Lalonde, M. (1974). *A new perspective on the health of Canadians: A working document.* Ottawa, Canada: Ministry of National Health and Welfare.

Landau, S. I. (Ed.). (1979). *Funk and Wagnalls standard desk dictionary.* New York: Funk and Wagnalls.

Livingood, W. C. (1996). Becoming a health education profession: Key to societal influence—1995 SOPHE presidential address. *Health Education Quarterly, 23*(4), 421–430.

Marx, E., & Wooley, S.E. (Eds.), with Northrop, D. (1998). Health is academic: A guide to coordinated school health programs. New York: Teachers College Press, Columbia University.

Mason, J. O., & McGinnis, J. M. (1990). Healthy people 2000: An overview of the national health promotion disease prevention objectives. *Public Health Reports, 105*(5), 441–446.

Mausner, J. S., & Kramer, S. (1985). *Epidemiology—An introductory text.* Philadelphia: W. B. Saunders.

McGinnis, J. M. (1985). The limits of prevention. *Public Health Reports, 100*(3), 255–260.

McGinnis, J. M., & Foege, W. H. (1993). Actual causes of death in the United States. *Journal of the American Medical Association, 270*(18), 2207–2212.

McKenzie, J. F., & Pinger, R. R. (1997). *An introduction to community health* (Web enhanced edition). Sudbury, MA: Jones and Bartlett.

McKenzie, J. F., & Smeltzer, J. L. (1997). *Planning, implementing, and evaluating health promotion programs: A primer.* Boston, MA: Allyn & Bacon.

McManus, M. C. (Ed.) (1988). Services to minority populations: Cross cultural competence continuum. *Focal Point, 3*(1), 1–4. Portland, OR: Research and Training Center, Regional Research Institute for Human Services, Portland State University.

Montagu, A. (1968). *Man observed.* New York: G. P. Putnam.

Moss, B. (1950). Joint Committee on Health Education Terminology. *Journal of Physical Education, 21,* 41.

Murray, C. J. L., & Lopez, A. D. (Eds.). (1996a). *Summary of the global burden of disease: A comprehensive assessment of mortality and disability from diseases, injuries, and risk factors in 1990 and projected to 2020.* Geneva, Switzerland: World Health Organization.

Murray, C. J. L., & Lopez, A. D. (Eds.). (1996b). *The global burden of disease: A comprehensive assessment of mortality and disability from diseases, injuries, and risk factors in 1990 and projected to 2020.* Geneva, Switzerland: World Health Organization.

National Center for Health Statistics (NCHS). (1995). *Health, United States, 1994.* (DHHS Publication No. (PHS) 95-1232). Hyattsville, MD: Public Health Service.

National Commission for Health Education Credentialing, Inc. (NCHEC). (1996). *A competency-based framework for professional development of certified health education specialists.* Allentown, PA: Author.

Raphael, D., Brown, I., Renwick, R., & Rootman, I. (1997). Quality of life: What are the implications for health promotion? *American Journal of Health Behavior, 21*(2), 118–128.

Rugen, M. (1972). *A fifty year history of the public health section of American Public Health Association; 1922–1972.* Washington, DC: American Public Health Association, Inc.

Ubbes, V. A., & Watts, P. R. (1995). Terminology, tolerance, and flexibility: Communication challenges for health education. *Journal of Health Education, 26*(4), 251–253.

Upton, L. A. (1970). *A study of secondary school counselors' perceptions of school counseling as a profession and their desires for professionalization of school counseling.* Doctoral dissertation. State University of New York at Buffalo.

U.S. Department of Health, Education, and Welfare (Public Health Service) (USDHEW). (1979). *Healthy people: The Surgeon General's report on health promotion and disease prevention.* (Publication No. 79-55071). Washington, DC: U.S. Government Printing Office.

U.S. Department of Health, Education, and Welfare (USDHEW). (1980). *Promoting health/ preventing disease: Objectives for the nation.* Washington, DC: U.S. Government Printing Office.

U.S. Department of Health and Human Services (DHHS). (1990a). *Healthy People 2000: National health promotion and disease prevention objectives* (DHHS pub. no. PHS 90-50212). Washington, DC: U.S. Government Printing Office.

U.S. Department of Health and Human Services (DHHS). (1990b). *Prevention '89/'90.* Washington, DC: U.S. Government Printing Office.

U.S. Department of Health and Human Services (DHHS). (1991). *Health status of minorities and low-income groups* (3rd ed.). Washington, DC: U.S. Government Printing Office.

U.S. Department of Health and Human Services (DHHS). (1997). *Issues brief: Development of healthy people 2010 objectives.* (On-line). Available—www: http://odphp.osophs.dhhs.gov/pubs/hp2000/2010.htm

Wallerstein, N., & Bernstein, E. (1988). Empowerment education: Freier's ideas adapted to health education. *Health Education Quarterly, 15*(4), 379–394.

Williams, J. F. (1934). Report of the Health Education Section of the American Physical Education Association: Definitions of terms in health education. *Journal of Physical Education, 5*(16–17), 50–51.

World development report 1993: Investing in health. (1993). New York: Oxford University Press (for the World Bank).

World Health Organization (WHO). (1947). Constitution of the World Health Organization. *Chronicle of the World Health Organization 1.* Geneva, Switzerland: Author.

Yoho, R. (1962). Joint Committee on Health Education Terminology: Health education terminology. *Journal of Physical Education and Recreation, 33*(Nov.), 27–28.

2 The History of Health and Health Education

CHAPTER OBJECTIVES

After reading this chapter and answering the questions at the end, you should be able to

1. Discuss health beliefs and practices from earliest humans to present day.
2. Identify the dual roots of modern health education.
3. Explain why a need for professional health educators emerged.
4. Trace the history of public health in the United States.
5. Relate the history of school health from the mid-1800s to the present.
6. Identify important governmental publications from 1975 to the present, and describe how these publications have impacted health promotion and education.

KEY TERMS

A New Perspective on the Health of Canadians
Asclepiads
Asclepius
atomic theory
bacteriological period of public health
caduceus
Code of Hammurabi
comprehensive school health instruction
comprehensive school health program

coordinated school health program
Health literacy
Healthy People
Healthy People 2000
Hippocrates
Hygeia
life expectancy
Medicaid
Medicare
miasmas theory

Panacea
Promoting Health/Preventing Disease: Objectives for the Nation
School Health Education Evaluation Study
School Health Education Study
Smith Papyri
social ecology

Introduction

While the history of health education as an emerging profession is only a little over one hundred years old, the concept of educating about health has been around since the dawn of humans. This chapter will chronicle human beings' knowledge of health and health care from the earliest records to the present. It will focus primarily on Northern Africa and Europe, as these were the areas that had the greatest influence on the development of health knowledge and health care in the United States. This should not be construed to mean that other parts of the world such as the Far East, Central America, and South America did not contribute to the history of health and health care. However, to review the history of all societies is beyond the scope of this book and would not be as directly relevant to the history of health, health care, and health education in the United States as is the health history of Western societies.

As one reads through this chapter, it should become clear that the need for professional health educators emerged as human beings' knowledge of health and health care increased. Particular emphasis will be placed on the history of health education during the past 150 years as it evolved to its present status from the dual roots of school health and public health.

This information should be of particular interest to the new health education student, as one cannot fully appreciate the profession without understanding its origin. Historical study allows one to see progress made and ascertain trends over time. It clearly depicts the difficulties and obstacles faced by those persons interested in promoting health throughout the years and enhances appreciation of their efforts. "At the same time, historical study shows us that despite the difficulties, change is possible, given dedication, organization and persistence. . . . Historical case studies may be able to teach us useful lessons about successful strategies used by public health reformers in the past" (Fee & Brown, 1997, p. 1763).

Early Humans

It must be assumed that the earliest humans learned by trial and error to distinguish those things that were good for them and would enhance health from those that were harmful and would impair health. Goerke and Stebbins (1968) noted, "By observing animals he learned that bathing not only cooled and refreshed his body, but helped remove external parasites; he learned that application of mud assuaged insect bites; and by determining the actions of certain herbs, he learned their various medicinal or poisonous characteristics" (p. 5).

It does not stretch the imagination too far to begin to see how health education first took place. Someone may have eaten a particular plant or herb and became ill. That person would then warn (educate) others against eating the same substance. Conversely, someone may have ingested a plant or an herb that produced a desired effect. That person would then encourage (educate) others to use

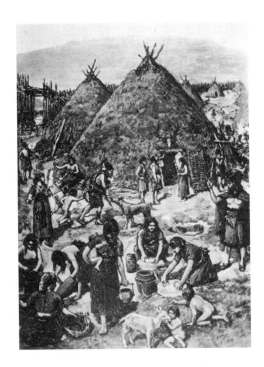

People have always been concerned about their health. This picture shows a reconstruction of life on the Sussex Downs in the late Bronze Age. (Corbis-Bettmann)

this substance. Through observation, trial, and error other types of health-related knowledge would be discovered. Eventually, this knowledge would be transformed into rules or taboos for a given society. Rules about preserving food and how to bury the dead may have been implemented. Perhaps taboos against defecation within the tribe's communal area or near sources of drinking water were established (McKenzie & Pinger, 1997). Over time and as knowledge increased, there would be less need for the trial and error method, which undoubtedly produced serious illness and even death among some of these early humans. Knowledge would be passed from one generation to the next, thus preventing at least some of the potential ill effects of everyday life.

There was still much more that was unknown than was known about how to protect health. Disease and death were probably much more common than health and longevity. To early humans, it was puzzling when disease and death occurred for no apparent reason. In an attempt to make these events seem more rational, "disease and infirmity were believed to be caused by the influence of magic or malevolent spirits that inhabited streams, trees, animals, the earth and the air. Purposively or accidentally provoking any of the spirits, it was thought, would result in dire consequences for the individual or his/her community" (Goerke & Stebbins, 1968, p. 5). To prevent disease, sacrifices were made to the gods, taboos were obeyed, amulets were worn, and haunted places were avoided.

Charms, spells, and chants were also used to protect one from disease (Duncan, 1988). Again, it is not too hard to imagine that there was some form of rudimentary health education taking place to inform people about what they needed to do to keep from provoking the spirits and, thus, prevent disease.

Early Efforts at Community Health

Evidence of broad-scale community health activity has been found in the very earliest of civilizations. In India, sites excavated at Mohenjo-Daro and Harappa dating back four thousand years indicate that bathrooms and drains were common. The streets were broad, paved, and drained by covered sewers (Rosen, 1958). Archeological evidence also shows that the Minoans (3000–1430 B.C.) and Myceneans (1430–1150 B.C.) built drainage systems, toilets, and water flushing systems (Pickett & Hanlon, 1990). The oldest written documents related to health care are the **Smith Papyri,** dating from 1600 B.C., which describe various surgical techniques. The earliest written record concerning public health is the **Code of Hammurabi,** the king of Babylon. It contained laws pertaining to health practices and physicians, including the first known fee schedule (Rubinson & Alles, 1984).

Egyptians

The medical lore of the distant past was handed down from generation to generation. In virtually every culture for which there are documented historical accounts, it appears there existed some type of a physician or medicine man to which people turned for health information, treatments, and cures (Green & Simons-Morton, 1990). In Egypt, as in many other cultures, this role was held by the priests. Eventually, the various incantations, spells, exorcisms, prescriptions, and clinical observations were compiled into written format, some of which survive in our museums and libraries (Libby, 1922).

Due at least in part to the conservatism of the priest-physicians, "Egyptian medicine never advanced far beyond primitive medicine with its simple faith in magic spells and the virtue of a rich pharmacopoeia, and its belief that the cause of disease was the malice of a demon, the justice of an avenging god, the ill-will of an enemy, or the anger of the dead" (Libby, 1922, p. 4). Some of the more disgusting substances the Egyptians used as remedies included "dung of the gazelle and the crocodile, the fat of a serpent, mammalian entrails and other excreta, tissues and organs. In some cases the object seems to have been to wheedle, in other cases to repel, the evil spirits that had taken possession of the patient" (Libby, 1922, p. 6).

Still, the Egyptians made substantial progress in the area of public health. They possessed a strong sense of personal cleanliness and were considered to be the healthiest people of their time. They used numerous pharmaceutic preparations and

BOX **2.1**

The Rights and Duties of the Surgeon of 2080 B.C.:
From the Code of Hammurabi

"If a physician operate on a man for a severe wound (or make a severe wound upon a man), with a bronze lancet, and save the man's life; or if he open an abscess (in the eye) of a man, with a bronze lancet, and save the man's eye, he shall receive ten shekels of silver (as his fee)."

"If he be a freeman,* he shall receive five shekels."

"If it be a man's slave, the owner of the slave shall give two shekels of silver to the physician."

"If a physician operate on a man for a severe wound, with a bronze lancet, and cause the man's death; or open an abscess (in the eye) of a man with a bronze lancet, and destroy the man's eye, they shall cut off his hands."

"If a physician operate on a slave of a freeman for a severe wound, with a bronze lancet, and cause his death, he shall restore a slave of equal value."

"If he open an abscess (in his eye), with a bronze lancet, and destroy his eye, he shall pay silver to the extent of one half of his price."

"If a physician set a broken bone for a man or cure his diseased bowels, the patient shall give five shekels of silver to the physician."

"If he be a freeman,* he shall give three shekels."

"If it be a man's slave, the owner of the slave shall give two shekels of silver to the physician."

"If a veterinary physician operate on an ox or ass for a severe wound and save its life, the owner of the ox or ass shall give the physician, as his fee, one sixth of a shekel of silver."

"If he operate on an ox or an ass for a severe wound, and cause its death, he shall give to the owner of the ox or ass one fourth its value."

*"Freeman" indicates a rank intermediate between that of "man" (or gentleman) and that of "slave."

Source: From R. F. Harper, The Code of Hammurabi, 1904, Chicago.

---

constructed earth privies for sewage, as well as public drainage pipes (Pickett & Hanlon, 1990).

The Hebrews of about 1500 B.C. extended Egyptian hygienic thought and formulated in the biblical book of Leviticus what is probably the world's first written hygienic code. It dealt with a wide variety of personal and community responsibilities, including cleanliness of the body, protection against the spread of contagious diseases, isolation of lepers, disinfection of dwellings after illness, sanitation of campsites, disposal of excreta and refuse, protection of water and food supplies, and specific hygiene rules for menstruating women and women who had recently delivered a child.

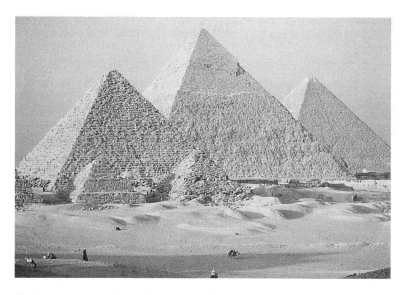

The Egyptians were known for their cleanliness and were considered the healthiest people of the time. (Hugh Sitton/Tony Stone Images)

Greeks

The history of health and health care in the Greek culture (1000–400 B.C.) is intriguing as well as relevant to modern health care philosophy. The Greeks were perhaps the first people to put as much emphasis on prevention of disease as on the treatment of disease conditions. The concept of balance among the physical, mental, and spiritual aspects of the person was emphasized. Religion played an important role in health care for early Greeks, but eventually the role of physician began to take shape, and a more scientific view of medicine emerged.

In the early stages of Greek culture, as represented in the *Iliad* and the *Odyssey*, the priesthood played a role in the healing arts. In the *Iliad*, **Asclepius** was a Thesalian chief who had received instruction in the use of drugs. By the beginning of the eighth century B.C., tradition had endowed him as the god of medicine. He had two daughters, who were also given health-related powers. **Hygeia** was given the power to prevent disease, while **Panacea** was given the ability to treat disease. Of the two daughters, Hygeia was the more prominent and was often pictured with her father in sculptures and illustrations of the time (Schouten, 1967). The words *hygiene* and *panacea* can be traced back to these daughters of Asclepius (Libby, 1922).

Eventually, hundreds of elaborate temples were built throughout Greece to worship Asclepius. These temples were typically on beautiful sites overlooking the sea or beside healing fountains. The temple priests practiced their healing arts, which often involved fraud. The priests played on the superstitions of the

BOX **2.2**

The Story of Asclepius

"According to Greek mythology, Asclepius, the son of Apollo, was a god of healing whose powers were so great that he could bring the dead back to life. When Hades, the god of the dead, jealously complained to Zeus that Asclepius was cheating the kingdom of the dead, Zeus agreed with Hades that Asclepius had violated a basic law of nature by saving mortals from death. Consequently, Asclepius was killed with a thunderbolt. Before he died, however, he gave his healing powers to two of his daughters: Panacea, goddess of healing, who administered medication to the sick, and Hygeia, goddess of health, who taught mortals to live wisely and preserve their bodies."

Source: Bates, I. J., & Winder, A. E. *Introduction to Health Education,* 1984, Mayfield Publishing.

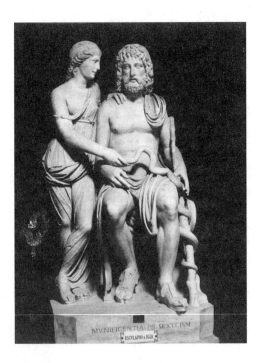

Asclepius and Hygieia. (Museo Vanticano/Art Resource)

sufferers through the use of sacrificial rites and purifications, tame snakes, and dream interpretation. In fact, sleep and dreams were a major aspect of the Asclepian temples. Sufferers were often allowed to sleep near the temple. Priests would impersonate Asclepius and appear to the sufferers while they slept. Those who believed they had benefited from the suggestions and worship left tablets

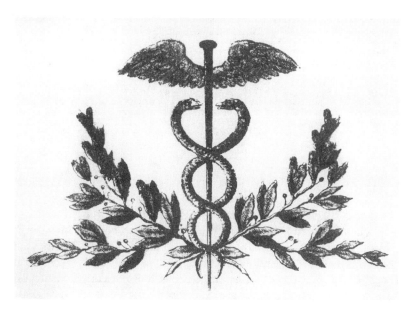

Illustration of a caduceus, a symbol which shows two snakes braided around a staff. It is representative of the medical profession and has its earliest association with Asclepius, the Greek healer. (Corbis-Bettmann)

telling of their cure or other remembrances such as gold, silver, or marble models of the cured body part. The priests always made sure all knew of the therapeutic value of a substantial fee (Libby, 1922). These ancient temples of Asclepius left their symbol as a permanent reminder of the past—the staff and serpent of the physician, known as the **caduceus** (Rubinson & Alles, 1984).

The temple priests should not be confused with the **Asclepiads**. The Asclepiads were a brotherhood of men present at the temples who initially claimed decent from Asclepius. While some of the Asclepiads probably helped the priests with their chicanery, others broke away from the priests and began to practice medicine based on more rational principles.

The famous Greek physician **Hippocrates,** came from the Asclepian tradition. He lived from about 460 B.C. until 377 B.C. He developed a theory of disease causation consistent with the philosophy of nature held by leading philosophers of his day. Essentially, he believed all things were composed of different combinations of particles too small to be seen. These particles were called "atoms"; thus, his theory became known as the **atomic theory.** Hippocrates believed there were only four kinds of atoms: earth, air, fire, and water. Each atom retained two of the four qualities of wetness, dryness, warmth, and coldness. Earth was cold and dry; air was hot and wet; water was cold and wet; and fire was hot and dry. Hippocrates further believed that the human body was made up of four substances, which he called the four "humours." The humours were blood, phlegm, yellow bile, and black bile. Each humour was made up of one type of atom. Blood

TABLE 2.1 Hippocrates' Atomic Theory

Body Parts	Atoms	Properties
Blood	Air	Hot and wet
Phlegm	Water	Cold and wet
Yellow bile	Fire	Hot and dry
Black bile	Earth	Cold and dry

was made up of air and possessed the properties of being hot and wet; phlegm was made up of water and was cold and wet; yellow bile was fire, so it was hot and dry; and black bile was earth, which meant it was cold and dry (Duncan, 1988). A visual depiction of Hippocrates' theory can be seen in Table 2.1.

Hippocrates taught that health was the result of balance of the four humours; conversely, disease was the result of an imbalance of the four humours. An excess of hot, wet blood, for example, resulted in fever, sweating, and diarrhea and could be treated by bleeding the sufferer. Colds, which were associated with cold, wet phlegm, were treated with hot, spicy foods and applications of mustard or other irritants to the chest to produce a feeling of warmth. Excess phlegm or black bile, both cold, could be sweated out in a steam bath or eliminated by vomiting. Excess yellow bile could be eliminated by enemas (Duncan, 1988).

In the Greek world, the ideal person was perfectly balanced in mind, body, and spirit. Thus, study and practice related to philosophy, athletics, and theology were all important to maintain balance. To do this, however, took a tremendous commitment of time and energy. Each day required physical activity, study, and philosophical discussion while maintaining proper nutrition and rest. Very few people could afford to lead such a life. Those who did were the aristocratic upper class leading a life of leisure supported by a slave economy (Rosen, 1958). The ideal Greek human being that is so often mentioned was, in fact, a very small percentage of the Greek population.

Hippocrates holds an important place in the history of medicine. While his atomic theory seems simplistic and of little value in today's world of modern medicine, it is important to remember that the atomic theory was still being taught in American medical schools as a valid theory of disease causation as recently as the first quarter of the twentieth century. Hippocrates, however, did more than just theorize about disease. He carefully observed and recorded associations between certain diseases and such factors as geography, climate, diet, and living conditions. Duncan (1988) noted, "One of his [Hippocrates'] most noteworthy contributions is the distinction between 'endemic' diseases, which vary in prevalence from place to place, and 'epidemic' diseases, which vary in prevalence over time" (p. 12). The traditional Hippocratic Oath is still used today and is the basis for medical ethics. Hippocrates and the Asclepiads moved health care away from religion and priests and attempted to establish a more rational basis to explain health and disease. Hippocrates' concept of balance in life is still promoted today as the best means for maintaining health and well-being.

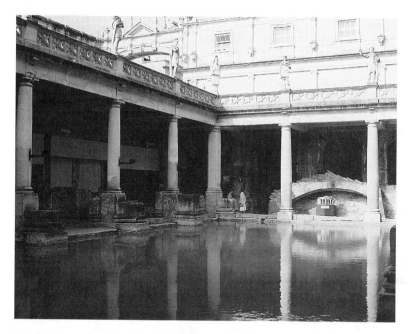

The Romans enjoyed a system of public baths that were supplied with fresh water. This picture shows the Roman baths in Bath, England. (Pierre Berger/Photo Researchers)

Hippocrates has been credited as being the first epidemiologist and the father of modern medicine (Duncan, 1988). It is not hard to imagine that he was also a health educator. One can easily see Hippocrates educating his friends and patients about diet, exercise, rest, and the importance of balance in preventing disease and promoting health.

Romans

The Romans conquered the Mediterranean world, including the Greeks. In doing so, however, the Romans did not destroy the cultures they conquered but learned from them. The Romans accepted many of the Greek ideas, including those related to health and medicine. "As clinicians, the Romans were hardly more than imitators of the Greeks, but as engineers and administrators, as builders of sewerage systems and baths, and as providers of water supplies and other health facilities, they set the world a great example and left their mark in history" (Rosen, 1958, p. 38).

The Roman Empire (500 B.C.–A.D. 500) built an aqueduct system that was both extensive and efficient. "Evidence of some 200 Roman aqueducts remains today, from Spain to Syria and from northern Europe to North Africa" (McKenzie & Pinger, 1997, p. 11). It has been estimated that the total capacity of the thirteen aqueducts delivering water to the city of Rome was 222 million gallons per twenty-four hours. At the height of the empire, this would have been enough water to provide each citizen of Rome with at least forty gallons of fresh water per day. In addition, attention was paid to water purity. At specific points along the aqueduct, generally near the middle and end, settling basins were located, in which sediment might be deposited (Rosen, 1958).

The Romans also developed an extensive system of underground sewers. These served to carry off both surface water and sewage. To demonstrate the size of this system, where the main Rome sewer emptied into the Tiber River, it was 10 feet wide and 12 feet high. This is still part of the sewer system of Rome today (Rosen, 1958).

The Romans had a great appreciation for hygiene and developed an extensive system of private and public baths. Rosen (1958) notes,

> A census of baths was taken by Agrippa in 33 B.C. At that time there were 170. The number grew steadily and later approached a thousand. The fee generally charged was about half a cent and children entered free. Up to the time of Trajan, mixed bathing was not formally prohibited, although there were **balneae** exclusively for women. Sometime between 117 and 138, Hadrian issued a decree separating the sexes in the baths. (p. 48)

The Romans made other health advancements. They learned to locate new towns on salubrious sites, giving considerable attention to the position, orientation, and drainage of dwellings. The Romans observed the effect of occupational hazards on health, and they were the first to build hospitals. By the second century A.D., a public medical service was constituted whereby physicians were appointed to various towns and institutions. A system of private medical practice also developed during the Roman era (Rosen, 1958).

The Romans furthered the work of the Greeks in the study of human anatomy and the practice of surgery. Some Roman anatomists even dissected living human beings to further their knowledge of anatomy (Libby, 1922). In quoting Latin writer Cornelius, Libby found that these anatomists "procured criminals out of prison, by royal permission, and dissecting them alive, contemplated, while they were still breathing, the parts which nature had before concealed, considering their position, color, figure, size, order, hardness, softness, smoothness, and asperity" (Libby, 1922, p. 54). While some opposed this hideous practice, others supported it, holding "it is by no means cruel as most people represent it, by the tortures of a few guilty, to search after remedies for the whole innocent race of mankind in all ages" (Libby, 1922, p. 54).

Middle Ages

The period of time from the collapse of the Roman Empire to about A.D. 1500 has become known as the Middle Ages or Dark Ages. This was a time of political and social unrest, when many of the advancements related to health were lost. Rosen

(1958) notes that "the problem that confronted the medieval world was to weld together the culture of the barbarian invaders with the classical heritage of the defunct [Roman] Empire and with the beliefs and teachings of the Christian religion" (p. 52). This proved to be no easy task.

With the Roman Empire no longer able to protect the settlements, each city had to be prepared to defend itself against its enemies. Security rested on its citizens and its encircling fortifications. To be safe, one had to live within the walls of the city. Domesticated animals were also kept inside the city. Many public health problems were simply the result of too many people and animals living within a confined area. As the population grew, expansion was difficult and overcrowding common (Rosen, 1958). The public health advancements of the Roman Empire were lost. Lack of fresh water and sewage removal was a major problem for many of these medieval cities.

To make matters worse, there was little emphasis on cleanliness or hygiene. The new religion, Christianity,

> found its disciples among the lower classes, where personal hygiene was not practiced, and as a consequence, an entirely different attitude toward the human body developed. Excessive care of the body, that is, man's earthly and mutable part, was unimportant in the Christian dualistic concept, which separated body from soul. For some Eastern churchmen and holy men, living in filth was regarded as evidence of sanctity: cleanliness was thought to betoken pride, and filthiness humility. (Goerke & Stebbins, 1968, p. 9)

Fortunately, as Christianity matured so did its concept of the human body. Eventually, Christians came to understand that the body is the abode for the soul while one is on earth, therefore permitting one to preserve and take care of it.

Early Christians also reinforced the earlier notion that disease was caused by sin or disobeying God. This propelled the priests and religious leaders back into the position of preventing and treating disease. The health-related advancements of the Greco-Roman era were abandoned and shunned. Entire libraries were burned, and knowledge about the human body was seen as sinful.

The Middle Ages were characterized by great epidemics. Perhaps the cruelest of these was leprosy, a disease characterized by severe facial disfigurement. It is highly contagious and virulent. All Western countries issued edicts against anyone suspected of having leprosy and regulated every aspect of the sufferer's life. In some communities lepers were given the last rites of the church and were forced to leave the city, were made to wear identifying clothing, and were required to carry a rod identifying them as lepers. Some were even forced to wear a bell around their necks and to ring it as a warning when others came near. Such isolation usually brought about a relatively quick death due to hunger and exposure (Goerke & Stebbins, 1968). Eventually, leprosy hospitals were founded to treat the inflicted. It has been estimated that by A.D. 1200 there were 1,900 leper houses and leposaria in Europe (Rosen, 1958).

The bubonic plague, known as the Black Death, may have been the most severe epidemic the world has ever known. The death toll was higher and the disruption of society greater than from any war, famine, or natural disaster in history. "At Constantinople, the plague raged with such violence that 5000, and even 10,000 persons are said to have died in a single day" (Donan, 1898, p. 94). Estimates of casualties vary from 20 to 35 million, with Europe losing a quarter to a third of its entire population. In Avignon, where 60,000 people died, the pope was forced to consecrate the Rhone River in order that bodies might be thrown into it, because the churchyards could no longer absorb the dead (Goerke & Stebbins, 1968).

Imagine what it must have been like to live through the plague. Literally one out of every three or four people you knew would have contracted the disease and died. The cause of the disease was unknown; thus, fear and superstition were rampant. Often religious leaders and doctors would be some of the first victims, as they would be exposed to the disease early in the epidemic through their contact with infected sufferers. This could leave a community with no religious or medical leadership as the death toll continued to rise.

Goerke and Stebbins (1968) note, "Many people reacted to the plague either by becoming licentious and hedonistic or by becoming severely ascetic, such as those who formed the sect known as the Flagellants. Jews were burned or exiled not so much because they were thought to have caused the epidemic, but rather because the nobles and communities were heavily indebted to them, and the deteriorated moral and ethical practices which accompanied the plague sanctioned escaping the debts in this way" (p. 11).

The Brotherhood of the Flagellants was a group of religious zealots who believed the plague could be avoided by admitting to their sins and then ritualistically beating themselves in atonement. Today, such a group would most likely be labeled a religious cult. Members of this group marched in long, two-column lines from city to city. In each city, they would chant a litany and conduct their ritualistic ceremony. At a signal from the group's master, the Flagellants would strip to the waist and march in a circle until they received another signal from the master. Upon receiving the second signal, they would throw themselves to the ground with their position indicating the specific sin they had committed. The master would move among the bodies thrashing those than had committed certain sins or had offended the discipline of the Flagellants in some way. This would be followed by a collective flagellation whereby each group member would rhythmically beat their own backs and breasts with a heavy scourge made of three or four leather thongs tipped with metal studs. According to eye witness accounts, the Flagellants lashed themselves until their bodies became swollen and blue, and blood dripped to the ground. Further complicating the health consequences of such punishment was a rule prohibiting bathing, washing, or changing clothes. When joining the Brotherhood, group members had to pledge to scourge themselves three times daily for thirty-three days and eight hours, which represented one day for each year of Christ's earthly life (Ziegler, 1969).

Much debate existed during this time concerning the cause of the plague. Jehan Jacme, the author of one treatise on the subject, wrote in 1348 that the disease was caused by five factors: the wrath of God, the corruption of dead bodies, waters and vapors formed in the interior of the earth, unnatural hot and humid winds, and the conjunction of stars and planets (Winslow, 1944). Despite the disagreement that existed on the cause of the disease, some people of the time began to believe that the disease was contagious. In other words, it was passed from person to person in some unknown way. While this concept of contagion had been around for many years and was discussed in the Bible, it was not until the Middle Ages and the epidemics of leprosy and bubonic plague that it started to become more universally accepted. The contagion concept opened the door to new interest in science and severely weakened the argument of those promoting the sin-disease theory.

The Middle Ages also saw epidemics of other communicable diseases, including smallpox, diphtheria, measles, influenza, tuberculosis, anthrax, and trachoma. The last major epidemic disease of this period was syphilis, which appeared in 1492. As with other epidemics, syphilis killed thousands of people (McKenzie & Pinger, 1997).

While there were no professional health educators during the Middle Ages, education about health continued to exist. It seems priests, medical doctors, and community leaders all had ideas about health and, in particular, the prevention of disease. They proceeded to "educate" all those who would listen and who agreed with their point of view. Given the rudimentary level of health knowledge and the lack of consensus on prevention and causation of disease, a professional health educator would probably have contributed little to the health of the populous in the Middle Ages.

Renaissance

The Renaissance, which means rebirth, was roughly from A.D. 1500 to 1700. It is characterized by a gradual rebirth of thinking about the world and humankind in a more naturalistic and holistic fashion. Science again emerged as a legitimate field of inquiry, and numerous scientific advancements were made.

It must be stressed, however, that progress was slow. The world did not change overnight from the superstitious and backward beliefs of the Dark Ages to a completely enlightened society in the Renaissance.

Disease and plague still ravaged Europe and overall medical care was still rudimentary. Bloodletting was a major form of treatment for everything from the common cold to tuberculosis. Popular remedies included crabs' eyes, foxes' lungs, oil of anise, oil of spiders, and oil of earthworms. A major means of diagnosing a patient's condition consisted of examining the urine for changes in color. The inspection of a patient's urine by a true physician was known as "water casting." For many years, this was the principal occupation of the medical profession. This technique was combined with crude estimates of the balance of four "humours," or fluids, in the body as had originally been theorized by Hippocrates (Hansen, 1980).

Much surgery and dentistry was performed by barbers, because they had the best chairs and sharpest instruments available. Some barbers took their role as physician seriously and dispensed health information, as can be seen in the following example from a Danish barber-surgeon: "It is very good for persons to drink themselves intoxicated once a month for the excellent reasons that it frees their strength, furthers sound sleep, eases the passing of water, increases perspiration, and stimulates general well-being" (Durant, 1961, pp. 495–496). Unfortunately, few were probably so continent as to restrict their binges to once a month.

Rosen (1958) notes that, while the Renaissance "is characterized by the rapid growth and spread of science in various fields, public health as a practiced activity received very little, if any, direct benefit from these advances " (p. 84). Evidence of the poor public health conditions is this note describing the average English household floor of the sixteenth century:

> As to floors, they are usually made with clay, covered with rushes that grow in the fens and which are so seldom removed that the lower part remains sometimes for twenty years and has in it a collection of spittle, vomit, urine of dogs and humans, beer, scraps of fish and other filthiness not to be named. (Pickett & Hanlon, 1990, p. 25)

While living conditions among the English royalty were certainly better than for those of the laboring class, health-related problems still were prevalent. Disposal of human waste was a major problem. Those who lived in old castles located their latrines in large projections on the face of walls. The excrement was discharged from these projections into deep-walled pits, moats, or streams near the walls of the castle. Those less fortunate used chamber pots and simply tossed their contents out the nearest window (Hansen, 1980).

Basic hygiene among royalty left much to be desired. Beneath the elaborate and costly garments of royalty was often a severe condition of uncleanliness. Few monarchs bathed more frequently than once a week. Much of the material used in royal apparel, such as silk, velvet, and ermine, could not be washed; thus, it simply accumulated dirt and perspiration. Cloaking scents were used to try to renew the clothing, but it was not terribly effective (Hansen, 1980).

Health problems resulting from sexual indiscretions were prevalent among royalty. It was common practice for the kings and queens of the sixteenth century to look outside of marriage to satisfy their sexual appetites. There were several reasons for this; one of which was they simply had the power and money to do so. Beyond this, it must be remembered that royal couples were matched without regard for personal compatability or mutual attraction. Language and cultural differences must have strained sexual relations. There was also tremendous pressure on these couples to produce royal offspring; thus, the royal bedroom was a place where duty and responsibility were carried out instead of a place for love and passion. Further, it has been noted that many of the royal family were not physically attractive. Hansen (1980) was blunt in his description of royalty when he noted, "Another problem was the extreme ugliness, even deformity, of the marriageable progeny of sixteenth-century royal families. The portraits we have do not tell the true story, painted as they were to the satisfaction of the royal subject" (p. 262). The deformities, as well as mental retardation, were probably the result of marrying within family bloodlines over many generations.

No doubt this overall lack of physical attraction and personal appeal, combined with power and money, contributed to extramarital sexual affairs, which in turn contributed to the incidence of sexually transmitted diseases. "Venereal disease was as common as the flux at most royal courts, and the malady ruined many a promising prince. . . . It was a horrible, virulent, disfiguring, and chronic malady" (Hanson, 1980, p. 260).

Disfigurement also was caused by the use of caustic cosmetics, which were actually suppose to improve looks:

> On top of natural, exculpable flaws, the princesses of Europe defiled themselves further with the most scarifying cosmetics. The ingredients of these paints were harmful; "fucus," a red paint, was actually mercuric sulfide. This ate into flesh and left trenches if used heavily, which it often was. "Cerusa," a whitening agent, was still more toxic, being white lead. Heavy use of this substance, quite popular in an era that held pallor in the highest regard, mummified the skin, turned hair white, and caused intestinal problems. Many a young woman's early death was at least partly attributable to lead poisoning. (Hansen, 1980, p. 263)

On the positive side, the Renaissance was a period of exploration and expanded trade. The search for knowledge characteristic of the Greek and Roman eras was revitalized. Superstitions of the Middle Ages were slowly replaced with a more systematic inquiry into cause and effect. A great impetus toward the revival of learning was Johann Gutenberg's invention of the printing press in the middle of the fifteenth century. This allowed the great classical works of Hippocrates and Galen to be reproduced and distributed to larger audiences (Gordon, 1959).

Many scientific advancements were made during the Renaissance. The human body was again considered appropriate for study, and realistic anatomical drawings were produced. John Hunter, father of modern surgery, undertook a more orderly exploration of the workings of the human body. Leeuwenhoek discovered the microscope and proved there were life forms too small for the human eye to see. These life forms, however, were not yet associated with disease. John Graunt forwarded the fields of statistics and epidemiology. Through studying the *Bills of Mortality*, published weekly in London, "he determined the excess of male over female births, the high rate of mortality during the earlier years of life, the approximate numerical equality of the sexes, and the excess of urban over the rural death rate" (Goerke & Stebbins, 1968, p. 16).

In Italy, numerous cities had originally instituted health boards to fight the plague. It did not take long, however, for their responsibilities to be expanded. By the middle of the sixteenth century, numerous matters had fallen under the control and jurisdiction of the health boards. These included "the marketing of meat, fish, shellfish, game, fruit, grain, sausages, oil, wine and water; the sewage system; the activity of the hospitals; beggars and prostitutes; burials, cemeteries, and pesthouses; the professional activity of physicians, surgeons and apothecaries; the preparation and sale of drugs; the activity of hostelries and the Jewish community" (Cipolla, 1976, p. 32).

Age of Enlightenment

The 1700s was a period of revolution, industrialization, and growth of cities. Both the French and American revolutions took place during this period. Plague and disease still continued to be a problem. Science had not yet discovered that these diseases were produced by microscopic organisms. Terrible epidemics were still frequent. It was the general belief that disease was formed in filth and that epidemics were caused by some type of poison that developed in the putrefaction process. The vapors, or "miasmas," rising from this rotting refuse could travel through the air for great distances and resulted in disease when inhaled. This was known as the **miasmas theory,** and it remained popular throughout much of the nineteenth century. As preventive measures, herbs and incense were often used to perfume the air supposedly filling the nose and crowding out any miasmas (Duncan, 1988). It was still not known that contaminated water could cause disease infection.

Scientific advancements continued throughout the period. Dr. James Lind, a Royal Navy surgeon, discovered that scurvy could be controlled on long sea voyages by having sailors consume lime juice. To this day, British sailors are known as limies. Edward Jenner discovered a vaccine procedure against smallpox. Bernardino Ramazzini wrote on trade and industrial diseases. Theorists of the time conceived of the mind and body not as separate entities but as dependent on one other. Eighteenth century philosophers such as Diderot, Locke, Rousseau, and Voltaire, all "promoted the worth of each human life and the importance of individual health for the well being of society" (Rubinson & Alles, 1984, p. 5).

Much progress was made during this time, yet health education per se still did not emerge as a profession. With the state of medical knowledge in the sixteenth, seventeenth, and even eighteenth centuries, there would have been little for a health educator to do other than promote the misconceptions and half-truths that predominated the time period; however, with the increases in scientific and medical knowledge and the development of health boards, which were the forerunner of today's health departments, the roots of modern health education had been planted, and the first sprouts would soon emerge.

The 1800s

Very little happened in the first half of the 1800s to improve the public's health. In England, the streets of London were filthy with animal and human waste. Overcrowding and industrialization greatly added to the problem. These conditions, under which so many people lived and worked, had dire results. Smallpox, cholera, typhoid, tuberculosis, and many other diseases reached exceedingly high endemic levels (Pickett & Hanlon, 1990).

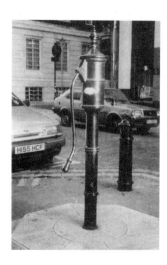

By removing the handle of this pump, which is still in place on Broad Street in London, John Snow interrupted a cholera epidemic. (Robert Hardy Picture Library Ltd., London)

In 1842, a momentous event occurred in the history of public health when Edwin Chadwick published his *Report on an Inquiry into the Sanitary Conditions of the Labouring Population of Great Britain*. In the report, he documented the deplorable living conditions of the laboring class in Great Britain, made a strong case that these conditions were the cause of much disease and suffering, and called for government intervention. This report eventually led to the formation of a General Board of Health for England in 1848 (Goerke & Stebbins, 1968).

Extraordinary advancements in biology and bacteriology were beginning to take place by the middle of the nineteenth century in England and throughout Europe. In 1849, Dr. John Snow, who laboriously studied epidemiological data related to a cholera epidemic in London, hypothesized that the disease was caused by microorganisms in the drinking water from one particular water pump located on Broad Street. He removed the pump's handle to keep people from using the water source and the epidemic abated. Snow's action was remarkable, as it predated the discovery that microorganisms cause disease and was in opposition to the miasmas theory prevailing at the time.

In 1862, Louis Pasteur of France proposed his germ theory of disease. After this, advancements in bacteriology greatly accelerated. Over the next twenty years, Pasteur discovered how microorganisms reproduce, he introduced the first scientific approach to immunization, and he developed a technique to pasteurize milk. Robert Koch, a German scientist, developed the criteria and procedures necessary to establish that a particular microbe, and no other, caused a particular disease. Joseph Lister, an English surgeon, developed the antiseptic method of treating wounds by using carbolic acid, and he introduced the principle of asepsis to surgery. These are just a few of the tremendous advancements in bacteriology made during the second half of the nineteenth century. So great were these advancements in the study of bacteria that the period from 1875 to 1900 has become known as the **bacteriological period of public health** (McKinzie & Pinger, 1997).

Public Health in the United States

During the 1700s, health conditions in the United States were much the same as they were in Europe—deplorable. Diseases such as smallpox, cholera, and diphtheria were prevalent. In addition, diseases such as yaws, yellow fever, and malaria were common in southern states, being brought to the region via the slave trade (Marr, 1982). Large numbers of immigrants were entering the ports, cities were growing, overcrowding was common, and the industrial revolution was on the verge of getting started.

The primary means of controlling disease at this time were quarantine and regulations on environmental cleanliness. For example, as early as 1647, the Massachusetts Bay Colony enacted regulations to prevent pollution of Boston Harbor. In 1701, Massachusetts passed laws allowing for the isolation of smallpox patients and for ship quarantine, to be used whenever needed. The problem with such laws was that there was no overseeing body or agency to enforce compliance.

In an attempt to address health problems, some cities formed local health boards (Pickett & Hanlon, 1990). These boards were made up of prominent citizens who were to advise elected officials on health-related matters. They had no paid staff, no budget, and no authority to enforce regulations. Tradition has it that the first health board was formed in Boston in 1799, with Paul Revere as its chairman. This is contested, however, by other cities claiming earlier health boards, including Petersburg, Virginia (1780), Baltimore (1793), Philadelphia (1794), and New York (1796).

One measure of health status for a given population is **life expectancy,** which is defined as "the average number of years a person from a specific cohort is projected to live from a given point in time" (McKenzie & Pinger, 1997, p. 674). The first life expectancy tables were developed for the United States in 1789 by Dr. Edward Wigglesworth (Ravenel, 1970). A copy of Wigglesworth's table can be seen in Table 2.2. It provides strong evidence of the prevailing health conditions in that, in 1789, life expectancy at birth was only 28.15 years, as compared with life expectancy at birth in 1996, which was 76.1 (Births & Deaths: United States, 1996).

From 1800 to 1850, there was little improvement in health status. The conditions of overcrowding, poverty, and filth worsened as the industrial revolution encouraged more and more people to move to the cities. Epidemics of smallpox, yellow fever, cholera, typhoid, and typhus repeatedly infected people. Tuberculosis and malaria also reached exceptionally high levels. For example, in Massachusetts in 1850, the tuberculosis death rate was 300 per 100,000 population, and infant mortality was about 200 per 1,000 live births. Indeed, the conditions were so bad that life expectancy actually decreased in some cities during this period of time. In Boston, average age at death dropped from 27.85 years in 1820–1825 to 21.43 in 1840–1845. In New York during the same period of time, the average age of death decreased from 26.15 to 19.69 (Shattuck, 1850).

Public health reform in the United States was slow in getting started. It is interesting to note, however, that a major report helped jump start the public health reform movement in the United States, just as Chadwick's landmark report stimulated public health reform in Britain. In the United States, the impetus was

TABLE 2.2 Expectation of Life According to Wigglesworth
Life Table—1789

Expectation	Years
At birth	28.15
At age 5	40.87
At age 10	39.23
At age 15	36.16
At age 20	34.21
At age 25	32.32
At age 30	30.24
At age 35	28.22
At age 40	26.04
At age 45	23.92
At age 50	21.16
At age 55	18.35
At age 60	15.43
At age 65	12.43
At age 70	10.06
At age 75	7.83
At age 80	5.85
At age 85	4.57
At age 90	3.73
At age 95	1.62

Lemuel Shattuck's *Report of the Sanitary Commission of Massachusetts.* His report contained remarkable insight into the public health problems of Massachusetts and equally remarkable foresight as to how these problems should be approached and solved. In describing the content of this famous report, Pickett and Hanlon (1990) noted:

> Among the many recommendations made by Shattuck were those for the establishment of state and local boards of health; a system of sanitary police or inspectors; the collection and analysis of vital statistics; a routine system for exchanging data and information; sanitation programs for towns and buildings; studies of the health of school children; studies of tuberculosis; the control of alcoholism; the supervision of mental disease; the sanitary supervision and study of problems of immigrants; the erection of model tenements, public bathhouses, and washhouses; the control of smoke nuisances; the control of food adulteration; the exposure of nostrums; the preaching of health from pulpits; the establishment of nurses' training schools; the teaching of sanitary science in medical schools; and the inclusion of preventive medicine in clinical practice, with routine physical examinations and family records of illness. (p.31)

The significance of this report can best be appreciated when one considers that there were no national or state public health programs at the time, and local

MILESTONES OF PUBLIC HEALTH IN AMERICA

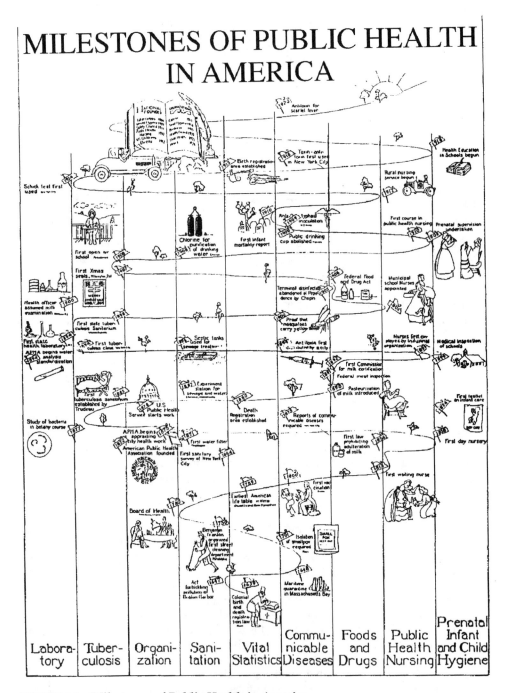

FIGURE 2.1   Milestones of Public Health in America.

Source: American Journal of Public Health (Dec. 1985) 75(15):1361–1504.

health agencies that existed were functioning at a minimal level. Still, Shattuck visualized what was needed to improve the public's health. "Of the 50 recommendations which Shattuck listed, 36 have become accepted principles of public health practice" (Goerke & Stebbins, 1968, p. 28).

In no way should the publication of Shattuck's report be construed to mean an end to the public health problems in the United States. In fact, the report went basically unnoticed for nineteen years until 1869, when the State of Massachusetts established a state board of health made up of physicians and laymen exactly as Shattuck had envisioned. Virginia and California, following the lead of Massachusetts, formed their own state boards of health one year later in 1870 (Ravenel, 1970). By 1900, thirty-eight states had established state boards of health. Today, every state in the United States has a state board or department of health.

Shortly after the formation of state boards of health, it was realized that state-level health departments could not meet health needs on a more local level. There was simply too much to do and neither enough time nor enough personnel to accomplish what needed to be done. As a result the first full-time county health departments were formed in Guilford County, North Carolina, and Yakima County, Washington, in 1911. Some sources have cited Jefferson County, Kentucky, as the first county health department, set up in 1908 (Pickett & Hanlon, 1990).

At about the same time as states were initiating boards of health, the American Public Health Association was founded. (See Chapter 8 for more information on the APHA.) Following a series of national conventions on quarantine held from 1857 through 1860, "Stephen Smith invited a group of 'refined gentlemen' to discuss informally the possibility of a national sanitary association" (Bernstein, 1972, p. 2). Smith's suggestion of an association for health officials and interested citizens was well received by those men who responded to his invitation. A decision was made to establish a committee to work on permanent organization. One year later, in 1873, the first annual meeting was held in Cincinnati, and seventy new members were elected.

In addition to the state and county departments of health, the federal government had in operation the beginnings of what is now known as the U.S. Public Health Service. The history of this illustrious organization dates back to 1798, when Congress passed the Marine Hospital Service Act. Up to this point, the sailors in the merchant marine had nowhere to turn for health care. They paid no local or state taxes and generally were not particularly welcomed in any port city where they happened to become ill or were injured. The Marine Hospital Service Act required the owners of every ship to pay the tax collector twenty cents per month for every seaman they employed. The money was used to build hospitals and provide medical services in all major seaport cities. This is of particular importance, as "it represented the first prepaid medical and hospital insurance plan in the world, under the administrative supervision of what eventually became a public health agency" (Pickett & Hanlon, 1990, p. 34).

The scope of the Marine Hospital service was gradually expanded by successive legislation throughout the nineteenth century until 1902, when Congress retitled it the Public Health and Marine Hospital Service and provided it with a definite organizational form under the direction of the surgeon general. In 1912,

Marine Hospital was dropped from the name and the service became the U.S. Public Health Service.

In 1879, Congress created the National Board of Health. The board was comprised of seven members appointed by the president, including representatives of the army, navy, Marine Hospital Service, and Justice Department. Its functions were to obtain information on all matters related to public health and to provide grant-in-aid to state boards of health. The National board also provided money to university scientists to conduct research on topics of health-related interest. Unfortunately, the board was short-lived. In administering quarantine functions, the board had incurred opposition from state agencies and private shipping concerns. Others in positions of power were not in favor of the research grant program and felt such expenditures were extravagant. Thus, in 1882, the board's appropriations were transferred to the Marine Hospital Service, which carried on with the quarantine functions but discontinued the grant program (USDHEW, 1976). With this, "the National Board of Health died, and the United States has never had a cabinet level health department or an official comparable to the minister of health in most other countries" (Pickett & Hanlon, 1990, p. 36)

The period from 1900 to 1920 has been called the reform phase of public health (McKenzie & Pinger, 1997). This period was marked by a growing concern for the many social problems facing America. Cities had continued to grow, and many people lived and worked in deplorable conditions. To address these concerns, federal regulations were passed concerning the food industry; states passed workers' compensation laws; the U.S. Bureau of Mines was created, as was the U.S. Department of Labor; and the first clinic for occupational diseases was established. By the end of this period, the movement for healthier conditions in the workplace had become well established.

It was also during this period that the first national voluntary agencies were formed. These were agencies designed to address a specific health problem and were run primarily by volunteers. The National Association for the Study and Prevention of Tuberculosis was established in 1902, and the American Cancer Society, Inc., was founded in 1913. Today, volunteer agencies continue to be important players in the prevention of disease and the promotion of health (McKenzie & Pinger, 1997).

The 1920s was a relatively quiet period in public health. Progress continued, but at a slower pace. By the end of the decade, average life expectancy had risen to 59.7 years. Of importance to health education professionals is that the Public Health Education Section of the American Public Health Association was founded in 1922 (Bernstein, 1972).

The need for health education was certainly present in the early years of the twentieth century. Moore (1923) included an entire chapter of his book on public health in the United States to "nostrums and quackery" and another chapter to health activities he described as "more or less misdirected." One of the most interesting examples involved a cure-all product known as Tanlac (see Photo 2.1). The May 11, 1917, edition of the *Holyoke Daily Transcript* contained both an advertisement for Tanlac featuring a testimonial by a Fred Wicks and Mr. Wicks's obituary (Moore, 1923, pp. 173–174).

About this time, the first evidence appeared of differences between those people more concerned with treatment and those more concerned with prevention. Moore (1923) related a story about a town in which public health work had banished malaria. A physician was asked how his profession had been affected by this public health advancement. He replied, "If it hadn't been for the influenza, I'd have gone broke. That saved us" (p. 373). As this off-handed and jocular reply suggests, there is a clash between preventive medicine and curative medicine in the United States that has existed since at least the early part of the twentieth century.

In explaining the emphasis on treatment over prevention in a more rational manner, Newsholme (1936) noted three reasons that treatment formed a larger part of public health efforts and why it would continue to do so in the future. First, the knowledge to prevent "a large proportion of the total sickness and mortality in the community is only partial" (p. 169). Second, "even when knowledge exists which if applied would reduce avoidable illness, it has not become vitally realized by most of us, and many among us are completely ignorant concerning it. Many more are unwilling to live in accord with this knowledge or are so circumstanced that their knowledge cannot be applied in their lives" (p. 169). Third, "physicians, hygienists, and Public Health Authorities find themselves confronted by an embarrassing multitude of sick people needing immediate aid; and their primary duty obviously is to give adequate and complete treatment of already existent sickness. Ambulance work must precede work to prevent future accidents, though no ambulance work is fully satisfactory which does not include thorough investigation of the origin of the accident and the full application of the conclusions from inquiry to the prevention of recurrent accidents" (pp. 169–170). Many of the same arguments are used today to account for the emphasis on traditional medical interventions instead of prevention.

The period from 1930 through World War II saw an expanded role for the federal government in social programs. Prior to the Great Depression of 1929, medical services were dependent on relatives and friends, as well as on religious organizations and some voluntary agencies. During the depression, however, it became clear that private resources could not meet the needs of all the people requiring assistance. In 1933, President Franklin D. Roosevelt created numerous agencies and programs as part of his "New Deal," to improve the plight of the disadvantaged. Much of the money was used for public health efforts, including the control of malaria, the building of hospitals, and the construction of municipal water and sewage systems.

The Social Security Act of 1935 was a real milestone and the beginning of the federal government's involvement in social issues, including health. The act provided support for state health departments and their programs. Funding was made available to develop sanitary facilities and to improve maternal and child health.

Two major public health agencies were formed during this period. On May 26, 1930, the Ransdell Act converted the Hygienic Laboratory to the National Institute of Health (now called the National Institutes of Health), with a broad mandate to ascertain the cause, prevention, and cure of disease (USDHEW, 1976). The National Institutes of Health is now one of the premiere, if not the premiere, medical research facilities in the world. During World War II, the Communicable Disease Center was established in Atlanta, Georgia. Now called the National Centers for Disease Control and Prevention (CDC), it has become one of the world's leading epidemiological centers and a major training facility for health communications and educational methods (Pickett & Hanlon, 1990).

Following World War II, there was concern over the number of health care facilities and the adequacy of the care they provided. In 1946, Congress passed the National Hospital Survey and Construction Act, also known as the Hill-Burton Act. This legislation was crafted to improve the distribution and enhance the quality of hospitals. From the passage of the Hill-Burton Act through the 1960s, new hospital construction occurred at a rapid rate. Little thought, however, was given to planning. As a result, some of these hospitals were built too close together and provided overlapping and unnecessary services (McKenzie & Pinger, 1997).

In 1965, the federal government again passed major legislation designed to improve the health of Americans. While major improvements had been made in health facilities and the quality of health care, there were still many people that were underserved. Most of these people were either poor or elderly. In response to these problems, Congress passed the Medicare and Medicaid bills, which were amendments to the Social Security Act of 1935. **Medicare** was created to assist in the payment of medical bills for the elderly, while **Medicaid** did the same for the poor. These bills provided medical care for millions of people who could not otherwise have obtained such services. Unfortunately, these bills also created an influx of federal dollars to the health care system, with the ultimate result of increasing the cost of health care for everyone.

By the 1970s it had become clear that providing facilities and access to care was not enough to significantly influence the health status of the U.S. population. The greatest potential for improving health and reducing health care costs lied in prevention. The first national effort to promote the health of citizens through a more preventive approach took place in Canada. In 1974, the Canadian Ministry of Health and Welfare released a publication entitled *A New Perspective on the Health of Canadians* (Lalonde, 1974). This document, often called the Lalonde Report, presented the epidemiological evidence supporting the importance of lifestyle and environmental factors to health and sickness and called for numerous national health promotion strategies to encourage Canadians to become more responsible for their own health. (See Chapter 1 for information on the Health Field Concept associated with this publication.) This report was highly influential in persuading numerous American health professionals to rethink current assumptions based on high-technology, treatment-focused medicine. So important was this report that Bates and Winder (1984) likened it to a reemergence of Hygeia and the beginning of the second public health revolution (p. 24).

In the United States, the first major recognition of the importance of lifestyle in promoting health and well-being came in the form of a governmental publication entitled *Healthy People* (U.S. Public Health Service, 1979). This was the

American version of Canada's *A New Perspective on the Health of Canadians.* It contained strong support for the need to shift emphasis away from the traditional medical model and toward lifestyle and environmental strategies which could help prevent many modern-day illnesses.

In 1980, another federal document called ***Promoting Health/Preventing Disease: Objectives for the Nation*** was released. This document contained 226 health objectives for the United States, which were divided into three areas: preventive services, health protection, and health promotion. These goals provided the framework for public health efforts during the 1980s. They allowed public health professionals to focus their attention on those areas that were most important and provided baseline data so progress could be measured (USDHHS, 1980).

By the end of the decade, only about half of the objectives had been met or were close to being met. Nevertheless, the planning and evaluation process used in developing the 1980 objectives demonstrated the value of setting goals and listing specific objectives as a means of measuring progress in the nation's health and health care services. Thus, the process was repeated in the late 1980s, and a new publication was released in 1990 titled *Healthy People 2000: National Health Promotion and Disease Prevention Objectives.* Its purpose was to commit the nation to the attainment of three broad goals: (1) Increase the span of healthy life for Americans, (2) reduce health disparities among Americans, and (3) achieve access to preventive services for all Americans. To guide the process of meeting these goals, 332 specific objectives were written in twenty-two priority areas (USDHHS, 1990).

As this book is being written, the process is already underway of developing objectives for the year 2010. According to the USDHHS (1997), which is developing the objectives,

> This next set of national objectives will be distinguished from Healthy People 2000 by the broadened prevention science base; improved surveillance and data systems; a heightened awareness and demand for preventive health services and quality health care; and changes in demographics, science, technology, and disease spread that will affect the public's health into the 21st century. (p. 5)

The preliminary vision of the proposed framework for the 2010 objectives can be seen in Figure 2.2. To learn more about ***Healthy People 2000*** and to follow the progress of *Healthy People 2010,* attach to the Healthy People web site at the following address: http://158.72.20.10/pubs/hp2000/

The latest important event in the history of health education occurred on October 27, 1997, when the Standard Occupational Classification (SOC) Policy Review Comittee approved the creation of a new, distinct classification for the occupation of health educator (Auld, 1997/1998). This has been a goal pursued by health educators for over 25 years. Until now health educators were included in the category "Instructional Coordinator." This was a broad, primarily education-related category that failed to consider the many varied and unique responsibilities of health educators. Approval of health education as a separate occupational

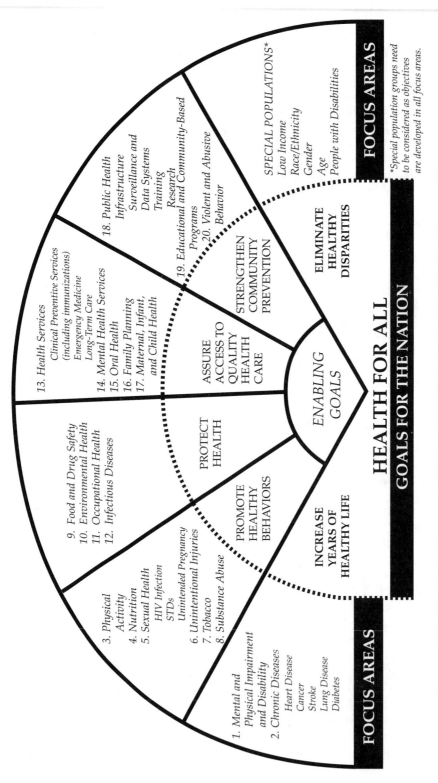

FIGURE 2.2 Proposed Healthy People Framework. Vision of 2010: Healthy People in Healthy Communities.

Source: Data from U.S. Department of Health & Human Services, Office of Disease Prevention and Health Promotion, *Developing Objectives for Healthy People 2010.* September 1997. http://web.health.gov/healthypeople/

classification means that the Department of Labor's Bureau of Labor Statistics, Department of Commerce's Bureau of the Census and all other federal agencies that collect occupational data will now collect data on health educators. In addition, many state and local governments will follow suit and maintain data on health education as well. For the first time, it will be possible to determine the number of health educators employed and the outlook for future health education positions. This approval is one more sign that health education is beginning to gain the respect and recognition it deserves.

As future health educators look back on public health in the 1990s, it may be known as the period of **social ecology.** To date, many health promotion efforts to alter individuals' behavior have fallen short. This may be due, in part, to the emphasis on the "individual" to change without considering the various social, political, and economic factors impacting the individual. The ecological perspective takes into account the social, political, and economic milieu in which people exist. Conceptually, the social ecological approach is more complex than focusing on individual behaviors, and the strategies are not as well defined, yet it would appear that this approach recognizes important behavioral supports and requires health educators to address them. (For a more detailed description of the social ecological perspective, see Chapter 4.)

School Health in the United States

Life in early America was hard, and there was little time for education. Days were filled with the labor of building homes, clearing forests, tilling fields, hunting, preparing food, and existing under primitive conditions. Settlements were few and far apart. Travel and transportation were costly, slow, and limited to foot, horseback, boat, or wagon.

In the mid-1600s, as communities became more established, the call for education was soon heard. Religion had always been an important part of life in America, and it was the religious leaders who led the drive for education. It was their belief that Satan benefited when people were illiterate, because they could not read the Scriptures. Therefore, Massachusetts' "Old Deluder" law was passed in 1647 to prevent Satan from deluding the people by keeping them from reading the Bible. The law specified that a town with fifty families should establish an elementary school and a town with one hundred households a Latin grammar secondary school (Means, 1962).

The curriculum in these early schools was largely derived from the educational practices in England. Essentially, reading, as the avenue to religious understanding, was the primary subject. Writing, spelling, grammar, and arithmetic supplemented reading. Later, geography and history were added, but the teaching of health was not part of the early education system in the United States.

Since only boys attended these early schools and working for the family was still a major concern, daily sessions were by necessity of short duration, and the length of the school term was usually only a few months. Teachers were lacking in preparation, with their basic qualifications as being able to (1) read, (2) know more of the Bible than the students, (3) work cheap, and (4) keep the students under control. Teachers were totally dependent on the rod for classroom management (Means, 1962).

School buildings were typically inadequate. They were poorly built, inaccessible, and sometimes temporary structures. Their interiors were inadequately lighted, were furnished with uncomfortable seating, had no sanitary facilities, and were heated with wood-burning stoves. These schools were not even close to meeting modern standards for school construction (Means, 1962).

The schools and their curricula remained much the same until the 1800s. By the mid-1800s, most schools had become tax supported, and attendance had become compulsory. Those concerned about public health pointed to numerous health and safety problems in the schools. These concerns helped bring attention to the conditions of the schools and ultimately paved the way for health instruction in the curriculum (Means, 1962).

Horace Mann, whose writings and speeches helped promote the importance of education in general, was perhaps the first spokesperson for teaching health in schools. Mann was elected secretary of the Massachusetts State Board of Education in 1837. Beginning in 1837 with the publication of his *First Annual Report* and continuing through the publication of the *Sixth Annual Report* in 1843, Mann called for mandatory programs of hygiene that would help students understand their bodies and the relationship between their behaviors and health (Rubinson & Alles, 1984).

Another momentous event in the development of school health occurred in 1850, when Lemuel Shattuck from Massachusetts wrote his *Report on the Sanitary Commission of Massachusetts* (1850). This is the same report discussed earlier in reference to public health. While the report has become a classic in the field of public health, it also provided strong support for school health (Means, 1975). In the report, Shattuck (1850) eloquently supports the teaching of physiology, as the term *health education* had yet to be coined:

> It has recently been recommended that the science of physiology be taught in the public schools; and the recommendation should be universally approved and carried into effect as soon as persons can be found capable of teaching it. . . . Every child should be taught early in life, that to preserve his own life and his own health and the lives and health of others; is one of the most important and constantly abiding duties. By obeying certain laws or performing certain acts, his life and health may be preserved; by disobedience, or performing certain other acts, they will both be destroyed. By knowing and avoiding the causes of disease, disease itself will be avoided, and he may enjoy health and live; by ignorance of these causes and exposure to them, he may contract disease, ruin his health, and die. Every thing connected with wealth, happiness and long life depend upon health; and even the great duties of morals and religion are performed more acceptably in a healthy than a sickly condition. (pp. 178–179)

Aside from local and state attempts to promote the teaching of health-related curricula in the schools, there was no concerted national effort until the Women's Christian Temperance Union. Originally founded in 1874, the union expounded on the evils of alcohol, narcotics, and tobacco through every conceivable means. It was one of the most effective lobbying organizations ever (Means, 1962). Between 1880 and 1890, every state in the union passed a law requiring instruction concerning the effects of alcohol and narcotics due to stimulus from the Temperance Movement (Turner, Sellery, & Smith, 1957).

Other national movements soon followed. In 1915, the National Tuberculosis Association introduced the "Modern Health Crusade" as a device for promoting the health of school children. It was based on promotion to "knighthood" on the basis of having followed certain health habits. The Child Health Organization of America encouraged the nation to adopt more functional health education programs. One of the active leaders of this organization, Sally Lucas Jean, was ultimately responsible for changing the name from hygiene education to health education (Means, 1962). With this name change, the focus of health education was also to change from that of physiology and hygiene, which was factual and unrelated to everyday living, to an emphasis on healthy living and health behavior.

Despite these advancements, health education from 1900 to 1920 was generally characterized by inconsistency and awkward progress. It took World War I to provide the impetus for widespread acceptance of school health education as a field in its own right (Turner, Sellery, & Smith, 1957). Out of 2,510,706 men who were examined to be drafted into the military at the time of World War I, 730,756 were rejected on physical grounds. A large portion of these physical deficiencies could have been prevented if the schools had been doing their part to train children concerning health and fitness (Andress & Bragg, 1922). In the immediate postwar years, sixteen states required hygiene instruction in their public schools, and twelve of these states made provisions for the preparation of health teachers in the teacher training schools supported by the state (Rogers, 1936).

Significant research and demonstration projects related to school health education were conducted in the 1920s and 1930s. There was the Malden, Massachusetts, project, which was done in cooperation with the Massachusetts Institute of Technology; the Mansfield, Ohio, project supported by the American Red Cross; the Fargo, North Dakota, project sponsored by the Commonwealth Fund; and the Cattaraugus County, New York, project financed by the Milband Memorial Fund. According to Turner, Sellery, and Smith (1957), "these programs showed that habits could be changed and health improved through health education" (p. 27).

In the 1930s, the impetus for health education from the public seemed to wane. Since there were no major wars or conflicts to concern people, the emphasis on physical fitness and health that had resulted from World War I was not present to the same extent it had been in the postwar years. Health education continued to address the major health issues of the time but without fanfare. Notable research studies supplemented authoritative opinion in helping to point out difficulties and offer solutions related to the teaching of health education. Several important conferences were held on health education and youth health (Means, 1962). The profession was moving forward.

Several professional organizations emerged during this time that are still in existence today. School health education, long associated with physical education, received official recognition in 1937, when the American Physical Education Association became the American Association for Health and Physical Education. One year later, recreation was added to the association, and the name changed to the American Association for Health, Physical Education and Recreation (AAHPER).

The American Association of School Physicians, founded in 1927, had greatly expanded its functions, interests, and scope of activity. As a result, it broadened its membership to include school health personnel other than physicians. In 1938, the name was changed to the American School Health Association to reflect these changes.

The American Public Health Association had long been an organization interested in and supportive of school health. In fact, many of the earliest supporters of health education in the schools had been leaders in public health. It was therefore appropriate that the organization establish a separate section within its administrative structure to focus on school health interests. In 1942, the School Health Section of the American Public Health Association was formed. (See Chapter 8 for more detailed information on these professional associations.)

With the bombing of Pearl Harbor, on December 7, 1941, the United States found itself at war. Once again the nation turned its focus to physical fitness and health. With no major threats of war in the previous twenty years, the physical status of young American men had again degenerated. Of the approximately 2 million men examined for induction into the nation's armed forces, almost 50 percent were disqualified. Of those disqualified, 90 percent were found to be physically or mentally unfit (American Youth Commission, 1942). This unfortunate situation helped greatly to stimulate the interest in the health of high school students and provided strong impetus for health education classes.

Following the war years, there were again many demonstration projects and studies completed to examine more carefully the impact of health education. The Massachusetts High School Study, the Astoria Study, The New York City Study, and the Denver Study were just a few of the efforts that provided valuable information on school health education (Means, 1975).

One of the more important studies was the **School Health Education Evaluation Study** of the Los Angeles Area. The purpose of the study was to evaluate the effectiveness of school health work in selected schools and colleges of the area. More specifically, the project aimed at the appraisal of the entire school health program, including administrative organization, school health services, health instruction, and healthful school environment. Further, the students' health knowledge, attitudes, and behavior were examined. The study resulted in eleven conclusions and seventeen important recommendations for the field. Of equal importance, the study's planning, design, and operational process established a research pattern which provided a model for the development of subsequent similar studies (Means, 1975).

The **School Health Education Study** was another study of significance to health education. Directed by Dr. Elena M. Sliepcevich, the study included 135 randomly selected school systems involving 1,460 schools and 840,832 students in thirty-eight states. Health behavior inventories were administered to students in grades 6, 9 and 12. Results were "appalling." The prevalence of health misconceptions among students at all levels was apparent. Further questionnaires were distributed to school administrators throughout the country to obtain data on organizational procedures and instructional practices related to health education. Again the results indicated major problems in the organization and administration of health programs. Cortese (1993) noted, ". . . some health topics were omitted while others were repeated grade after grade at the same level of sophistication. No logical rationale placed learning exercises at various grade levels, and a need existed for a challenging and meaningful curriculum" (p. 21).

As a second phase of the School Health Education Study, a curriculum writing team was established to develop a health education curriculum based on needs identified from phase one of the study. The team consisted of many prominent names in health education, including Gus T. Dalis, Edward B. Johns, Richard K. Means, Ann E. Nolte, Marion B. Pollock, and Robert D. Russell (Means, 1975). Over the next eight years, the writing team developed a comprehensive curriculum package that still influences school health curricula today.

After World War II, health education continued to grow as a profession. As Means (1975) observed, "This period from 1940 into the 1970's was one of appraisal, re-evaluation, and consolidation with respect to research accomplished in school health education. During this time leaders in the field attempted to look back, review, and take stock of what was known as a determinant of future action" (p. 107).

School health programs continued to evolve from the mid-1970s to the present time. Several important events and trends have impacted school health education as well as the overall school health programs. In 1978, the Office of Comprehensive School Health was established within the Department of Education. The primary purpose of the office was policy development for health education issues that affected children and youth. Having such a presence in the Department of Education held great promise for school health education efforts. Unfortunately, the office was never fully funded. A director was named, Peter Cortese, but the office was deactivated with the advent of the Reagan administration's budget cuts (Rubinson & Alles, 1984).

The 1980s saw the advent of two important concepts: comprehensive school health programs and comprehensive school health education. A **comprehensive school health program** "is an organized set of policies, procedures, and activities designed to protect and promote the health and well-being of students and staff which traditionally included health services, healthful school environment, and health education. It should also include, but not be limited to, guidance and counseling, physical education, food service, social work, psychological services and employee health promotion" (Joint Committee on Health Education Terminology, 1991, p. 181). Ideally, these eight components should function in concert to promote the health of the faculty, students, staff, and community as a whole. Professional staff involved with any aspect of the program should work as an integrated team. Further, there needs to be some coordination and integration of these components for programs to succeed.

It was Allensworth and Kolbe (1987) who proposed the expanded concept of a comprehensive school health program as previously described. Interestingly, the concept of a team effort to improve school health involving multiple program components was not new. A similar idea was proposed in 1957 by Turner, Sellery, and Smith. They described the school health team as including classroom teachers, administrators, physicians, school nurses, physical educators, nutritionists, dentists, dental hygienists, supervisors of health education, health coordinators, the health chairperson in elementary schools, and the school custodian. They also spoke of the importance of maintaining the health of the staff. Little was done with this concept in the thirty years after it was first proposed.

Comprehensive school health instruction (or education) "refers to the development, delivery, and evaluation of a planned curriculum, preschool through 12, with goals, objectives, content sequence, and specific classroom lessons which includes, but is not limited to the following major content areas: community health, consumer health, environmental health, family life, mental and emotional health, injury prevention and safety, nutrition, personal health, prevention and control of disease, and substance use and abuse" (Joint Committee on Health Education Terminology, 1991, p. 182). Therefore, comprehensive school health instruction is one part of the comprehensive school health program.

In 1995, another milestone event occurred when the Joint Committee on National Health Education Standards published the National Health Education Standards (see Table 2.3). The committee was comprised of representatives from the major professional associations and the American Cancer Society. The standards were designed to promote **health literacy,** the capacity of individuals to access, interpret, and understand basic health information and services and the skills to use the information and services to promote health. Their purpose was to serve as a framework for organizing knowledge and skills into curricula at the state and local levels. They were not intended to be a federal mandate for a specific health curriculum (Joint Committee on Health Education Standards, 1995).

Since 1987, the concept of a comprehensive school health program has dominated the school health arena. At first glance, it would seem that schools would be excited to initiate comprehensive school health programs. How could one oppose a concept that would bring together multiple components of the school in an integrated attempt to improve the health of faculty, staff, students, and the community? A healthy child taught by a healthy teacher in a health-conscious community should forward the school's overall mission to provide each child with the best education possible. Unfortunately, the full potential of comprehensive school health programs has never been realized in the vast majority of school districts. This is probably due to many factors, such as the low priority placed on

TABLE 2.3   National Health Education Standards

1. Students will comprehend concepts related to health promotion and disease prevention.
2. Students will demonstrate the ability to access valid health information and health promoting products and services.
3. Students will demonstrate the ability to practice health-enhancing behaviors and reduce health risks.
4. Students will analyze the influence of culture, media, technology, and other factors on health.
5. Students will demonstrate the ability to use interpersonal communication skills to enhance health.
6. Students will demonstrate the ability to use goal-setting and decision-making skills to enhance health.
7. Students will demonstrate the ability to advocate for personal, family, and community health.

Source: From Joint Committee on National Health Education Standards: Achieving Health Literacy. Available from the American School Health Association, American Association for Health Education, or the American Cancer Society.

health by many school administrators, a lack of leadership to coordinate and oversee comprehensive school health programs, and adverse reactions from conservative groups that perceive comprehensive school health as a means of incorporating sex education into the curriculum. As a result of these negative responses to the concept of "comprehensive," it has largely been replaced by the concept of "coordinated," which better describes the intent of such programs. Thus readers will see "coordinated school health programs" in future references to this movement.

Summary

The history of health and health education is important to professional development in health education. Only by understanding the past can students appreciate the present and evolve into future leaders in this emerging profession.

The concept of health education as understood today is a relatively new concept dating back only to the middle to late 1800s. From the times of earliest intelligence, however, humans have been searching for ways to keep themselves healthy and free of disease. Without knowledge of disease causation or medical treatment, it was only natural to rely on superstition and spiritualism for answers. The concept of prevention was intriguing, but the knowledge and skills to prevent disease were unknown.

As one examines the great civilizations of Egypt, Greece, and Rome, progress in preventing and treating disease can be seen. The realization that humans had to have sound minds and sound bodies was conceived by these early cultures. Systems of rudimentary pharmacology and advancements in the areas of waste disposal and the provision of safe drinking water were among some of the most noteworthy advancements.

During the Middle Ages, much of what had been learned was lost. It was as if society took a giant step backward. Science and knowledge were shunned, while religion gained new favor as the preferred means of preventing and treating disease. Great epidemics struck the European continent, and millions of people lost their lives.

The Renaissance witnessed a rebirth of interest in knowledge. Science again flourished, and advancements were made in health care. Understanding of disease, however, was still rudimentary, and treatment was often worse than the effects of the disease. Sanitary conditions were deplorable and would remain so through the 1800s. The emergence of health education as a profession was still more than a century away.

The era of Enlightenment saw tremendous growth in cities as the industrial movement got underway in both England and the United States. Unfortunately, this population growth compounded sanitation problems related to overcrowding. Epidemics were still prevalent. In addition, the employment conditions of the working class were frequently unsafe and unhealthy.

By the mid-1850s, conditions were ripe for the birth of public health in the United States. The contagion theory of disease was emerging, and early reformers called for the government to step in and take control of environmental conditions that led to disease. The first city and state departments of health were established. These were soon followed by county health departments in the early 1900s. Health departments began to monitor and regulate food safety, water safety, and waste disposal. Professional organizations for health personnel emerged, and voluntary agencies were formed. Major pieces of legislation were passed as government sought to improve working conditions and took greater responsibility for the poor and infirm. During the mid-1900s, emphasis was placed on building new medical facilities and enhancing the technology required to treat disease.

By the 1970s the cost of medical treatment had escalated, and concern had shifted to prevention. This set the stage for the development of national health objectives for the decades of the 1980s and 1990s. Health education made great strides as an emerging profession.

In the mid-1800s, as public health was starting to make important strides, school health education was also emerging. In addition to reading, writing, and arithmetic, early pioneers saw the need to educate students about health-related matters. In the early 1900s, groups such as the National Tuberculosis Association, the American Cancer Society, and the Women's Christian Temperance Union were strongly supporting the need to educate school children about health. Both World War I and World War II provided important impetus for health-related instruction and physical training in the schools.

The 1960s and 1970s saw several important studies completed that supported the need for health education and documented its effectiveness.

Comprehensive school health programs emerged in the 1980s and are still an important focus for school health although they are now known as coordinated school health programs.

While health and health education have made great strides since the first humans contemplated how to treat and prevent disease, there is still a long way to go. Both in the United States and worldwide there are many people who do not have access to medical care or the important information and skills of professionally trained health educators. Heart disease, cancers, diabetes, and HIV are prevalent in developed countries, while the traditional infectious diseases continue to affect those in developing countries.

As in the past, health professionals must envision what can be and strive to make that vision a reality. Turner, Sellery, and Smith (1957) noted,

> As society looks ahead, it can conceive the hope that some day almost every human being will be well, intelligent, physically vigorous, mentally alert, emotionally stable, socially reasonable and ethically sound. At least, society must concern itself with progress toward that goal. (p. 18)

Health educators must be important players in this process.

REVIEW QUESTIONS

1. Describe the earliest efforts at health care and informal health education.

2. Compare and contrast the great societies of Egypt, Greece, and Rome. How are these cultures similar in relation to health? How are they different?

3. What were the major epidemics of the Middle Ages? Why were they so feared? What factors contributed to their spread? What were some strategies people used to prevent these diseases?

4. Discuss the Renaissance and why it is important to the history of health and health care.

5. Who wrote the *Report of the Sanitary Commission of Massachusetts* (1850)? Explain how this report was important to the history of both school health and public health.

6. Identify at least five major groups or events that forwarded school health programs.

7. What Canadian publication and its United States counterpart helped focus attention on the importance of disease prevention and health promotion?

8. What are "national health objectives"? Where can they be found? Why are they so important?

9. Describe the initiatives that have shaped school health education programs over the past ten years.

10. Explain why it is important for health education professionals to understand the history of health, health education, and health care.

ACTIVITIES

1. Develop a timeline using one hundred-year increments from the early Egyptians to the year 2000. Mark all of the important health-related events as they occurred along the timeline.

2. Imagine what it would have been like to live through an outbreak of the Black Death in the Middle Ages. Write a thirty-day personal diary, with daily entries depicting what you might have seen or heard and how you might have felt.

3. Interview several individuals who are at least eighty years old concerning the health care they received as young children. Ask them to describe any health education they can remember. When was it? Where did it take place? Who provided the education? Was it effective?

REFERENCES

Allensworth, D., & Kolbe, L. (1987). The comprehensive school health program: Exploring an expanded concept. *Journal of School Health, 57,* 409–412.

American Youth Commission. (1942). *"Health and fitness," youth and the future.* Washington, DC: American Council on Education.

Andress, M.J., & Bragg, M.C. (1922). *Suggestions for a program for health teaching in the elementary schools.* U.S. Department of the Interior, Bureau of Education, Health Education No. 10, Washington, DC: U.S. Government Printing Office.

Auld, E. (Winter 1997/1998). Executive edge. *SOPHE News & Views,* 24 (4), 4.

Bates, I.J., & Winder, A.E. (1984). *Introduction to health education.* Palo Alto, CA: Mayfield.

Bernstein, N. R. (1972). *APHA: The first one hundred years.* Washington, DC: American Public Health Association.

Births & Deaths: United States. (1996). *Monthly Vital Statistics Report, 46* (1–S2).

Cipolla, C.M. (1976). *Public health and the medical profession in the Renaissance.* Cambridge, England: Cambridge University Press.

Cortese, P.A. (1993). Accomplishments in comprehensive school health education. *Journal of School Health, 63* (1), 21–23.

Donan, C. (1898). *The Dark Ages 476–918.* London: Rivingtons.

Duncan, D. (1988). *Epidemiology: Basis for disease prevention and health promotion.* New York: Macmillan.

Durant, W. (1961). *The Age of Reason begins.* Volume VII in Durant, *The story of civilization.* New York: Simon and Schuster.

Fee, E., & Brown, T.M. (1997). Editorial: Why history? *American Journal of Public Health, 87* (11), 1763–1764.

Goerke, L.S., & Stebbins, E.L. (1968). *Mustard's introduction to public health* (5th ed.). New York: Macmillan.

Gordon, B. (1959). *Medieval and Renaissance medicine.* New York: Philosophical Library.

Green, W.H., & Simons-Morton, B.G. (1990). *Introduction to health education.* Prospect Heights, IL: Waveland Press.

Hansen, M. (1980). *The royal facts of life.* Metuchen, NJ: The Scarecrow Press.

Joint Committee on Health Education Standards. (1995). *National health education standards: Achieving health literacy.* Atlanta, GA: American Cancer Society.

Joint Committee on Health Education Terminology. (1991). Report of the 1990 Joint Committee on Health Education Terminology. *Journal of Health Education, 22*(3), 173–184.

Lalonde, M. (1974). *A new perspective on the health of Canadians.* Ottawa: Government of Canada.

Libby, W. (1922). *The history of medicine in its salient features.* Boston: Houghton Mifflin.

Marr, J. (Winter, 1982). Merchants of death: The role of the slave trade in the transmission of disease from Africa to the Americas. *Pharos, 31.*

McKenzie, J.F., & Pinger, R.R. (1997). *An introduction to community health.* Boston: Jones and Bartlett.

Means, R.K. (1962). *A history of health education in the United States.* Philadelphia: Lea & Febiger.

Means, R.K. (1975). *Historical perspectives on school health.* Thorofare, NJ: Charles B. Slack.

Moore, H.H. (1923). *Public health in the United States.* New York: Harper & Brothers.

Newsholme, A. (1936). *The last thirty years in public health.* London: George Allen & Unwin.

Pickett, G., & Hanlon, J.J. (1990). *Public health administration and practice* (9th ed.). St. Louis: Times Mirror/Mosby.

Ravenel, M.P. (Ed.). (1970). *A half century of public health.* New York: Arno Press & The New York Times.

Rogers, J.F. (1936). *Training of elementary teachers for school health work.* U.S. Department of the Interior, Office of Education, Pamphlet No. 67. Washington, DC: U.S. Government Printing Office.

Rosen, G. (1958). *A history of public health.* New York: MD Publications.

Rubinson, L., & Alles, W.F. (1984). *Health education foundations for the future.* St. Louis: Times Mirror/Mosby.

Schouten, J. (1967). *The rod and serpent of Asclepius.* Amsterdam: Elsevier.

Shattuck, L. (1850). *Report of the Sanitary Commission of Massachusetts.* Boston: Dutton and Wentworth.

Turner, C.E., Sellery, C.M., & Smith, S.A. (1957). *School health and health education* (3rd ed.). St. Louis: Mosby.

U.S. Department of Health and Human Services (USDHHS). (1980). *Promoting health/preventing disease: Objectives for the nation.* Washington, DC: U.S. Government Printing Office.

U.S. Department of Health and Human Services. (USDHHS) (1990). *Healthy people 2000: National health promotion and disease prevention objectives* (DHHS pub. no. PHS 90–50212). Washington, DC: U.S. Government Printing Office.

U.S. Department of Health and Human Services (USDHHS). (1997). *Developing objectives for healthy people 2010.* Washington, DC: U.S. Government Printing Office.

U.S. Department of Health, Education, and Welfare (USDHEW). (1976). Health in America: 1776–1976. Washington, DC: U.S. Government Printing Office. DHEW Pub. No. (HRA) 76-616).

U.S. Public Health Service. (1979). *Healthy people: The surgeon general's report on health promotion and disease prevention.* Washington, DC: U.S. Department of Health, Education, and Welfare. Superintendent of Documents, U.S. Government Printing Office.

Winslow, C.A. (1944). *The conquest of epidemic disease.* Princeton, NJ: Princeton University Press.

Ziegler, P. (1969). *The Black Death.* New York: Harper & Row.

3 Philosophical Foundations

CHAPTER OBJECTIVES

After reading this chapter and answering the questions at the end, you should be able to

1. Define the terms *philosophy, humanism, wellness, holistic, and symmetry* and explain the differences between them.

2. Discuss the importance of having a personal philosophy about life.

3. Compare and contrast the advantages and disadvantages of having a life philosophy and an occupational philosophy that are similar.

4. Formulate a statement that describes your personal philosophy of life and identify the influences that account for your philosophy.

5. Identify and explain the differences between
   a. behavior change philosophy
   b. cognitive-based philosophy
   c. decision-making philosophy
   d. freeing/functioning philosophy
   e. social change philosophy
   f. eclectic health education philosophy

6. Explain how a health educator might use each of the five health education philosophies to address a situation in a scenario.

7. Create and defend your own philosophy of health education.

KEY TERMS

behavior change philosophy
cognitive-based philosophy
decision-making philosophy
eclectic health education
   philosophy

freeing/functioning
   philosophy
holistic philosophy
humanism

philosophy
philosophy of symmetry
social change philosophy
wellness

Introduction

When considering the meaning of the phrase "health education philosophy," it seems almost imperative to begin by asking questions. This chapter will explore answers to questions such as

- What is a philosophy?
- Why does a person need a philosophy?
- What are some of the philosophies or philosophical principles associated with the notion of "health"?
- What are the philosophical viewpoints related to health education of some of today's leading health educators?
- How is a philosophy developed?
- What are the predominate philosophies used in the practice of health education today?
- How will adopting any one of the health education philosophies impact the way health educators might approach their job?

The purpose of discussing the development of a health education philosophy is not to provide a treatise on "the nature of the world," so to speak, but to emphasize the importance of a guiding philosophy on the practice of any profession. Although the term *philosophy* seems to imply to many an almost ethereal, esoteric dimension, in actuality, development of a well-considered philosophy provides the underpinnings that support the bridge between theory and practice.

What Is a Philosophy?

The word *philosophy* comes from Greek and literally means "the love of wisdom" or "the love of learning." The term **philosophy** in the context of this chapter means a statement summarizing the attitudes, principles, beliefs, values, and concepts held by an individual or a group. In an academic setting, a philosopher studies the topics of ethics, logic, politics, metaphysics, theology, and/or aesthetics. It is certainly not an imperative that a person be a philosophy professor to have a philosophy. All of us have convictions, ideas, learnings, values, experiences, and attitudes about one or more of the areas listed above as they apply to life. These are the building blocks (sometimes known as principles) that make up any philosophy. Therefore, the probability is high that you have already developed certain philosophical viewpoints or notions about what is real and what is true in the world as you know it. The manner in which you consistently act toward other people is often a reflection of your philosophy concerning the importance of people in general. The fact that you are studying to become a health educator also says something about your philosophical leanings in terms of a career. For

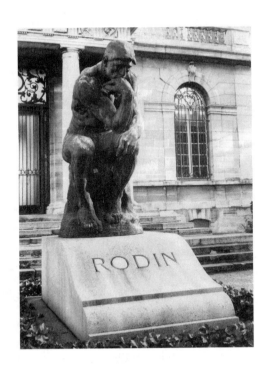

Rodin's sculpture, The Thinker, *illustrates the philosopher in all of us. (Art Resource)*

example, the profession of health education is considered a helping profession. Those who work in the profession should value helping others.

In today's society there are many examples of the use of a philosophical stance. Corporations, for example, create slogans espousing their purported philosophy (of course, they are also trying to sell a product or service at the same time). Many of us recognize certain companies by phrases such as "Just do it!" (Nike), "The good hands people" (Allstate), or "A message of caring" (Blue Shield Health Insurance). The use of caring slogans and catchy phrases is meant to convey to the public that the company is in business solely because it is interested in the welfare of people everywhere and responsive to their needs. The fact of the matter is that any corporation is in business to make money, or it will cease to exist. This comment is not meant to give a bad rap to the businesses that use these slogans. Life is better for many of us because of the products and services they provide.

Just as often, insight into a person's philosophy can be gained by hearing, reading, or analyzing quotes or sayings by that person. For example, the following quote attributed to Scottish poet Robert Burns is most certainly a reflection of his life philosophy: "The purpose of life, is a life of purpose." After reading his words, there is little doubt that he valued a life's work that was well considered and of benefit not only to him, but to others as well. As Bedworth and Bedworth (1992) state, "Philosophy is a wisdom of the nature of things—a comprehension of nature and of reality, a body of knowledge that defines the perimeters of life and living" (p. 10).

The thoughts stated above are well summarized by Loren Bensley (1993), one of the leading health educators of our time, who wrote,

> Philosophy can be defined as a state of mind based on your values and beliefs. This in turn is based on a variety of factors which include culture, religion, education, morals, environment, experiences, and family. It is also determined by people who have influenced you, how you feel about yourself and others, your spirit, your optimism or pessimism, your independence and your family. It is a synthesis of all learning that makes you who you are and what you believe. In other words, a philosophy reflects your values and beliefs which determine your mission and purpose for being, or basic theory, or viewpoint based on logical reasoning. (p. 2)

As can be seen, a philosophy does not have to be abstract. Pondering the reason for being gives people a chance to integrate their past, present, and future into a coherent whole that guides them through life.

Why Does One Need a Philosophy?

The answer to the question "Why Does One Need a Philosophy?" is both simple and complex. Each of us already has a way we look at the world—our philosophy. This image helps shape the way we experience our surroundings and act toward others in our environment. In other words, people's philosophies help form the basis of reality for them.

Of course, some philosophical change is probably inevitable. New experiences, new insights, and new learnings create the possibility that a retooling of some of the tenets comprising the philosophy might occur. This is a normal part of growth. Most people's philosophical views are altered somewhat as they study and experience the world in different ways.

Usually a person's philosophy (e.g., determining how to treat others, what actions are right or wrong, and what is important in life) needs to be synchronous in all aspects of life. This means that a person's philosophical viewpoint holds at home, at school, in the workplace, and at play. If an incongruency develops between a person's philosophy and the philosophy of the leaders in the workplace, problems can occur.

As an example, consider the career of a community health educator working in HIV/AIDS prevention education who is employed by a state department of education. Assume that this individual has a philosophical view that all human life is sacred and education is the best source of prevention. Also assume that the person's work both on and off the job reflects a consistency and a commitment to those ideals. In other words, the person's actions are synonymous with the aforementioned philosophy. As long as the administration in the state department of education, and family and friends remain supportive of the role and philosophy of the HIV/AIDS educator, chances are that all will be well with this person. If, however, leadership in the state department changes and the new superintendent is not at all amenable to the idea that individuals infected with HIV are worth saving (because they chose their behaviors) or refuses to allow the term *condom* to be mentioned as a secondary source of prevention, the health educator will have a difficult time remaining in that environment. The reason is because this educator is now not allowed to act according to her beliefs, ideals, and knowledge. There is a disharmony between the philosophical stance and the ability to act in concert with that stance.

Certainly, there are exceptions to this rule. Health educators might hold philosophies on how they might personally live, yet they might be called on to educate those who have made choices that are in opposition to their belief system. This situation begins to cross the bounds of a general philosophy and get into ethics (right behavior) (see Chapter 5). Although a possible moral-philosophical conflict seems apparent in this situation, health educators need to keep in mind that their primary concern is to protect and enhance the health of those within their jurisdiction. Health is not a moral issue. The health of any one of us affects the health of all of us in some manner (legally, monetarily, physically, or emotionally). At the very least, the health educator should refer this situation to another trained individual who can fulfill the obligation to the public.

Former Surgeon General C. Everett Koop was confronted with the same dilemma when he was in office. Although he was a strong conservative Christian leader and against the use of drugs or the initiation of sex before marriage, he championed the cause of HIV/AIDS education by stressing that the epidemic was

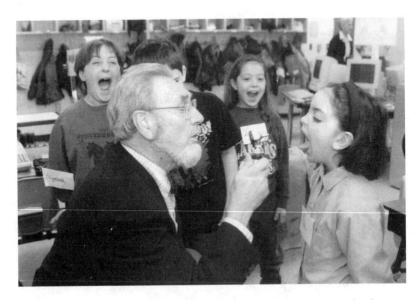

Former Surgeon General C. Everett Koop remains a staunch advocate for the value of health education as the key to prevention. (AP Photo/Valley News, Medora Hebert)

a health problem needing a health-based prevention message. Through the power of his office, he insisted that HIV/AIDS prevention education include the merits of abstinence, the dissemination of needles to inner-city addicts, and the increased availability of condoms to those individuals who chose to be sexually active or promiscuous.

A final example that illustrates the impact of a philosophy comes from Judy Drolet (1993), health education professor at Southern Illinois University. She comments that her philosophy of health education has served to guide her "present commitments and choices in practice, research, and programs" (p. 31). The emphasis she places on the areas of teaching, research, and service is a direct reflection of the personal and professional philosophical foundation she formed over the years.

In summary, the formation of a philosophy is one of the key determining factors behind the choice of an occupation, a spouse, a religious conviction, and friends. A philosophical foundation serves as a beacon that lights the way and provides guidance for many of the major decisions in life.

Principles and Philosophies Associated with Health

In Chapter 1, the meaning of the term *health* was discussed. Recall that, while the term *health* is elusive to define, almost all definitions include the idea of a multi-dimensional construct that most people value, particularly when health deteriorates. Over the past thirty to fifty years, educators have identified several philosophies or philosophical principles that tend to be associated with the establishment and maintenance of health. These philosophies help provide a set of guiding principles that help create a framework to better understand the depth of the term *health.*

Rash (1985) mentions that, while health is often not an end in itself, good health does bring a richness and enjoyment to life which will make service to others more possible. He feels that those who seek to enhance the health of others through education should espouse a **philosophy of symmetry;** that is, health has physical, emotional, spiritual, and social components, and each is just as important as the others. Health educators should seek to motivate their students or clients toward a symmetry (balance) among these components.

Oberteufer (1953) rejected the notions of a dualistic (human = mind + body) or a triune (human = mind + body + spirit) nature for humanity. Instead, he embraced the ideal of a **holistic philosophy** of health when he stated, "The mind and body disappear as recognizable realities and in their stead comes the acknowledgment of a whole being . . . man is essentially a unified integrated organism" (p. 105). Thomas (1984) is convinced that the holistic view of health produces health professionals who are more passionate about creating a society in which the promotion of good health is seen as a positive goal.

Bedworth and Bedworth (1992) propose that **humanism,** one of the underlying theories of education, is worthy of consideration for each potential health

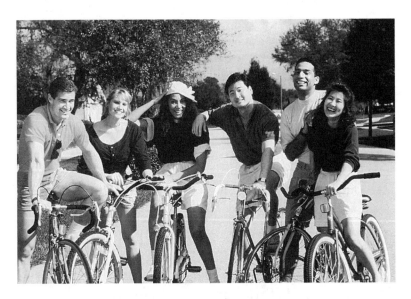

Total health allows people to function at their best. (Bill Cachmann, Photo Researchers)

educator to include in formulating a philosophy of health. They note that humanism is characterized by a concern for humanity. Humanism also "promotes the basic premise of the worth of human life and the ability of individuals to achieve . . . self fulfillment" (p. 5).

Finally, Greenberg (1992) and Donatelle and Davis (1996), among others, have elevated the construct of wellness to the level of a philosophy. **Wellness,** always a positive quality (as opposed to illness being always a negative) is visualized as the integration of the spiritual, intellectual, physical, emotional, environmental, and social dimensions of health to form a whole "healthy person." Those who subscribe to this philosophy believe that all people can achieve some measure of wellness, no matter what limitations they have, and that achieving optimal health is an appropriate journey for everyone. The optimum state of wellness occurs when people have developed all six of the dimensions of health to the maximum of their ability. (See Figures 3.1. and 3.2.)

The philosophies previously mentioned are not meant to be all inclusive. The purpose for discussing them is to help provide a framework to further assist the reader in developing a philosophy about health and, ultimately, health education.

Leading Philosophical Viewpoints

The December 1993 edition of *The Eta Sigma Gamma Monograph Series* was entitled "Reflections: The Philosophies of Health Educators of the 1990's." In order to

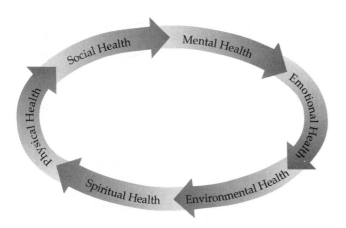

FIGURE 3.1   The Six Dimensions of Health.

Source: From Donatelle and Davis, *Health: The Basics,* 2nd edition.
Copyright © 1997 by Allyn & Bacon. Reprinted by permission.

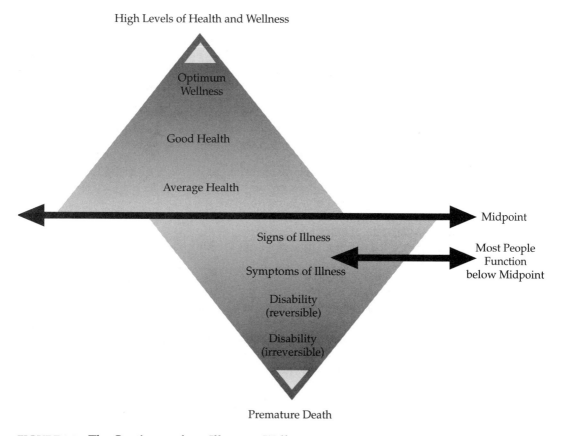

FIGURE 3.2   The Continuum from Illness to Wellness.

Source: From Donatelle and Davis, *Health: The Basics,* 2nd edition. Copyright © 1997 by Allyn & Bacon.
Reprinted by permission.

assist you in formulating your own health education philosophy, we believe it is instructive to present a representative sample of the philosophies expressed in this volume. As has been previously mentioned, one of the ways a philosophical approach is developed is through the influence of role models, or mentors. The viewpoints that follow may help stimulate your thoughts and provide guidance as you consider a career in health education.

Loren Bensley (1993)

I believe health education offers an individual an invitation to be and to become—to affirm the self and become committed to the development of individual potential through decision making and action. I am committed to the philosophy of existentialism (the existential health educator sees his/her function as one of awakening learners to their own capacities and of providing opportunities for them to be responsible for their own learning opportunities and/or ignorance—(Shirreffs, 1976) as an approach to health education (p. 3) . . . I also believe the ultimate goal of health education is to provide learning experiences from which one can develop skills and knowledge to make better informed decisions which will maintain or better their health, or the health of others (p. 4).

Joyce Fetro (1993)

I believe health education is an "ongoing process"—meaning that something is "going on." It implies continuous movement. The content and process of health education should change as individuals and current health issues change. To me, health education is an invitation to a smorgasbord. Health educators make the curriculum and program selections, arrange them in a way that is most meaningful, and appealing to their students, and replenish them when necessary (p. 59). . . . Critical to the health education feast is a forum that promotes openness and acceptance of individual differences (p. 63). . . .

Fetro concludes with this quote from Rosenstock (1960), "We must keep constantly in mind that an individual's behavior is determined by his motives and his beliefs, regardless of whether the motives and beliefs correspond to our notion of reality and what is good for him.

Marian Hamburg (1993)

Eta Sigma Gamma's invitation to contribute has given me the chance to expound on a few of my beliefs about health education.

1. You can't plan everything. Unexpected opportunities appear and it is important to be ready to take advantage of them (p. 68).
2. I believe in mentorship. Its power incorporated into health education programming has enormous strength for influencing positive health behaviors (p. 70).
3. I believe that effective health education programming requires appropriate inter-sectoral cooperation, and that health educators, regardless of the source of their professional preparation, must be its facilitators. School-community can be one world (p. 71).
4. I believe that we need to put more of our resources into joint efforts and coalition building. Much of health education's future as a profession depends upon the support that health educators, regardless of their specialized training, provide for the maintenance and expansion of certification (p. 73).

5. It is not surprising to me that the concept of networking has become an important basis for health education practice. We bring together people with common problems to seek solutions through the sharing of feelings and information (p. 73).

John Seffrin (1993)
I believe the most fundamental outcome of health education is the enabling of individuals to achieve a level of personal freedom not very likely to be obtained otherwise. Freedom means being able to avoid any unnecessary encumbrance on one's ability to make an enlightened choice (p. 110). . . . we need to be resourceful and open to change. In doing so, however, we need to change in ways that do not violate certain basic principles:

1. appreciation for each individual's uniqueness;
2. respect for ethnic and cultural diversity;
3. protection for individual and group autonomy;
4. promotion and preservation of free choice; and
5. intervention strategies based on good science (p. 114).

Philosophies are as individual as the people themselves, yet some common themes seem to emerge and hold true regardless of the health educator. Let us now examine how these philosophies are actually applied in the practice of health education.

Developing a Philosophy

Now that it is clear that a philosophy is not some abstraction that is used only by individuals such as the Dali Lama or Gandhi, let us explore the ways in which a philosophy is formed. In previous sections, it was noted that most practicing professionals and many organizations have developed certain philosophical stances that serve as a road map and guide for living and working in the world. What provides the basis for forming a philosophy?

Assume that you are asked to analyze this quote from a famous movie star: "Tomorrow is the most important thing in life. Comes to us at midnight very clean. It's perfect when it arrives and puts itself in our hands. It hopes we learned something from yesterday." How would you describe the perspective of the person who made that statement? What would she be using as a basis for those thoughts?

A possible answer to the first question might be that the person loves life and the opportunities and challenges it presents. She sees each day as a gift and hopes to use what she learned the day before to make the next day even better. It might also reflect an attitude that what occurred the previous day cannot be changed, so time and energy spent in worry about yesterday are wasted.

Answering the second question helps provide guidance as to how a philosophy is developed. The person most likely would have arrived at the conclusion that tomorrow is most important through (1) experience, (2) education or study,

(3) guidance from teachers, religious leaders, and mentors, and (4) learnings from friends and relatives. She then pieces together all of this information and synthesizes it into a way of thinking, acting, or viewing the world that works for her. That is the same way any philosophical viewpoint is attained. Reading about and thinking about what is important, learning about life by being involved in and experiencing and examining the pros and cons of certain actions, having mentors and role models, and speaking with friends and relatives and learning from their experiences and teaching help mold and develop a way of thinking—a philosophy.

Please note, however, that using these four avenues (studying, experiencing, having a mentor or role model, and learning from friends and family) to formulate a philosophy does not guarantee that the philosophy will remain stable. As a matter of fact, there is a strong likelihood that some changes will occur because of new learnings, activities, and experiences (e.g., working in a different culture, experiencing the premature death of a child or spouse, losing a job as a result of downsizing). A philosophy results from the sum of knowledge, experience, and principles from which it was formed.

As a further aid to formulating a philosophy statement about health and health education, we would like to conclude this section with three short vignettes illustrating several concepts or principles that need to be considered when formulating a philosophy statement about life, health, and health education practice. The first comes from Mongolia.

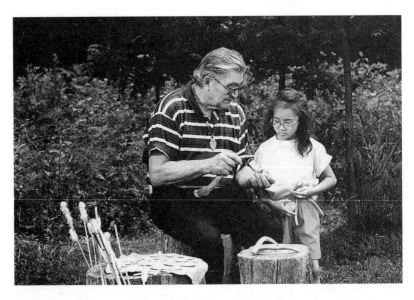

Family members, friends, mentors, and role models help shape our philosophy.
(Lawrence Migdale/Stock, Boston)

A farmer had a teenage son who caused trouble from time to time. The neighbors constantly criticized the farmer for having such a son. One day the farmer went to town and purchased a wild horse in the hope that he could tame it and use it for transportation to and from town. That evening the son sneaked out and attempted to get on the horse. It escaped. On learning of the circumstances surrounding the horse's escape, the neighbors berated the farmer for his son and the bad luck he caused. The farmer, however, responded that maybe the horse's escape was bad; maybe it wasn't. The next day, to everyone's amazement, the horse reappeared with fifteen other wild horses. The farmer and the neighbors could not believe the good fortune.

That night the son tried to ride one of the wild horses, was thrown off, and broke his leg. The neighbors were quick to seize the opportunity to point out this misfortune as well. Again, the farmer responded that maybe the son's breaking his leg was bad, but maybe it wasn't. The next day the Mongols declared war on a country far away, and soldiers came to the village and conscripted every able-bodied son from every family. Of course, because of his broken leg the farmer's son was not taken. He grew to live a long, healthful, and prosperous life and became a mayor of the village.

How things turn out is many times a matter of how they are perceived. A personal philosophy is often a reflection of the individual's perspective of the world and how and why it seems to work that way.

The second story comes from the United States.

One Saturday in late spring a family decided to visit the local zoo. As they entered, it was noted that the feature attraction for that day was a flea circus. Now, the father, being a skeptic, had heard of flea circuses before but thought them to be fictional. Approaching the area where the flea circus was supposedly housed, he was amazed to find a large piece of plywood complete with fleas jumping around. Nearby was a young woman who wore a suit with the tag "flea trainer" conspicuously inscribed on it. The father went up to the woman and asked her (tongue in cheek) how she was able to train the fleas. She responded that training them was actually quite easy. She went on to explain that a flea can jump higher for its size than any living creature. Her method involved placing the fleas in a three-inch-high box with a lid on it. At first the fleas jump and hit the lid. After a few minutes, however, they learn to jump just short of the top. When she determines that they have reached that level of training (she can no longer hear them hitting the inside of the box lid), she removes the lid and places them on the plywood. Although they have not lost any of their ability to jump, they never again go any higher than the height of the box lid.

Too many times, in determining abilities, people set their sights and dreams too low. A personal philosophy needs to incorporate the realization that life sometimes dishes out bumps and bruises. The awareness of this fact helps prevent any of us from becoming too limiting in the assessment of our place in the world.

The third idea is really more a factor to consider when examining one's potential and what is valued in life.

Never compare yourself with others. There is always someone better than you in anything you might try. The key is that no one person is better than you are in all aspects of life. Having role models is valuable. Just make certain to be realistic about your abilities and to realize that no one has the same combination of talents that you do.

Remember, the formation of a philosophy whether personal or occupational requires basically three steps. First, individuals need to answer the following questions in reference to themselves: What is important? What is most valued? What ideals are held? Second, they need to identify ways the answers to the first questions influence the way they believe and act. Third, after carefully considering and writing down the answers to these questions, a philosophy statement can be formulated. The statement (usually about a paragraph in length—250 words) reflects and identifies those factors, principles, ideals, and influences that help shape reality for those individuals.

As previously mentioned, these steps can be used to formulate any type of philosophy statement. However, for those who are studying health education, there is one more important question to answer: Is this philosophy statement consistent with being a health educator? If the answer is yes, then for that person health education is a profession worthy of further consideration.

Predominate Health Education Philosophies

Butler (1997) accurately points out that, even though there are several definitions for *health education,* there are recurring themes in many of the definitions that allow for a general agreement as to the meaning of the phrase "health education." He notes, however, that the methods used to accomplish health education are less clear. The manner in which a person chooses to conduct health education can be demonstrated to be a direct reflection of that person's philosophy of health education. With that in mind, have any predominate philosophies of health education emerged? If so, what are they?

Welle, Russell, and Kittleson (1995) conducted a study to determine the philosophies favored by health educators. As part of the background for their study, they conducted a literature review and identified five dominant philosophies of health education that have emerged during this half-century. Those identified were behavior change, cognitive-based, decision-making, freeing/functioning, and social change:

1. The **behavior change philosophy** involves a health educator using behavioral contracts, goal setting, and self-monitoring to try to foster a modification in an unhealthy habit in an individual with whom he is working. The nature of this approach allows for the establishment of easily measurable objectives, thus enhancing the ability to evaluate outcomes.
2. A health educator who uses a **cognitive-based philosophy** focuses on the acquisition of content and factual information. The goal is to increase the

knowledge of the person or group so that they are better armed to make decisions about their health.

3. In using the **decision-making philosophy,** a health educator presents simulated problems, case studies, or scenarios to students or clients. Each problem, case, or scenario requires decisions to be made in seeking a "best approach or answer." By creating and analyzing potential solutions, the students develop skills needed to address many health-related decisions they might face. An advantage of this approach is the emphasis on critical thinking and lifelong learning.

4. The **freeing/functioning philosophy** was proposed by Greenberg (1978) as a reaction to the fact that he felt traditional approaches of health education ran the risk of blaming people for practicing health behaviors that were often either out of their control or not seen as in their best interests. The health educator who uses this philosophical approach has the ultimate goal to free people to make the best health decisions possible based on their needs and interests—not necessarily on the interests of society.

5. The **social change philosophy** emphasizes the role of health education in creating social, economic, and political change that benefits the health of individuals and groups. Health educators espousing this philosophy are often at the forefront of the adoption of policies or laws that will enhance the health of all.

The previously listed philosophies of health education are the products of nearly fifty years of study, experimentation, and dialogue within the profession. The research conducted by Welle, Russell, and Kittleson (1995) alluded to earlier found that the first preference of a philosophy by both health education practitioners and academicians was decision making. Both groups listed behavior change as a second choice, and both agreed that their least favorite was cognitive-based. The fact that health educators who are employed in the academic setting and those who are employed as practitioners in the field agreed on these choices as predominate philosophies speaks well for the interface between preparation programs and practice.

Another interesting finding from the study occurred when, as a part of the survey, the health educators were given health education vignettes to address or solve. In many cases, the respondents changed the philosophical approach they used, depending on the setting (school, community, worksite, medical). The responding health educators had earlier identified a specific health education philosophy they favored. These results indicate that health educators are adaptable and resourceful, and they will use any health education approach that seems to be appropriate to the situation. The possibility exists that in practice health educators use an **eclectic health education philosophy**

The results are not surprising, because in any list of philosophies there is always the possibility of one philosophy overlapping with another, so in practice not all is as clean as it might seem. Actually using the principles inherent in only one of these philosophies is not easy. The next section will explore how adoption

BOX **3.1**

Practitioner's Perspective

Name:	Kristy L. Jones
Current Position/Title:	Health Education Specialist/Cancer Prevention and Control Supervisor
Employer:	Idaho Department of Health and Welfare
Major(s):	B.S. Public Health—Utah State University
Minor(s):	Community Health

Primary job responsibilities: I am the program manager for the Tobacco Prevention and Control Program and supervise the Breast and Cervical Cancer Screening Program. My job includes duties such as working with state and local tobacco coalitions, local health departments, American Heart and Lung Associations, and the American Cancer Society, as well as other partners to plan and implement projects and promotions. My responsibilities include writing grant applications and reports, monitoring program budgets, assessing program needs and planning programs to meet statewide health objectives, supervising and evaluating program staff, planning and conducting health education trainings for health district staff, and developing and monitoring contracts for services.

How I obtained my position: Through networking I learned that the position of health education specialist was open. I applied, was placed on the state register, was interviewed, and was hired. I had some prior local health department experience, which enabled me to understand how to relate to local health departments and other contractors—a bonus in a state-level position.

My philosophy of health education: Health education and health education programs should be broad-based and population-focused. We need to move from looking at individuals within a community to looking at the entire community. My philosophy would advocate using strategies that impact the most people with the strongest intervention at the least cost.

What I like most about my position: I enjoy leading and collaborating on projects from conception through planning, implementing, and evaluation. Creating statewide projects includes working with a number of people and with all types of people. This can be challenging yet rewarding. I also like to collaborate with partners on media campaigns.

What I like least about my position: Political constraints associated with working with a bureaucracy can be frustrating. Paperwork takes much time, and I miss the opportunity to work more with local organizations and people from around the state on a face-to-face basis.

My recommendations for health education students who would someday like a job like mine: A quality internship is a very important job prerequisite and can mean the difference in whether or not the applicant is hired. Students should apply to state and local health departments, hospitals, and voluntary health organizations such as the American Heart Association. Quality internships should include practice in needs assessment, program planning and evaluation, survey development, report writing, and public interaction. Also, round out your studies by taking courses generally found outside of health education such as statistics, accounting, business administration, marketing, human resources, and behavioral psychology.

of any or all of these philosophies might impact the way a person practices health education.

Impacting the Delivery of Health Education

This section will use scenarios to help focus on the methods health educators might use, depending on their philosophical stance. The decision to use any philosophy involves understanding and accepting the foundation that helped create the philosophy in the first place. To this end, Welle, Russell, and Kittleson (1995) state,

> Health educators must remember that every single educational choice carries with it a philosophical principle or belief. Educational choices carry important philosophical assumptions about the purpose of health education, the teacher, and also the learner. Thus, health educators should take the time necessary for individual philosophical inquiry, in order to be able to clearly articulate what principles guide them professionally. . . . Different settings may produce the need for different philosophies. Every health educator should be aware of which elements of their individual philosophies they are willing to compromise. (p. 331)

At the outset, it is important to remember that one of the overriding goals of any health education intervention is the betterment of health for the person or the group involved. All of the philosophies have that goal. They differ in how to approach that objective.

Consider the case of Anne, a forty-year-old mother of two, who smokes, does not exercise regularly, and has a family history of heart disease. Anne is enrolled in a required health education course at a local university. She is going back to school to become an elementary school teacher. Because a health appraisal is a required part of the class, she has come in to visit the health education office. Three health educators (Sam, Carla, and Alice) are employed in the center. Each one has a different philosophy of health education. How will their approaches differ? Here is a possible intervention scenario.

Sam has adopted the philosophy of behavior change. As a proponent of this approach, he believes that all people are capable of adapting their health behavior if they can be shown the steps to success. He would use a behavior change contract method to get Anne to try to eliminate one or two of her negative health behaviors. As a part of this process, some preliminary analysis would be done in an attempt to identify the triggers that cause her to practice the negative health behaviors. He would help her identify short-term and long-term goals. Together they would establish objectives to reach those goals, and strategies to reach the objectives. He would also try to ensure that she receives some appropriate reward for every objective and goal she accomplishes.

Carla, on the other hand, is an advocate of the health education philosophy known as decision-making. This means that she believes in equipping her clients with problem-solving and coping skills, so that they make the best possible health choices. Initially, she might sit down with Anne and hypothesize some situations that would necessitate Anne thinking through the rationale behind the negative health behaviors she practices. Carla also would most likely try to get Anne to see that some of her behaviors impact more people than just herself. The goals are to get Anne to see that some of her health behaviors need to be changed and to help her identify the reasons that changing them would make her life better.

Finally, Alice advocates a freeing/functioning philosophy of health education. She feels that, too often, health educators fail to find out the needs and desires of the client. They simply "barge in" and either overtly or covertly blame the client for any negative health behaviors. Alice would advocate change only if the behavior were infringing on the rights of others. In the beginning, Alice would confer with Anne and find out "how her life was going." She would ask Anne to identify any behaviors she wanted to change, making certain that Anne had all of the information necessary to make an informed decision. Although Alice might believe that Anne should stop smoking and start exercising, she would help Anne change only those behaviors Anne wanted to change.

One sidelight needs to be mentioned at this time. The facts that Anne was required to take a health education course in her teacher preparation program and that the instructor required a health assessment illustrate at a microlevel the social change philosophy at work. If health were not a state requirement (legislation) in the first place, she might not have considered changing any of her negative health behaviors.

Anne's situation illustrates a point made earlier—in practice, there often is a natural mixing of some of the philosophies. For example, all of the approaches mentioned used portions of the cognitive-based health education philosophy. To reiterate, this philosophy is based on the premise that persons need to be provided with the most current information that impacts their health behaviors, and the acquisition of that information should create a dissonance and cause change.

The fifth philosophy, social change, is probably not as well suited to addressing the health behaviors of individuals one on one. Proponents stress changes in social, economic, and political arenas to impact the health of populations. Of course, populations are made up of individuals, so changing the environment of an inner-city neighborhood to be healthier (for example, creating jobs, assuring adequate and safe housing and safe schools, providing health care coverage for all) ultimately impacts the health of people at the individual level as well.

Summary

The term *philosophy* means a statement summarizing the attitudes, principles, beliefs, and concepts of an individual or a group. Forming both a personal and an occupational philosophy requires reflection and the ability to identify those factors, principles, ideals, and influences that help shape your reality. The decision to use any philosophy involves understanding and accepting the foundation that helped create the philosophy in the first place. A sound philosophical foundation serves as a guidepost for many of the major decisions in life.

The five predominate philosophies of health education that were identified in the chapter are behavior change, cognitive-based, decision-making, freeing/functioning, and social change. Health educators might disagree on which philosophy works best. They might even use an eclectic or a combination philosophical approach, depending on the setting or situation. However, it is important to remember that one of the overriding goals of any health education intervention is the betterment of health for the person or group involved. All of the philosophies have that goal. They simply differ in how to approach that objective.

REVIEW QUESTIONS

1. Define each of the following and explain their relationship to one another;
   - philosophy
   - humanism
   - wellness
   - holistic
   - symmetry

2. Why is it important to have a personal philosophy about life?

3. What four primary avenues or influences help in formulating both a personal and a professional philosophy?

4. Compare and contrast the value of having a personal life philosophy and an occupational life philosophy that are similar.

5. Define and explain the differences among
   - behavior change philosophy
   - cognitive-based philosophy
   - decision-making philosophy
   - freeing/functioning philosophy
   - social change philosophy
   - eclectic health education philosophy

6. Explain how a person might use each of the five health education philosophies to address a societal problem that can be addressed by health education (e.g., smoking, seat belt use, air pollution).

ACTIVITIES

1. Reread the story of the Mongolian farmer. How would you describe the farmer's philosophy of life? What values or ideals are found by the farmer that helped form the basis of his philosophy? What life experiences do think he had that helped shape his philosophy?

2. After reexamining the philosophies of health, write a paragraph that could be used to explain your philosophy of health to a friend or colleague.

3. Interview a school or community health educator in your community. Ask his or her philosophy of health education. Then ask about the influences that helped the educator form his or her philosophy. Summarize the interview in a one-page paper.

4. Use any three of the five philosophical approaches to health education discussed in the chapter and address the following situation:

In the past week in your community, two teenagers have been killed in separate incidents while riding bicycles. In neither case was the person wearing a helmet. A local citizens group has asked you and two of your health education colleagues to attend a meeting concerning what to do about this issue.

REFERENCES

Bedworth, D. A. & Bedworth, A. E. (1992). *The profession and practice of health education.* Dubuque, IA: Wm. C. Brown.

Bensley, L. B. (1993). This I believe: A philosophy of health education. *The Eta Sigma Gamma Monograph Series, 11*(2),1–7.

Butler, J. T. (1997). *The Principles and practices of health education and health promotion.* Englewood, CO: Morton.

Donatelle, R. J, & Davis, L. G. (1996). *Health: The basics* (2nd ed.). Boston, MA: Allyn and Bacon.

Drolet, J. C. (1993). Pondering a professional philosophy. *The Eta Sigma Gamma Monograph Series, 11*(2), 26–38.

Fetro, J. S. (1993). Health education: A smorgasbord of life. *The Eta Sigma Gamma Monograph Series, 11*(2), 56–66.

Greenberg, J. S. (1978). Health education as freeing. *Health Education, 9*(2), 20–21.

Greenberg, J. S. (1992). *Health education: Learner centered instructional strategies* (2nd ed.). Dubuque, IA: William C. Brown.

Hamburg, M. V. (1993). Would I do it all over! *The Eta Sigma Gamma Monograph Series, 11*(2), 67–74.

Hills, M. D. & Lindsey, E. (1994). Health promotion: A viable curriculum framework for nursing education. *Nursing Outlook, 42*(4), 158–162.

Oberteufer, D. (1953). Philosophy and principles of school health education. *The Journal of School Health, 23*(4), 103–109.

O'Rourke, T. (1989). Reflections on the directions in health education: Implications for policy and practice. *Health Education, 28*(6), 4–14.

Pigg, R. M. (1993). Three essential questions in defining a personal philosophy. *The Eta Sigma Gamma Monograph Series, 11*(2), 94–101.

Rash, J. K. (1985). Philosophical bases for health education. *Health Education, 16*(3), 48–49.

Rosenstock, I. M. (1960). *Decision-making by individuals.* Paper presented at the Annual Meeting of the Society for Public Health Educators, October 29, San Francisco, CA.

Seffrin, J. R. (1993). Health education and the pursuit of personal freedom. *The Eta Sigma Gamma Monograph Series, 11*(2), 109–118.

Shirreffs, J. (Spring, 1976). A philosophical approach to health education. *The Eta Sigma Gamman,* 21–23.

Thomas, S. B. (1984). The holistic philosophy and perspective of selected health educators. *Health Education, 15*(1), 15–20.

Timmreck, T. C.,et al. (1987). Health education and the health promotion movement: A theoretical jungle. *Health Education, 18*(5), 24–28.

Timmreck, T. C., et al. (1988). Health education and health promotion: A look at the jungle of supportive fields, philosophies, and theoretical foundations. *Health Education, 18*(6), 23–28.

Welle, H. M, Russell, R. D., & Kittleson, M. J. (1995). Philosophical trends in health education: Implications for the 21st century. *Journal of Health Education, 26*(6), 326–333.

4 Theoretical Foundations

CHAPTER OBJECTIVES

After reading this chapter and answering the questions at the end, you should be able to

1. Define and explain the difference among *theory, concept, construct, variable,* and *model.*
2. Explain the importance of theory to the health education discipline.
3. Distinguish between models of implementation and change process theories.
4. Distinguish between planning models and the theories and models focusing on behavior change.
5. Identify the planning models and their components used in health education/health promotion and briefly explain each:
   a. PRECEDE-PROCEED
   b. Model for Health Education Planning (MHEP)
   c. Comprehensive Health Education Model (CHEM)
   d. Model for Health Education Planning and Resource Development (MHEPRD)
   e. Generic Health and Fitness Delivery System (GHFDS)
   f. Generalized Model for Program Planning (GMPP)
6. Identify the theories and models focusing on behavior (change process theories) and their components used in health education/promotion and briefly explain each:
   a. health belief model
   b. transtheoretical model or stages of change
   c. theory of planned behavior
   d. social cognitive theory
   e. theory of diffusion

KEY TERMS

action stage
administrative and policy
   diagnosis
attitude toward the behavior
behavioral capability
behavioral diagnosis
change process theories

concepts
construct
contemplation stage
cue to action
diffusion theory
early adopters
early majority

ecological perspective
educational and
   organizational diagnosis
emotional-coping response
EMPOWER
enabling factor
environmental diagnosis

epidemiological diagnosis
expectancies
expectations
health belief model
impact evaluation
implementation
innovators
laggards
late majority
likelihood of taking action
locus of control
maintenance
model
outcome evaluation

perceived barriers
perceived behavioral control
perceived benefits
perceived
   seriousness/severity
perceived susceptibility
perceived threat
PRECEDE-PROCEED
precontemplation stage
predisposing factor
preparation stage
process evaluation
reciprocal determinism

reduction of threat
reinforcement
reinforcing factor
self-control (self-regulation)
self-efficacy
social diagnosis
subjective norm
theories/models of
   implementation
theory
theory of planned behavior
transtheoretical model
variable

As noted in Chapter 1, health education/health promotion is a multidisciplinary field of practice that has evolved from the theory and practice of a number of other biological, behavioral, sociological, and health science disciplines. As the profession has grown, the theoretical base on which it was formed has become more apparent. In this chapter, we will introduce the definitions of *theory, concept, construct, variable,* and *model;* explain why it is important to use theory in health education/promotion; provide an overview of the different theories and models that will be used in your future work; and leave you with a word of caution about the application of theories and models.

Definitions

In order to be able to understand the theoretical foundations presented in this chapter, it is important to be familiar with some key related words. Let us begin with theory. One of the most frequently quoted definitions of **theory** is one in which Glanz, Lewis, and Rimer (1997) modified an earlier definition written by Kerlinger (1986). It states, "A *theory* is a set of interrelated concepts, definitions, and propositions that presents a *systematic* view of events or situations by specifying relations among variables in order to *explain* and *predict* the events of the situations" (Glanz, Lewis, & Rimer, 1997, p. 21). Stated a little differently, "a theory is a systematic arrangement of fundamental principles that provide a basis for explaining certain happenings of life" (McKenzie & Smeltzer, 1997, p. 97). Thus, "the role of theory is to untangle and simplify for human comprehension the complexities of nature" (Green et al., 1994, p. 398). As applied to the profession of health education, a theory is a general explanation of why people act or do not act to maintain and/or promote the health of themselves, their families, organizations, and communities. The primary elements of theories are known as **concepts**

(Glanz, Lewis, & Rimer, 1997). When a concept has been developed, created, or adopted for use with a specific theory, it is referred to as a **construct** (Kerlinger, 1986). In other words, constructs are synthesized thoughts or key concepts of specific theories. The operational (practical use) form of a construct is known as a **variable.** Variables "specify how a construct is to be measured in a specific situation" (Glanz & Rimer, 1995, p. 11).

A **model** is a subclass of a theory (McKenzie & Smeltzer, 1997, p. 97). "Models draw on a number of theories to help people understand a specific problem in a particular setting or context" (Glanz, Lewis, & Rimer, 1997, p. 24). Models provide health educators with a framework on which to create plans for programs. Unlike theories, models do "not attempt to explain the processes underlying learning, but only to represent them" (Chaplin & Krawiec, 1979, p. 68).

Now consider how these terms are used in practical application. A personal belief is a *concept* that has been shown to relate to various health behaviors. Using a *theory* that includes the concept of personal beliefs helps explain why people fear being trapped in a burning vehicle if they use their safety belts. This personal belief of fear acts as a perceived barrier to safety belt use. Perceived barrier is a part of a specific theory and is referred to here as a *construct.* If a health educator develops a program around a theory to help people overcome this barrier and wear their safety belts, then safety belt use is the *variable* being studied. The health educator realizes that this theory, which emphasizes personal beliefs, will not explain all the reasons that people do not wear safety belts. Thus, other theories, which emphasize other concepts (i.e., knowledge, environment, incentives, comfort, convenience, etc.) need to be considered.

Eventually, all of these theories may be combined into a *model* that will explain, at least in part, why people wear safety belts. If a model were a perfect model, it would predict with 100 percent accuracy who would wear safety belts. Unfortunately, behavior is very complex and there are no perfect models in health education. It is therefore important for health educators to keep revising their models to improve their understanding of health behavior.

The Importance of Using Theory in Health Education/Promotion

Theory is important to the profession because it helps guide the practice of health educators. It can help during the various stages of planning, implementing, and evaluating a program (Glanz & Rimer, 1995). "Theories can provide answers to program developers' questions regarding *why* people aren't already engaging in a desirable behavior of interest, *how* to go about changing their behaviors, and *what* factors to look for when evaluating a program's focus" (van Ryn & Heaney, 1992, p. 326). Stated a little differently, "a theory based approach provides direction and justification for program activities and serves as a basis for processes that are to be incorporated into the health promotion program" (Cowdery et al., 1995, p. 248). Though not all health education/health promotion programs are successful, those that are based on sound theory are more likely to succeed than those that are not.

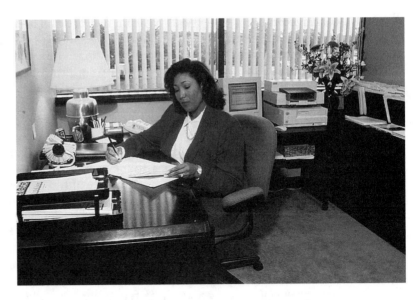

A theory-based approach provides direction and justification for program planners. (John Coletti)

An Overview of the Theories and Models Used in Health Education/Promotion

The remaining portions of this chapter present many of the theories and models that are often used in the discipline of health education/promotion. There are a number of ways that the theories and models could be organized and presented in this chapter. We will present the theories and models in two groups. The first are those used in planning, implementing, and evaluating health education/ promotion programs. Some have referred to these as the *theories/models of implementation*. To lessen the confusion of terminology, we will refer to them as planning models. The second group includes the theories and models that focus on behavior change. McLeroy and colleagues (1992) have referred to these theories as change process theories. *Change process theories* "specify the relationships among causal processes operating both within and across levels of analysis" (McLeroy et al., 1992, p. 3). In other words, change process theories help explain, through their constructs, how change takes place. For example, the change of getting a non-exerciser to exercise can be explained in part by change process theories.

Planning Models (Theories/Models of Implementation)

Good health promotion programs are not created by chance. They are the result of much hard work and are organized around a well-thought-out and well-conceived model. Models for planning provide health educators with a frame on which develop a plan. A number of models have been developed over the years. The models that are presented in this section have been used most frequently by health educators. Please note that the presentation of the models here is just to familiarize you with the names and components of the major planning models. It is assumed that you will obtain a working knowledge of the models in your upper-level health education classes. For more detailed explanations of the models, see the original publications of the models (Bates & Winder, 1984; Green & Kreuter, 1991; Patton et al., 1986; Ross & Mico, 1980; Sullivan, 1973) or other related works (Glanz, Lewis, & Rimer, 1997; Glanz & Rimer, 1995; McKenzie & Smeltzer, 1997).

PRECEDE-PROCEED.   Currently, the best-known and most often used theory of implementation is the **PRECEDE-PROCEED** model. PRECEDE is an acronym for Predisposing, Reinforcing, and Enabling Constructs in Educational/ Environmental Diagnosis and Evaluation, while PROCEED stands for Policy, Regulatory, and Organizational Constructs in Educational and Environmental Development (Green & Kreuter, 1991). The PRECEDE-PROCEED model was developed over a period of fifteen to twenty years, with the PRECEDE framework being conceived in the early 1970s (Green, 1974) and evolving into a planning model in the late 1970s (Green, 1975, 1976; Green, Levine, & Deeds, 1975; Green et al., 1978; Green et al., 1980). The PROCEED portion was developed in the early to mid-1980s (Green, 1979, 1980, 1981a, 1981b, 1982, 1983a, 1983b, 1984a, 1984b, 1984c, 1984d, 1986a, 1986b, 1986c, 1986d, 1986e, 1987a, 1987b; Green & Allen, 1980; Green & McAlister, 1984; Green, Mullen, & Friedman, 1986; Green, Wilson, & Lovato, 1986; Green, Wilson, & Bauer, 1983). It "is essentially an elaboration and extension of the administrative diagnosis step of PRECEDE, which was the final and least developed link in the PRECEDE framework" (Green & Kreuter, 1991, p. 25).

As is noted in Figure 4.1, PRECEDE-PROCEED is comprised of nine phases, or steps. The first five phases, which make up the PRECEDE portion of the model, are diagnostic in nature. The last four phases, the PROCEED portion, are implementation and evaluation (process, impact, and outcome) steps, with emphasis on the latter to improve the former (Glanz & Rimer, 1995). At first glance, the PRECEDE-PROCEED model appears overly complicated, but on close examination you will find that there is a very logical sequence to the nine phases that outline the health promotion planning process. "The underlying approach of this model is to begin by identifying the desired outcome, to determine what causes it, and finally to design an intervention aimed at reaching the desired outcome. In other words, PRECEDE-PROCEED begins with the final consequences and works backwards to the causes" (McKenzie & Smeltzer, 1997, p. 12). Table 4.1 provides an overview of the nine phases of the model.

Many of those who use the PRECEDE-PROCEED model for the first time find it difficult to use because of the many constructs that are included in it.

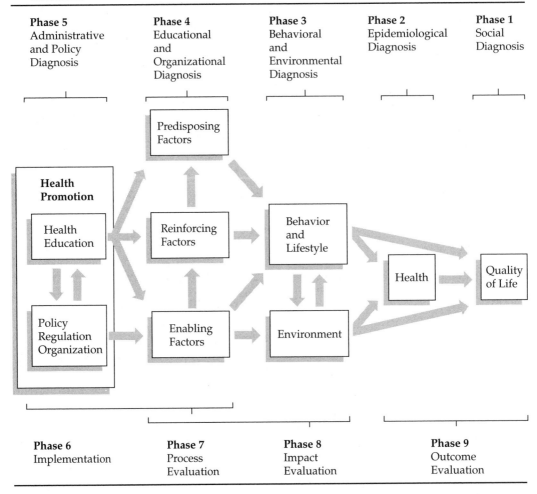

FIGURE 4.1   PRECEDE-PROCEED Model for Health Promotion Planning and Evaluation.

However, there is now a computer program available called **EMPOWER** (Expert Methods for Planning and Organization within Everyone's Reach) that allows users to work through a decision matrix based on the PRECEDE-PROCEED model (Gilbert & Sawyer, 1995). The program, which incorporates technology related to artificial intelligence and expert systems, was developed to help users design a community-based health promotion program for a diverse, high-risk population (Green et al., 1994). EMPOWER is available from Jones and Bartlett Publishers, 40 Tall Pine Drive, Sudbury, MA 01776, 1-800-832-0034.

TABLE 4.1   The Nine Phases of the PRECEDE-PROCEED Model

Phase 1. **Social diagnosis** is "the process of determining people's perceptions of their own needs or quality of life, and their aspirations for the common good, through broad participation and application of multiple information-gathering activities designed to expand understanding of the community" (Green & Kreuter, 1991, p. 45).

Phase 2. **Epidemiological diagnosis** is "the delineation of the extent, distribution, and causes of a health problem in a defined population" (Green & Kreuter, 1991, p. 431).

Phase 3. **Behavioral diagnosis** is the "delineation of the specific health-related actions that most likely effect, or could effect, a health outcome" (Green & Kreuter, 1991, p. 429), and **environmental diagnosis** is " a systematic assessment of factors in the social and physical environment that interact with behavior to produce health effects or quality-of-life outcomes" (Green & Kreuter, 1991, p. 432).

Phase 4. **Educational and organizational diagnosis** "identifies factors that must be changed to initiate and sustain the process of behavioral and environmental change" (Green & Kreuter, 1991, p. 151). **Predisposing factor** is "any characteristic of a person or population that motivates behavior prior to the occurrence of the behavior" (Green & Kreuter, 1991, p. 434); **reinforcing factor** is "any reward or punishment following or anticipated as a consequence of a behavior, serving to strengthen the motivation for the behavior after it occurs" (Green & Kreuter, 1991, p. 434); **enabling factor** is "any characteristic of the environment that facilitates action and any skill or resource required to attain a specific behavior" (Green & Kreuter, 1991, p. 431).

Phase 5. **Administrative and policy diagnosis** is "an analysis of the policies, resources and circumstances prevailing in an organizational situation to facilitate or hinder the development of the health promotion program" (Green & Kreuter, 1991, p. 429).

Phase 6. **Implementation** is "the act of converting program objectives into actions through policy changes, regulation and organization" (Green & Kreuter, 1991, p. 432).

Phase 7. **Process evaluation** is "the assessment of policies, materials, personnel, performance, quality of practice or services, and other inputs and implementation experiences" (Green & Kreuter, 1991, p. 434).

Phase 8. **Impact evaluation** is "the assessment of program effects on intermediate objectives including changes in predisposing, enabling, and reinforcing factors, and behavioral and environmental changes" (Green & Kreuter, 1991, p. 432).

Phase 9. **Outcome evaluation** is the "assessment of the effects of the program on the ultimate objectives, including changes in health and social benefits or quality of life" (Green & Kreuter, 1991, p. 433).

Model for Health Education Planning (MHEP). The MHEP (Ross & Mico, 1980) was first developed in 1966 by Mico and has been periodically updated since. It is comprised of six phases: initiate, needs assessment, goal setting, planning and programming, implementation, and evaluation. Within each phase, the model focuses on the three dimensions of content (subject matter), method (steps and techniques), and process (interactions). Table 4.2 provides an outline of this model.

TABLE 4.2   Model for Health Education Planning (MHEP)

Phase	Content Dimension	Method Dimension	Process Dimension
6. Evaluation	Understand evaluation; know problem and target population	Clarify measures; collect and analyze data; provide feedback; redefine problem	Come to agreement; communicate; reduce threat of results
5. Implementation	Know plan, subject, and content and problem solving; writing skills	Initiate activity; problem solve; report	Communicate with and help others; resolve conflict
4. Planning and programming	Understand planning techniques, system analysis, and political process	Develop an implementation plan; design management systems; negotiate commitments; create agreements	Understand and commit clarify roles; communicate; negotiate
3. Goal setting	Role of goals; nature of policy; manage by objectives; understand theory of change	Establish criteria for and set goals and objectives; link to policy development; determine strategies for implementation	Set agreement; understand process and roles
2. Needs assessment	Identify standards, criteria, and needed data	Review criteria; collect and analyze data; describe problem	Select starting point; open communication with appropriate people
1. Initiate	Gain knowledge of the problem and target population	Gain entry to the community; organize those concerned	Reduce threat of the unknown; build trust

Source: Data from H. S. Ross and P. R. Mico, *Theory and Practice in Health Education,* 1980, Mayfield Publishing, Palo Alto, CA.

Comprehensive Health Education Model (CHEM). The CHEM (Sullivan, 1973), like the MHEP, has six major components (see Table 4.3). However, these components are referred to as steps and use different labels: involve people, set goals, define problems, design plans, conduct activities, and evaluate results.

Model for Health Education Planning and Resource Development (MHEPRD). A lesser-known model of planning is the MHEPRD (Bates & Winder, 1984). This model is a bit different from those already presented, in that the graphic representation of the model is circular (see Figure 4.2). The developers of this model have indicted that it can be distinguished from others because it separates process from end results, and because of the continuous evaluation, which tests and validates program assumptions throughout the planning process (Bates & Winder, 1984). Each of the five major components of the model—health education plans, demonstration programs, operational programs, research programs, and information and statistics—represents an end result of the planning process.

TABLE 4.3   Comprehensive Health Education Model (CHEM)

Step	Description
1. Involve people	Identifying the target population and those needed to carry out the program; determining the roles of those involved; establishing the necessary relationships among the people
2. Set goals	Creating the ultimate goals related to health status, personal action, health education practices, and health education resources
3. Define problems	Conducting a needs assessment; determining the gaps between what is and what ought to be; deciding what problem to tackle
4. Design plans	Identifying the most appropriate approach for reaching the goals; setting operational objectives; defining timetables, activities, and resources; piloting the plans; developing evaluation procedures; getting approval for the plans; obtaining commitments for resources
5. Conduct activities	Obtaining the resources to implement; creating policies and procedures for implementation; carrying out the implementation
6. Evaluate results	Determining the overall worth of the program by comparing the results with the program objectives and goals in the context of the activities and resources used

Source: Data from D. Sullivan, "Model for comprehensive, systematic program development in health education" in *Health Education Report, 1*(1), 1973.

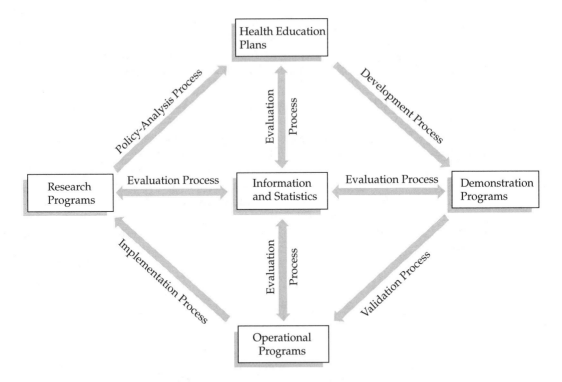

FIGURE 4.2   Conceptual Model for Health Education Planning and Resource Development (MHEPRD).

Generic Health and Fitness Delivery System (GHFDS).   The fifth model to be presented in this chapter is the GHFDS (Patton et al., 1986). As its title indicates, this model was not developed specifically for health education/promotion programs; however, it can easily be adapted to them. This goal-oriented planning model (see Table 4.4) is comprised of five steps—needs assessment, goal setting, planning, program implementation, and evaluation. Each of the steps has an education and a service component. The education component focuses on a cognitive experience, while the service component has a more psychomotor emphasis.

A Generalized Model for Program Planning (GMPP).   As can be noted in the five models presented so far, there are a variety of approaches and frameworks on which to develop a program. Each model seems to have its own characteristics, whether it is the terminology used (e.g., predisposing, enabling, and diagnosis or involve people or initiate), the number of components (e.g., nine phases versus six steps), or the progression through the phases or steps (e.g., circular, linear, or starting with the desired end and working backwards). In other words, there are a number of different ways of getting from point A to point B. However, on closer

TABLE 4.4   Generic Health and Fitness Delivery System (GHFDS)

Steps	Education Component	Service Component
Needs assessment ↑↓ input/feedback ↑↓	Educational needs	Behavioral needs
Goal setting ↑↓ input/feedback ↑↓	Learning goals and objectives	Behavioral goals and objectives
Planning ↑↓ input/feedback ↑↓	Learning intervention	Behavioral intervention
Program implementation ↑↓ input/feedback ↑↓	Of learning intervention	Of behavioral intervention
Evaluation	Educational assessments	Behavioral assessments

Source: Data from R. P. Patton, et al., *Implementing Health/Fitness Programs,* 1986. Human Kinetics Publishers, Champaign, IL.

examination in each of the five models previously presented, you will see that each revolves around the six primary tasks incorporated in the Generalized Model for Program Development (McKenzie & Smeltzer, 1997). The six tasks are

1. Assessing the needs of the target population
2. Identifying the problem(s)
3. Developing appropriate goals and objectives
4. Creating an intervention that considers the peculiarities of the setting
5. Implementing the intervention
6. Evaluating the results (see Figure 4.3)

To better understand the planning process in health education and the various models presented, consider the following scenario. A health educator was hired to develop health promotion programs in a corporate setting. Her first task was to assess the needs of the target population. She did this by reviewing the relevant literature, examining company health insurance claims, conducting a survey of employees, and holding focus groups with selected employees. In task two, she identified a target health problem based on the results of the needs assessment. In this company, the problem was a higher than expected number of breast

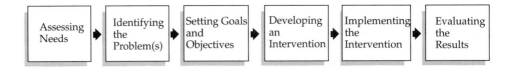

FIGURE 4.3 Generalized Model for Program Development.

Source: From J. F. McKenzie and J. L. Smeltzer, *Planning, implementing, and evaluating health promotion programs: A primer,* 1997. Copyright © 1997 by Allyn and Bacon. Reprinted by permission.

cancer cases in the target population. This was due in part to (1) the limited knowledge of employees about breast cancer, (2) the limited number of employees conducting breast self-examination (BSE), and (3) the low number of employees having mammograms on a regular basis.

In task three, the health educator created specific objectives to (1) increase the employees' knowledge of breast cancer from baseline to after program participation, (2) increase the number of women receiving mammograms by 30 percent and (3) increase the number of women reporting monthly breast self-examination by 50 percent. With these objectives in mind, the health educator developed multiple intervention activities in task four:

1. An information sheet to be distributed with employee paychecks on the importance of BSE and mammography
2. A mobile mammography van to be at the site every other month
3. Plastic BSE reminder cards that can be hung from the showerhead distributed to all female employees
4. An article in the company newsletter on the high rate of breast cancer in the company and the new program to help women reduce their risk
5. Posters and pamphlets from the American Cancer Society to be displayed in the lunchroom

In task five, all of the listed intervention activities were carried out. And, finally, in task six, the health educator completed an evaluation to determine if there was a increase in knowledge, mammograms, and monthly BSE.

As can be seen from this scenario, health education involves careful, systematic planning. The skills needed to conduct a program like the one described can be acquired in upper-division classes. For now, it is enough to see the type of work a health educator is involved in and to understand the importance of using planning models to achieve successful programs.

Theories and Models Focusing on Health Behavior Change (Change Process Theories)

As with planning models, there are a number of theories and models that health educators can use to design appropriate health education interventions to help those in the target populations with behavior change. And, as with planning models, each of these theories and models works better in some situations than in others, depending on which level of influence the health education program is being planned. However, before presenting the theories and models focusing on health behavior change, we need to present the concept of level of influence.

The concept of level of influence is included in the *ecological perspective* (McLeroy et al., 1988). This perspective includes five levels of influence on health-related behaviors and conditions:

1. Intrapersonal, or individual, factors
2. Interpersonal factors
3. Institutional, or organizational, factors
4. Community factors
5. Public policy factors

The ecological perspective "recognizes that health behaviors are part of the larger social system (or ecology) of behaviors and social influences, much like a river, forest or desert is part of a larger biological system (or ecosystem), and that lasting changes in health behaviors require supportive changes in the whole system, just as the addition of a power plant, the flooding of a reservoir, or the growth of a city in a desert produce changes in the whole ecosystem" (O'Donnell, 1996, p. 244).

Figure 4.4, which was created by Eng (1997), provides a visual representation of the ecological perspective. To apply this perspective to health education, let us look at how health educators can use it in assisting people to quit smoking. Health educators can provide the smoking cessation program that gives smokers important knowledge and skills necessary to quit. This is an individual strategy depicted in the center circle of Figure 4.4. Going beyond this individual approach, the health educators can also consider the social networks (friends and family) of the individuals and try to alter them to be more supportive. Family members can be provided information on how to help support the behavior change. This is the interpersonal level. Next the health educators can examine the institutions to which the individuals belong to encourage them to support the new behavior. This might include the smokers' religious community, social groups, or work environment. A strategy at this level would be to encourage worksites to be smoke free or churches to provide support and prayer groups for smokers trying to quit. Beyond this level are the communities in which the smokers reside. What are the prevailing attitudes toward smoking, and how can these attitudes be modified to help support nonsmoking behaviors? Will the community culture support a nonsmoking environment? Finally, the health educators might look beyond the local communities to the population or society as a whole. Is there support for public policy? Are people willing to push for appropriate laws limiting smoking, and can such laws be enforced?

In addition to the levels noted in Figure 4.4, there are four terms noted in bold print: *theory, practice, environments,* and *research.* Eng (1997) noted that, for the

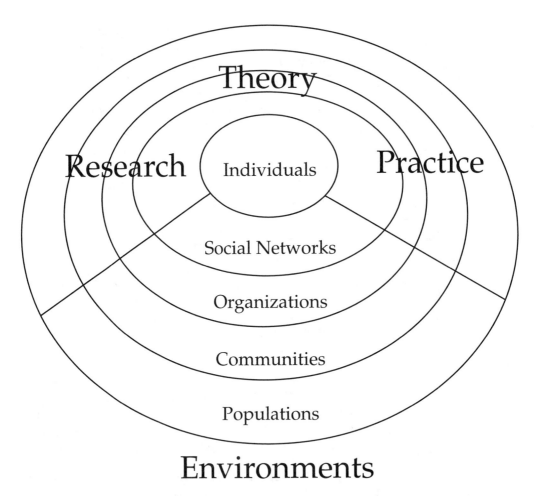

FIGURE 4.4   Social Ecological Framework.

ecological perspective to be successful, the theory must be placed into practice in multiple environments, where research can be conducted to determine its effectiveness.

Having presented the concept of level of influence as it is found in the ecological perspective, we are now ready to present the theories and models focusing on behavior change. For the purpose of this presentation, we are using a modification of the ecological perspective, whereby the final three levels—institutional, community, and public policy factors are combined into a single level called community. The modification was used earlier by Glanz and Rimer (1995). Please be aware that there are more theories and models that could be presented; however, we do not want to overwhelm you with too many at one time. We are assuming

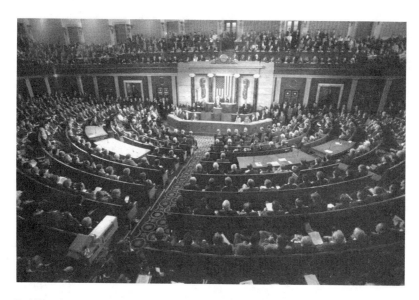

Public policy has become an important intervention strategy for health promotion.
(AP Photo/Ron Edmonds)

that you will have an opportunity to study these and other theories in greater detail in your upper level major courses. As with the theories of implementation, we refer you to the works of other authors (Ajzen, 1988; Bandura, 1977, 1986; Glanz, Lewis, & Rimer, 1997; Glanz & Rimer, 1995; McKenzie & Smeltzer, 1997; Rogers, 1983; Rosenstock, 1966; Rotter, 1954) for more detail on the theories associated with behavior change.

Intrapersonal (Individual) Theories. Intrapersonal theories focus on factors within individuals such as knowledge, attitudes, beliefs, self-concept, mental history, past experiences, motivation, skills, and behavior (Glanz & Rimer, 1995). The three theories that are useful in changing these factors are the health belief model, the transtheoretical model or stages of change, and the theory of planned behavior.

Health Belief Model. The *health belief model* "addresses a person's perceptions of the threat of a health problem and the accompanying appraisal of a recommended behavior for preventing or managing the problem" (Glanz & Rimer, 1995, p. 17). It was developed in the 1950s by a group of psychologists to help explain why people would or would not use health services (Rosenstock, 1966). A graphic representation of this model is presented in Figure 4.5. Refer to that figure as you read this example of why a person may or may not do self-screening for cancer. While reading a weekly news magazine, the person sees an advertisement about self-screening for cancer. This is a *cue to action* that gets the person thinking about his

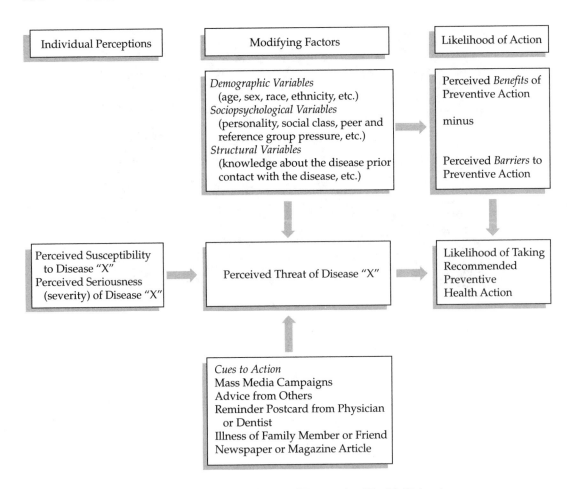

FIGURE 4.5   Health Belief Model as a Predictor of Preventive Health Behavior.

possibility of getting cancer. There may be some variables (demographic, sociopsychological, and structural) that cause the person to think about it a bit more. The person remembers his college health course, which included information about self-screenings and cancer. This person knows he is at a higher than normal risk for cancer because of family history, age, and less than desirable health behavior. Therefore, he comes to the conclusion that he is susceptible to cancer *(perceived susceptibility)*. The person also believes that, if he develops cancer, it can be very serious *(perceived seriousness/severity)*. Based on these factors, the person thinks that there is reason to be concerned about cancer *(perceived threat)*. This person knows that self-screening can help detect cancer earlier and thus reduce the severity *(perceived benefits)*. But self-screening takes time to do, and this person

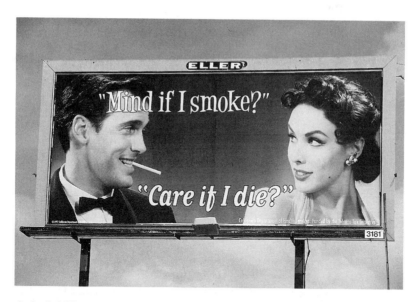

A single billboard along a highway can serve as a cue to action for many people.
(Stock, Boston)

does not always remember to do it *(perceived barriers)*. He must now analyze the difference between the benefits of self-screening and the barriers to self-screening *(reduction of threat)*. For this person, the *likelihood of taking action* (self-screening) will be determined by weighing the perceived threat against the reduction of threat.

Transtheoretical Model or Stages of Change Model. The *transtheoretical model* revolves around an "individual's readiness to change or attempt to change toward healthy behaviors" (Glanz & Rimer, 1995, p. 17). The model suggests that "people move from *precontemplation,* not intending to change, to *contemplation,* intending to change within 6 months, to *preparation,* actively planning change, to *action,* overtly making changes, and into *maintenance,* taking steps to sustain change and resist temptation to relapse" (Prochaska et al., 1994, p. 473). (See Figure 4.6.) The model was first used in psychotherapy and was developed by Prochaska (1979) after he completed a comparative analysis of a number of therapy systems and many therapy studies. Since its development, the model has been used by program planners with a variety of topics ranging from alcohol abuse to weight control.

Here is an example of applying the transtheoretical model to smoking cessation. In the **precontemplation stage,** smokers are not seriously thinking about stopping smoking in the next six months. "Many individuals in this stage are unaware or underaware of their problems" (Prochaska, DiClemente, & Norcross,

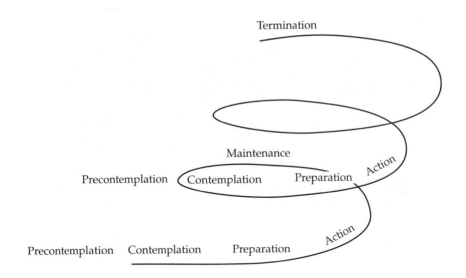

FIGURE 4.6 **Developmental Sequence for the Transtheoretical Model (Stages of Change).**

1992, p. 1103). In the **contemplation stage,** smokers know that smoking is bad for them and consider quitting, but they are not quite ready to do so. In the third stage, the **preparation stage,** the smokers have combined intention and behavioral criteria. "Individuals in this stage are intending to take action in the next month and have unsuccessfully taken action in the past year" (Prochaska et al., 1992, p. 1104). It is now that the smokers may have cut back on the number of cigarettes smoked, but they have not reached an effective criterion for effective action (Prochaska et al., 1992).

In the fourth stage, the **action stage,** smokers are overtly making changes in their behavior, experiences, or environment in order to stop smoking. This stage of the model reflects a consistent behavior pattern, is usually most visible, and receives the greatest external recognition (Prochaska et al., 1992). As the smokers make these changes, they are moving toward the fifth stage, maintenance. **Maintenance** is a continuation of the change that was started in the action stage. For smoking and other addictive behaviors, the beginning of this stage has been defined as six months after taking overt action to change these behaviors (Prochaska et al., 1992).

Please note that the representation of this model is spiral. The reason for this is that "for most health behavior problems the majority of people relapse and return to the precontemplation or contemplation stage of change, before eventually succeeding in maintaining change. In this model, relapse is not extraordinary, but a natural part of the change cycle" (Prochaska et al., 1994, p. 473).

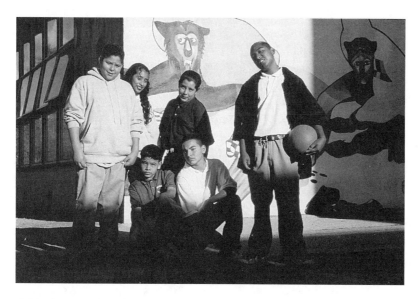

Subjective norm is an important construct to be considered when planning programs for adolescents. (Will Hart)

Theory of Planned Behavior.   According to the *theory of planned behavior*, individuals' intentions to perform a given behavior is a function of their attitude toward preforming the behavior, their beliefs about what relevant others think they should do, and their perception of the ease or difficulty of preforming the behavior. The theory of planned behavior (see Figure 4.7) is an extension of the theory of reasoned action (Fishbein & Ajzen, 1975). Unlike the theory of reasoned action, the theory of planned behavior addresses behaviors in which there is both complete and incomplete volitional control. To use the example of the use of spit tobacco as a behavior not fully under volitional control, the theory of planned behavior predicts that people intend to give up its use if they

1. Have a positive attitude toward quitting **(attitude toward the behavior)**
2. Think others whom they value believe it would be good for them to quit **(subjective norm)**
3. Perceive that they have control over whether or not they quit **(perceived behavioral control)**

Interpersonal Theories.   The category of interpersonal theories is comprised of theories that "include factors related to individuals' experience and perceptions of their environments in combination with their personal characteristics" (Glanz & Rimer, 1995, p. 22). Included in this category are theories dealing with social learning, social power, interpersonal communication, social networks, and social

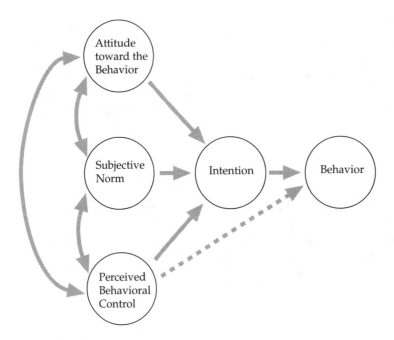

FIGURE 4.7   Theory of Planned Behavior.

support. Because of the importance of social learning to health education/ promotion and because of space limitations, the only theory we will discuss is the social cognitive theory.

The social cognitive theory (SCT) (Bandura, 1986) dates back to the 1950s (Bandura, 1977; Rotter, 1954), when it was known as the social learning theory (SLT). (Some still refer to it as the SLT today.) In brief, the SCT describes learning as a reciprocal interaction among an individual's environment, cognitive processes, and behavior (Parcel, 1983). Those who espouse the SCT believe that reinforcement contributes to learning, but it is the combination of reinforcement with an individual's expectations of the consequences of the behavior that determines the behavior. The SCT explains learning through its constructs. Those constructs that have been most often used in health education/promotion are presented in Table 4.5, along with an example of each.

Community Theories.   As noted earlier, this group of theories includes three categories of factors from the ecological perspective—institutional, community, and public policy. Institutional factors include such things as rules, regulations, and policies of an organization that can impact health behavior. Community factors include social networks and norms, while public policy includes legislation that can impact health behavior. Theories associated with these three factors include

TABLE 4.5   **Often-Used Constructs of the Social Cognitive Theory and Examples of Their Application**

Construct	Definition	Example
Behavioral capability	Knowledge and skills necessary to perform a behavior	If people are going to exercise aerobically, they need to know what it is and how to do it.
Expectations	Beliefs about the likely outcomes of certain behaviors	If people enroll in a weight-loss program, they expect to lose weight.
Expectancies	Values people place on expected outcomes	How important is it to people that they become physically fit?
Locus of control	Perception of the center of control over reinforcement	Those who feel they have control over reinforcement are said to have internal locus of control. Those who perceive reinforcement under the control of an external force are said to have external locus of control.
Reciprocal determinism	Behavior changes result from an interaction between the person and the environment; change is bidirectional (Glanz & Rimer, 1995).	Lack of use of vending machines could be a result of the choices within the machine. Notes about the selections from the nonusing consumers to the machine's owners could change the selections and change the behavior of the consumers to that of users.
Reinforcement (directly, vicariously, self-management)	Responses to behaviors that increase the chances of recurrence	Giving verbal encouragement to those who have acted in a healthy manner
Self-control, or **self-regulation**	Gaining control over own behavior through monitoring and adjusting it	If clients want to change their eating habits, have them monitor their current eating habits for seven days.
Self-efficacy	People's confidence in their ability to perform a certain desired task or function	If people are going to engage in a regular exercise program, they must feel they can do it.
Emotional-coping response	For people to learn, they must be able to deal with the sources of anxiety that surround a behavior.	Fear is an emotion that can be involved in learning, and people would have to deal with it before they could learn a behavior.

theories of community organization and organizational change, and the diffusion theory. It is this later theory that we will present here.

The **diffusion theory** provides an explanation for the diffusion of innovations in populations. In health education/promotion, innovations come in the form of new ideas, techniques, behaviors, and programs. When people become "consumers" of an innovation, they are referred to as adopters.

Rogers (1983) has categorized adopters on the basis of when they adopt innovations. They include innovators, early adopters, early or late majority, and laggards. The rate at which people become adopters can be represented by the bell-shaped curve (see Figure 4.8). **Innovators** are the first to adopt an innovation. They are venturesome, independent, risky, and daring. They want to be the first to do something. The second group consists of the **early adopters.** These people are very interested in innovation, but they do not want to be the first involved. Early adopters are respected by others in the social system and looked at as opinion leaders. Following the early adopters is the **early majority.** This group of people may be interested in the innovation but will need some external motivation to get involved. These people, along with those in the late majority, make up the largest portions of any group of people. The **late majority** is comprised of people who are skeptical and will not adopt an innovation until most people in the social system have done so. The last group, the **laggards,** will be the last to get involved

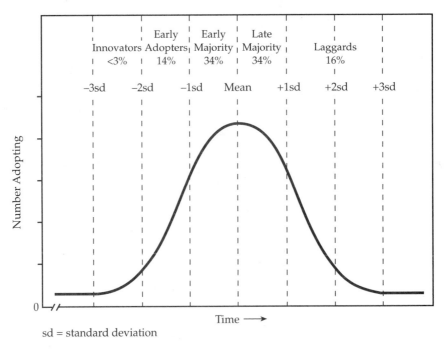

sd = standard deviation

FIGURE 4.8   Bell-Shaped Curve and Adopter Categories.

in an innovation, if they get involved at all. Let us look at an application of this theory. If the health education staff at the Walkup Health Maintenance Organization (HMO) is beginning a new series of health stress management classes for the HMO members, they can expect that about 3 percent of the target population (the innovators) will sign up and attend as soon as they hear about the series. Shortly thereafter, another 14 percent (early adopters) will probably get involved, possibly after reading about the merits of the program. At this point, the health education staff will have to get a little more aggressive in attracting the others to the program. It will take constant reminders to get the early majority involved, while buddy, peer, or mentoring programs might be needed to get the late majority involved. The laggards will probably not attend the series at all.

A Final Note about Theories and Models

Having spent a number of pages discussing the theories (and some models) commonly used in the profession, also note that there are some individuals in the profession who feel that the theories presented in this chapter, and some others not discussed, still are not as useful to health educators as they should or could be in helping move from theory to practice. Stated another way, these theories have limited usefulness in explaining (accounting for) the desired outcomes of health education/promotion programs. The criticism is that much of what is presented in this chapter is based on logical positivism. Logical positivism can be thought of as experimental, hypothesis-testing methodology, in which those "conducting" the experiment have a great amount of control over the process (Buchanan, 1994). It is an approach that has worked well in the natural sciences, but can it be assumed that it will work in the social sciences too? To do so, Buchanan (1992) states that it would have to be assumed

> that there is no essential differences between human behavior and the behavior of chemicals in a test tube, gases in a bubble chamber, or planets in space. Human behavior may be more complex, but in principle, it is no different from any [other] natural process. It is governed by immutable laws that are determined by very structured nature. Based on this assumption, positivists claim the methods and "language" (i.e., mathematics) of physics and chemistry are not only the best, but even more strongly, the only valid and reliable means to explain human behavior. (p. 129)

A question now facing the profession is whether the theories presently available to health educators are adequate and should continue to be used, or should there be a movement toward the development of new theories to help guide health educators' work? The need to expand the theoretical foundations of health education to go beyond logical positivism has been discussed by several authors (Buchanan, 1992, 1994; Burdine & McLeroy, 1992; Labonte, & Robertson, 1996; McLeroy et al., 1992; McLeroy et al., 1993). Some of the issues raised in these articles have been discussed and countered in another work (Green et al., 1994). Space does not permit to have a full discussion of this debate here. Though there may not be agreement on whether health educators can build on the theories and models that are in use now or whether they must be replaced, both sides agree that theories and models are necessary components in guiding the work of health educators.

Summary

Health education/health promotion is a multidisciplinary field of practice that has evolved from the theory and practice of a number of other biological, behavioral, sociological, and health science disciplines. The theories and models that are used in health education/promotion have also evolved from these other disciplines. This chapter presented an overview of the theoretical foundations of health education. Readers were introduced to the definitions of *theory, concept, construct, variable,* and *model.* A rationale was also provided to explain why it is important that health educators use theory in their work. Readers were then introduced to six planning models (theories/models of implementation) and five theories and models used in helping change health behavior (theories of change). The latter theories and models were presented within the five levels within the ecological perspective. The chapter concluded with a word of caution about the application of theories and models and what the future may hold for theories used by health educators.

REVIEW QUESTIONS

1. Define each of the following and explain how they relate to each other.
   - theory
   - concept
   - construct
   - variable
   - model

2. Why is it important to use theory in the practice of health education/promotion?

3. What is the difference between planning models and the theories and models focusing on behavior change (change process theories)?

4. Name the six planning models (theories/models of implementation) presented in this chapter and list one distinguishing characteristic of each.

5. Of the six planning models (theories/models of implementation) presented in this chapter, which one is most commonly used? Name the phases of this model.

6. What five or six components seem to be common to the the six planning models (theories of implementation) presented in this chapter?

7. What are the five levels within the ecological perspective? How do they relate to the theories of change (change process theories)?

8. Identify the five theories and models presented in this chapter that focus on health behavior change (change process theories). Briefly describe each of the theories or models and name their components.

9. Explain why it might be important that health educators have a good understanding of the transtheoretical model (stages of change).

ACTIVITIES

1. Interview a practicing health educator, asking about the theories and models the person has used in planning and implementing health education/promotion programs. Also ask why those theories and models were used. Also, find out if the health educator has run into any problems trying to use the theories and models. Summarize the interview in a one-page paper.

2. Choosing and selecting from the components found in the theories of implementation, create your own model. Draw a diagram of your model and, in two paragraphs, explain why you have included the components you did.

3. Pick one of the theories of change. Then choose a health behavior. In a one-page paper, explain how the theory can be applied to the health behavior you chose.

REFERENCES

Ajzen, I. (1988). *Attitudes, personality, and behavior.* Chicago: Dorsey Press.

Bandura, A. (1977). *Social learning theory.* Englewood Cliffs, NJ: Prentice-Hall.

Bandura, A. (1986). *Social foundations of thought and action.* Englewood Cliffs, NJ: Prentice-Hall.

Bates, I. J., & Winder, A. E. (1984). *Introduction to health education.* Mountain View, CA: Mayfield.

Buchanan, D. R. (1992). An uneasy alliance: Combining qualitative and quantitative research methods. *Health Education Quarterly, 19*(3), 117–135.

Buchanan, D. R. (1994). Reflections on the relationship between theory and practice. *Health Education Research, 9*(3), 273–283.

Burdine, J. N., & McLeroy, K. R. (1992). Practitioners' use of theory: Examples from a workgroup. *Health Education Quarterly, 19*(3), 331–340.

Chaplin, J. P., & Krawiec, T. S. (1979). *Systems and theories of psychology* (4th ed.). New York: Holt, Rinehart & Winston.

Cowdery, J. E., Wang, M. Q., Eddy, J. M, & Trunks, J. K. (1995). A theory driven health promotion program in a university setting. *Journal of Health Education, 26*(4), 248–250.

Eng, E. (1997). *Room with a view for a change.* Keynote address to the Annual Meeting of the National Society of Public Health Education, Indianapolis, IN.

Fishbein, M., & Ajzen, I. (1975). *Belief, attitude, intention and behavior: An introduction to theory and research.* Reading, MA: Addison-Wesley.

Gilbert, G. G., & Sawyer, R. G. (1995). *Health education: Creating strategies for school and community health.* Boston: Jones & Bartlett.

Glanz, K., Lewis, F. M., & Rimer, B. K. (Eds.). (1997). *Health behavior and health education: Theory, research, and practice.* San Francisco: Jossey-Bass.

Glanz, K., & Rimer, B. K. (1995). *Theory at a glance: A guide for health promotion practice* (NIH publication no. 95–3896). Bethesda, MD: National Institutes of Health, National Cancer Institute.

Green, L. W. (1974). Toward cost-benefit evaluations of health education: Some concepts, methods, and examples. *Health Education Monographs, 2* (Suppl. 1), 34–64.

Green, L. W. (1975). Evaluation of patient education programs. Criteria and measurement techniques. In *Rx: Education for the patient: Proceedings of the Continuing Education Institution, Southern Illinois University* (pp. 89–98). Carbondale, IL: Southern Illinois University Press.

Green, L. W. (1976). Methods available to evaluate the health education components of preventive health programs. In *Preventive Medicine,* USA (pp. 162–171). New York: Prodist.

Green, L. W. (1979). National policy on the promotion of health. *International Journal of Health Education, 22,* 161–168.

Green, L. W. (1980). Healthy people: The surgeon general's report and the prospects. In W. J. McNervey (Ed.), *Working for a healthier America* (pp. 95–110). Cambridge, MA: Ballinger.

Green, L. W. (1981a). Emerging federal perspectives on health promotion. In J. P. Allegrante (Ed.), *Health promotion monographs.* New York: Teachers College, Columbia University.

Green, L. W. (1981b). The objectives for the nation in disease prevention and health promotion: A challenge to health education training. In *Proceedings of the National Conference for Institutions Preparing Health Educators,* (DHHS Publication No. 81–50171) (pp. 61–73). Washington, DC: U.S. Office of Health Information and Health Promotion.

Green, L. W. (1982). Reconciling policy in health education and primary care. *International Journal of Health Education, 24* (Suppl. 3), 1–11.

Green, L. W. (1983a). New policies in education for health. *World Health,* (April-May), 13–17.

Green, L. W. (1983b). *New policies for health education in primary health care* (Background document for the technical discussions of the 36th World Health Assembly, May 1983.) Geneva: World Health Organization.

Green, L. W. (1984a). La educacion para la salud en el medio urbano. In *Conferencia InterAmericana de Educacion Para La Salud* (pp. 80–82). Mexico City: Sector Salud, SEP, and International Union for Health Education and World Health Organization.

Green, L. W. (1984b). Health education models. In J. D. Matarazzo, S.M. Weiss, & J. A. Herd (Eds.), *Behavioral health: A handbook of health enhancement and disease prevention* (pp. 181–198). New York: Wiley.

Green, L. W. (1984c). Modifying and developing health behavior. *Annual Review of Public Health, 5,* 215–236.

Green, L. W. (1984d). A triage and stepped approach to self-care education. *Medical Times, 111,* 75–80.

Green, L. W. (1986a, October). *Applications and trials of the PRECEDE framework for planning and evaluation of health programs.* Paper presented at the meeting of the American Public Health Association, Las Vegas, NV.

Green, L. W. (1986b). Evaluation model: A framework for the design of rigorous evaluation of efforts in health promotion *American Journal of Health Promotion, 1*(1), 77–79.

Green, L. W. (1986c). *New policies for health education in primary health care.* Geneva: World Health Organization.

Green, L. W. (1986d). Research agenda: Building a consensus on research questions. *American Journal of Health Promotion, 1*(2), 70–72.

Green, L. W. (1986e). The theory of participation: A qualitative analysis of its expression in national and international health policies. In W. B. Ward (Ed.), *Advances in health education and promotion* (pp. 211–236). Greenwich, CT: JAI Press.

Green, L. W. (1987a). How physicians can improve patients' participation and maintenance in self-care. *Western Journal of Medicine, 147,* 346–349.

Green, L. W. (1987b). *Program planning and evaluation guide for lung associations.* New York: American Lung Association.

Green, L. W., & Allen, J. (1980). *Toward a healthy community: Organizing events for community health promotion* (PHS Publication No. 80–50113). Washington, DC: USDHHS, Office of Disease Prevention and Health Promotion.

Green, L. W., Glanz, K., Hochbaum, G. M., Kok, G., Kreuter, M. W., Lewis, F. M., Lorig, K., Morisky, D., Rimer, B. K., & Rosenstock, I. M. (1994). Can we build on, or must we replace, the theories and models in health education? *Health Education Research, 9*(3), 397–404.

Green, L. W., Gold, R., Tan, J., & Kreuter, M. W. (1994). The EMPOWER/Canadian health expert system: The application of artificial intelligence and expert system technology to community health program planning and evaluation. *Canadian Medical Infamatics,* Nov./Dec., 20–23.

Green, L. W., & Kreuter, M. W. (1991). *Health promotion planning: An educational and environmental approach* (2nd ed.). Mountain View, CA: Mayfield.

Green, L. W., Kreuter, M. W., Deeds, S. G., & Partridge, K. B. (1980). *Health education planning: A diagnostic approach.* Palo Alto, CA: Mayfield.

Green, L. W., Levine, D. M., & Deeds, S. G. (1975). Clinical trials of health education for hypertensive outpatients: Design and baseline data. *Preventive Medicine, 4,* 417–425.

Green, L. W., & McAlister, A. L. (1984). Macro-intervention to support health behavior: Some theoretical perspectives and practical reflections. *Health Education Quarterly, 11,* 323–39.

Green, L. W., Mullen, P. D., Friedman, R. (1986). An epidemiological approach to targeting drug information. *Patient Education and Counseling, 8,* 255–268.

Green, L. W., Wang, V. L., Deeds, S. G., Fisher, A. A., Windsor, R., & Rogers, C. (1978). Guidelines for health education in maternal and child health programs. *International Journal of Health Education, 21* (suppl.), 1–33.

Green, L. W., Wilson, A. L., & Lovato, C. Y. (1986). What changes can health promotion achieve and how long do these changes last? The tradeoffs between expediency and durability. *Preventive Medicine, 15,* 508–521.

Green, L. W., Wilson, R. W., & Bauer, K. G. (1983). Data required to measure progress on the objectives for the nation in disease prevention and health promotion. *American Journal of Public Health, 73,* 18–24.

Kerlinger, F. N. (1986). *Foundations of behavioral research* (3rd ed.). Austin, TX: Holt, Rinehart & Winston.

Labonte, R., & Robertson, A. (1996). Delivering the goods, showing our stuff: The case for a constructivist paradigm for health promotion research and practice. *Health Education Quarterly, 23*(4), 431–447.

McKenzie, J. F., & Smeltzer, J. L. (1997). *Planning, implementing, and evaluating health promotion programs: A primer* (2nd ed.). Boston: Allyn and Bacon.

McLeroy, K. R., Bibeau, D., Steckler, A., & Glanz, K. (1988). An ecological perspective for health promotion programs. *Health Education Quarterly, 15*(4), 351–378.

McLeroy, K. R., Steckler, A., Goodman, R., & Burdine, J. N. (1992). Health education research, theory and practice: Future directions. *Health Education Research: Theory and Practice, 7*(1), 1–8.

McLeroy, K. R., Steckler, A., Goodman, R., Burdine, J. N., & Gottlieb, N. (1993). Social science theories in health education: Time for a new model? *Health Education Research: Theory and Practice, 8*(3), 305–312.

O'Donnell, M.P. (1996). Editor's notes. *American Journal of Health Promotion, 10*(4), 244.

Parcel, G. S. (1983). Theoretical models for application in school health research. *Health Education, 15*(4), 39–49.

Patton, R. P., Corry, J. M., Gettman, L. R., & Graff, J. S. (1986). *Implementing health/fitness proprams.* Champaign, IL: Human Kinetics.

Prochaska, J. O. (1979). *Systems of psychotherapy: A transtheoretical analysis.* Homewood, IL: Dorsey Press.

Prochaska, J. O., DiClemente, C. C., & Norcross, J. C. (1992). In search of how people change: Application to addictive behaviors. *American Psychologist, 47*(9), 1102–1114.

Prochaska, J. O., Redding, C. A., Harlow, L. L., Rossi, J. S., & Velicer, W. F. (1994). The transtheoretical model of change and HIV prevention: A review. *Health Education Quarterly, 24*(4),
471–486.

Rogers, E. M. (1983). *Diffusion of innovations* (3rd ed.). New York: Free Press.

Rosenstock, I. M. (1966). Why people use health services. *Milbank Memorial Fund Quarterly, 44,*
94–124.

Ross, H. S., & Mico, P. R. (1980). *Theory and practice in health education.* Palo Alto, CA: Mayfield.

Rotter, J. B. (1954). *Social learning and clinical psychology.* New York: Prentice–Hall.

Sullivan, D. (1973). Model for comprehensive, systematic program development in health education. *Health Education Report, 1*(1), 4–5.

van Ryn, M., & Heaney, C. A. (1992). What's the use of theory? *Health Education Quarterly, 19*(3),
315–330

5 Ethics and Health Education

CHAPTER OBJECTIVES

After reading this chapter and answering the questions at the end, you should be able to

1. Identify and define the three major areas of philosophy.
2. Define *ethics.*
3. Explain the difference between ethics and morality.
4. Explain why it is important to act ethically.
5. Explain and briefly describe the two major categories of ethical theories.
6. Identify principles that create a common ground for all ethical theories.
7. Outline a guide for making ethical decisions.
8. Identify ethical issues associated with the profession of health education.
9. Explain how a profession can ensure that its professionals will act ethically.
10. Define *code of ethics* and identify the sources of codes available for health educators.

KEY TERMS

beneficence
benevolence
code of ethics
consequentialism
epistemology
ethical
ethics

formalism (deontological or
    nonconsequentialism)
goodness (rightness)
individual freedom (equality
    principle, principle of
    autonomy)
justice (fairness)

metaphysics
moral
moral philosophy
nonmaleficence
truth telling (honesty)
value of life

In recent years, there has been an increasing interest in ethical questions in all walks of life. The interest has become so great that it is difficult to avoid the topic of ethics in everyday living. Newspapers and television networks are constantly covering stories that involve ethical issues, many of which are related to health. Examples include genetic engineering, abortion, the right to die, nuclear waste storage, the marketing of harmful products such as tobacco in developing countries, the reduction of welfare benefits, appropriate sexual behavior, and professional behavior, to name a few.

How is it that we determine what is ethical or unethical? By whose standards do we make such judgments? To answer these questions requires some background and perspective. In this chapter, we will provide the background and perspective to understand how ethics relates to the profession of health education. First, we will present key terms that relate to the study of ethics and examine the origin of ethics. Next we will look at reasons why people should work from an ethical base. We will then briefly look at the theories used to create ethical "yardsticks" and how these theories can be used to make ethical decisions. Within this context, a sampling of ethical issues facing health educators today will be presented. Finally, we will conclude with a discussion on how a profession, or an emerging profession, can ensure that its professionals will act ethically.

Key Terms and Origin

Ethics, the study of morality, is one of the three major areas of philosophy. The other two are **epistemology,** the study of knowledge, and **metaphysics,** the study of the nature of reality (Thiroux, 1995). Ethics, or **moral philosophy** as it is often stated, dates back two thousand plus years to Socrates (470–399 B.C.), "the ancient Greek philosopher, who spent his days in the Athenian marketplace challenging people to think about how they lived" (White, 1988, p. 7). Though philosophers do not sit in the marketplace (or malls) today to challenge people, the behavior, actions, and values of people are constantly being examined for their appropriateness.

You will note that the word *ethics* was described using the words *moral* and *morality*. " 'Ethics' and 'morals' come to us from two words in ancient Greek and Latin, *ethos* and *mores*; both mean 'character.' When we ask if an action is ethical, we can think, 'Is it the sort of thing somebody with a 'good character' would do?' " (White, 1988, p. 8). Thiroux (1995) has made a distinction between ethics and morals, saying that ethics "seems to pertain to the individual character of a person or persons, whereas morality seems to point to the relationships between human beings" (p. 3). Nevertheless, to avoid confusion throughout the rest of this chapter, we will use **ethical** and **moral** to mean the same thing. "The important thing to remember here is that moral, ethical, immoral, and unethical, essentially mean, good, right, bad, and wrong, often depending on whether one is referring to people themselves or to their actions" (Thiroux, 1995, p. 3).

White (1988) refers to the words *good, right, bad,* and *wrong* as the labels people use when making ethical judgments about human actions. Some authors have used these words to define ethics. Mellert (1995, p. 2) states, "Ethics is the study of making right choices. It is a discipline practiced by everyone who has ever wondered, 'why should I do this rather than that?'" Penland and Beyrer (1981, p. 6) define ethics as "the study of rightness and wrongness in human conduct." "Acting 'ethically' is connected *with* what a person is doing and *how* he or she is doing it" (White, 1988, p. 8).

Why Should People and Professionals Act Ethically?

Because ethics is one of the three major areas of philosophy, a philosophical answer to the question of why people should act ethically is that to act ethically brings meaning or purpose to the life of an individual (McGrath, 1994). It provides a standard by which to live. Ethical living, in turn, provides for a better society for all. It is the right thing to do for society and self.

From a more practical viewpoint, observation has shown "that those who are ethical tend to lead healthier (both physically and psychologically), more emotionally satisfying lives" (McGrath, 1994, p. 131). "In fact, the ethical life promises rewards for everyone involved. Your friends and associates will obviously feel better about life and about you if you treat them decently. And they'll probably reciprocate, treating you the same way, which will make your life better" (White, 1988, pp. 84–85). In short, the ethical person is more mature, stronger, healthier, and more advanced and has a more fully developed personality than those who are not ethical (White, 1988).

From a professional viewpoint, ethical behavior is expected from professionals. "Ethical conduct is particularly important to professional health educators, since we belong to a profession with a mission to serve the individual" (Pigg, 1994, p. iii). Health education is a profession with much human interaction. Dorman (1994) adds, "As writers, reviewers, and scientists we must insist on the highest of ethical practices in publication and research. As practitioners, we must seek to actively practice ethical behavior in our service and teaching. Individually, we must aspire for a reputation which reflects a life of personal integrity. The wisdom of King Solomon probably puts it best: '*A good name is more desirable than great riches; to be esteemed is better than silver or gold*'" (p. 4).

Ethical Theories

Philosophers do not speak with a common voice about the standards of morality. Depending on the ethical theory espoused, one philosopher may see a certain behavior as moral or ethical, while another may see the same behavior as immoral or unethical. For example, one philosopher may see corporal punishment as a moral action to punish a person for murder, while the second philosopher sees the taking of another life, for whatever reason, as immoral. The purpose of this section is not to present a detailed description of ethical theories—that has been done elsewhere (Mellert, 1995; O'Connell & Price, 1983)—but to categorize and summarize the better-known theories (see Table 5.1) and to suggest ways by which their content can be applied to health education practice.

The primary means by which ethical theories have been categorized has been to place them in the category of formalism (**deontological, or nonconsequentialism,** as some refer to it) or consequentialism (or teleological, as some refer to it). **Formalism** includes "those theories which look at the nature of the individual act and determine morality from whether that act is right or wrong in itself" (Mellert, 1995, p. 130). For example, a formalist would argue that lying to a client or patient is wrong even if it is done to help that person. According to this theory, the mere act of lying is wrong, regardless of the benefits it may bring. "What is moral or immoral is decided on some standard or standards of morality other than consequences" (Thiroux, 1995, p. 84)—that is to say, the end (the consequences) *does not* justify the means (the act).

Consequentialism, on the other hand, evaluates the moral status of an act by looking at its consequences (White, 1988). If the act produces good or happiness, it is morally okay; if it does not, it is immoral. Using the same example of lying to a patient/client, if the consequences turned out okay, the consequentialist would see this act as morally okay. In short, this category of ethical theories states that the end *does* justify the means.

As can be seen from these descriptions of formalism and consequentialism, the primary point of contention is whether or not the means justify the end. "Is there a way to reconcile these two approaches to ethics, or must we simply make a choice between them?" (Mellert, 1995, p. 133). Most people would say that neither category of ethical theory can answer all moral questions in their lives. There are times formalism provides guidance for the ethical way to act, while consequentialism is best in other situations. What this means is that each person must carefully study the ethical theory options, combine what is compatible and resolve what is inconsistent in those options, and attempt to work out a moral consensus for herself and society (Mellert, 1995). This is not an easy process. Many times, philosophical questions and problems are abstract or conceptual in nature. For example, is there ever a time when it is okay for a health educator to lie to his

TABLE 5.1   **Summary of Ethical Theories**

Category	Primary Reasoning	Examples of Such Theories
Formalism (also known as deontological or nonconsequentialism)	The end does not justify the means.	Natural law morality, deontological ethics, existentialism
Consequentialism	The end does justify the means.	Contractarian ethics, utilitarianism, pragmatism

supervisor? Such questions are answered through philosophical thought, using reason, logic, and argument. As such, the most important tool people can use to find these answers is the mind.

When analyzing an ethical problem, people need to depend more on thinking than feeling—using their minds and not their hearts (White, 1988). For example, if a person says, "I feel that abortion, no matter when it occurs, is morally wrong," that person is really saying there is something about abortion that makes her uneasy, unhappy, or distressed. This person is expressing a feeling, not a moral position. This person's feelings would be better stated if she were to say, "Abortion makes me feel upset." However, if a person states that abortion is immoral, then she should be prepared to provide specific reasons for holding this belief (White, 1988). It is for these reasons that answering ethical questions is a thinking, not a feeling, process. Or, as Penland and Beyrer (1981), have stated, "If ethics is to have personal meaning it demands thoughtful examination. The answers to ethical questions are found by looking within, examining our personal belief systems and values, and using our intelligence to integrate what we have learned and what we have experienced with what we believe and value" (p. 6).

Basic Principles for Common Moral Ground

As was shown in the previous section, formalists and consequentialists are not in agreement when it comes to the rationale to be used in making moral decisions. No single ethical theory can answer every ethical question to the satisfaction of all, yet, to live in a moral society, all must be able to work from a common moral ground. "We must search for a larger meeting ground in which the best of all these theories and systems can operate meaningfully with a minimum of conflict and opposition" (Thiroux, 1995, p. 172).

To help us with this common ground, Thiroux (1995) has identified five basic principles that can apply to human morality, regardless of the embraced theory. The first principle is the **value of life** principle. This is the most basic of principles. Without living human beings, there can be no ethics. Thiroux (1995), has specifically stated this principle as "human beings should revere life and accept death" (p. 180). This means that no life should be ended without very strong justification.

The second principle is the principle of **goodness, (rightness).** "Good" and "right" are at the core of every ethical theory. Theorists may disagree on what is good and bad and right and wrong, but they all strive for goodness and rightness. It should be noted that several others (Fox & Swazey, 1997; Jecker, 1997, to name a few) have presented this principle as two related principles: (1) the principle of **nonmaleficence** and (2) the principle of **beneficence,** or **benevolence.** "Briefly, nonmaleficence refers to the non-infliction of harm to others. The principle involves a moral obligation to 'above else, do no harm.' It encompasses bringing intentional harm to others as well as the risk of bringing harm that is non-intentional. It also encompasses harm which may result from both action and inaction—acts of omission and commission" (Balog et al., 1985, p. 91).

"Beneficence means simply doing good. It holds that we have the responsibility for taking positive steps to help others including acts which involve: doing good, removing evil and/or harm, and preventing harm or evil. Beneficence is generally thought to be more altruistic and more far reaching than nonmaleficence because it requires that we take positive steps to help others" (Balog et al., 1985, pp. 91–92). In the bioethical realm, nonmaleficence and beneficence make up the "benefit-harm ratio" in which, ideally, benefits outweigh costs and in which the "minimization of harm" rather than the "maximation of good" is more strongly emphasized (Fox & Swazey, 1997).

Thiroux's third principle is the principle of **justice, (fairness).** This principle states "that human beings should treat other human beings fairly and justly in distributing goodness and badness among them" (Thiroux, 1995, p. 184). Does this mean that all people will always get their fair share of goodness and badness? No, but it does mean everyone will have an equal chance at obtaining the good (Thiroux, 1995). "The bottom line is that one has indeed acted justly toward a person when that person has been given what she or he is due or owed" (Balog et al., 1985, p. 90).

The fourth principle of this common moral ground is the principle of **truth telling (honesty).** At the heart of any moral relationship is communication. A necessary component of any meaningful communication is telling the truth, being honest. This may be the most difficult principle to live by. This is not to say that people will never lie or that lying might be justified, but there is a need for a strong attempt to be truthful. In the end, morality depends on what people say and do (Thiroux, 1995).

The fifth principle is that of **individual freedom (equality principle** or **principle of autonomy).** "This principle means that people, being individuals with individual differences, must have the freedom to choose their own ways and means of being moral **within the framework of the first four basic principles**" (Thiroux, 1995, p. 187). This is to say that individual freedom is limited by the other four principles. This is a principle that health educators deal with on a regular basis, specifically as it relates to helping others engage in enhancing health behavior. Health educators need to respect the rights of others to deliberate, choose, and act (Balog et al., 1985).

With the grounding of the ethical theories and the establishment of these basic principles, let us examine the process of making ethical decisions.

Making Ethical Decisions

"Ethical decision making in health education, as in other areas, involves determining right and wrong within situations where clear demarcations do not exist or are not clearly apparent to the decision maker. . . . To be considered a professional health educator, one must possess requisite skill and knowledge in making individual decisions. And, in making decisions it is imperative that one has analyzed his or her decisions in terms of standards of right and wrong, good and bad"

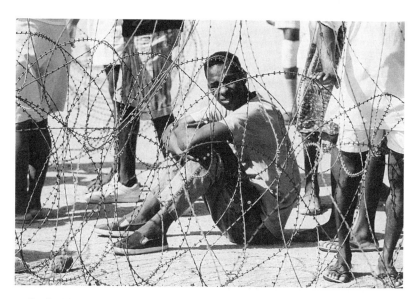

Individual freedom is an important principle of human morality.
(Steve Starr/Stock, Boston)

(Balog et al., 1985, p. 88). In order to decide and, in turn, act in an ethical manner, people must rely on their values, principles, and ethical thinking. Figure 5.1 traces this process. In short, Figure 5.1 notes that judgments about what ought to be done in particular situations "are justified by moral rules, which in turn are justified by principles, which ultimately are defended by an ethical theory" (Beauchamp & Childress, 1989, p. 7).

Though Figure 5.1 is easily read and understood, it is more difficult to put it into practice. To help with this process, several authors have presented guides to assist individuals in applying the theoretical concepts to make ethical decisions in their everyday lives. Because of the limitation of space, we are presenting just a single guide (Mellert, 1995) that practically applies what is presented in Figure 5.1. This guide is representative of several of the guides for making ethical decisions. We will present the guide and then give an example of its application.

The first step to take when confronted with an ethical decision is to "define the nature of the problem and seek answers to relevant informational questions" (Mellert, 1995, p. 156). Such questions include the following: What is possible and what is not? Does a decision have to be made? If so, by when and in what context? Are these decisions within the realm of your authority, or are they determined by someone else with other responsibilities/authority/resources? Balog et al. (1985) have referred to this step as analyzing the alternatives.

Second, "contemplate the ultimate goals and ideals for which you as a moral person are striving. What are the most noble human aspirations that pertain to this concrete situation?" (Mellert, 1995, p. 156). How should you as an ethical person want to act in this situation? Consider the ethical theory you embrace and the

Ethical theories
    ▲   Formalism
    ⋮   Consequentialism
Principles for common ground
    ▲   Value of life principle
    ⋮   Goodness or rightness
    ⋮   beneficence
    ⋮   nonmaleficence
    ⋮   Justice or fairness
    ⋮   Truth telling or honesty
    ⋮   Autonomy; Individual freedom
Moral rules/codes/values
    ▲   Keeping promises
    ⋮   Codes of ethics
    ⋮   Respecting others
    ⋮   Equal opportunity
Judgments/decisions and actions/behavior
        Keeping promises to clients
        Not sharing confidential information
        Providing same information to all
        Not coercing others

FIGURE 5.1   From Ethical Theory to Practice.

Source: From T. L. Beauchamp and J. F. Childress, *Principles of biomedical ethics*, 3rd edition, 1989, Oxford University Press, New York.

principles for common ethical ground (Figure 5.1). How do these goals and ideals apply to this decision? Ultimate goals and ideals do not always apply to every decision and sometimes may not be appropriate, but, to the extent they do apply, let them help with the decision.

Third, "consider the probable consequences of each alternative under reflection" (Mellert, 1995, p. 157). Look at both the short- and long-term consequences of each alternative. How will these consequences affect you, others, and the environment? In other words, weigh the strengths and weaknesses of the alternatives based on the consequences (Balog et al., 1985). Maybe the consequences are very different, or maybe they are not and, thus, may not be important in the final decision.

Fourth, "consider the nature of the alternatives" (Mellert, 1995, p. 157). Consider the formalist approach to the decision-making process in selecting an alternative. Does the alternative lead to an act or a behavior that is wrong, according to the natural law hypothesis? Would you be violating anyone's basic rights? Does it go against basic human ideals and intrinsic moral values? If you answer yes to these questions, you do not need to eliminate the alternative from further consideration but should give greater consideration to those alternatives that do not violate this portion of your reflection.

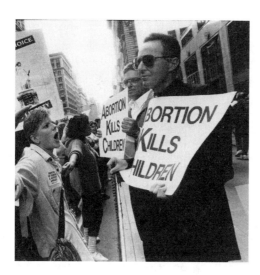

Social context plays an important role in ethical decision making.
(Hazel Hankin/Stock, Boston)

Fifth, "reflect on yourself" (Mellert, 1995, p. 157). What impact will a proposed course of action have on you as a moral person? Will it enhance or detract from your moral stature? If it detracts, then maybe other alternatives should be considered. If you cannot accept a course of action "as part of your inner self and as data for your own moral growth, then there must be something morally questionable about it" (Mellert, 1995, pp. 157–158).

Sixth, "reflect on your society and your environment" (Mellert, 1995, p. 158). Will your action mesh with that of society and the environment? Moral acts are unselfish acts in that they do not prefer one's own interests at the expense of the interests of others (Mellert, 1995). Will society in general see your action as morally correct?

Seventh, "apply the categorical imperative" (Mellert, 1995, p. 158). Would you want your course of action to be a role model for others? If others were faced with the same decision, is this how you would want them to act?

Eighth, choose your alternative (Balog et al., 1985) and "act courageously and decisively" (Mellert, 1995, p. 158). You have put a great deal of effort and thought into this conclusion. You have acted responsibly; you should have no regrets and feel no guilt over your decision.

In considering these components in Mellert's guide, it is important to note that Mellert realizes that moral decision making does not occur in a vacuum. If it were, every decision would be resolved with the "right" alternative for all. Each decision is surrounded by the context in which it must be made. Mellert feels that, when working through the guide, a person must consider and be aware of the context. When making ethical decisions, people must have a sense of

1. Place. Be aware of the appropriateness of an action in a particular environment. One action may be appropriate in one setting but not in another.

2. Time. Be aware of the history leading up to the decision and other similar decisions. Learn from past decisions.
3. Identity. Who am I? How does this moral decision relate to me?
4. Social relationships. Be aware that making moral decisions will impact social relationships. There is a good chance that not everyone will agree with your decision and action.
5. The ideal. When making a moral decision, aim for the most noble ideals of humanity.
6. The concrete. Never lose sight of the fact that choices arise from concrete events.
7. Seriousness. When making a moral decision, do so with an attitude that is appropriate to the situation.

Now let us see if we can apply Mellert's guide to the profession of health education. Consider the following ethical dilemma. You are the health educator responsible for the employee health promotion program of your organization. Based on the results of the health risk appraisals you administered, you are aware that one employee, "high up in the organization" (e.g., school principal, department manager), is a consistent abuser of alcohol. This person's supervisor is also aware of the situation but has decided to ignore it. The employee in question is well liked within the organization and is a good employee. To the best of your knowledge, alcohol has not impacted this person's work performance, but you feel it has the potential to do so. What should you do with this information? Consider the following questions:

A. Nature of the problem
   1. Do you have to do anything with this information?
   2. What are your alternatives?
   3. How soon do you need to make a decision? Are others in danger?
   4. Are there others who can help you with this decision?
B. The ultimate goals and ideals
   1. How does this situation fit with the ethical theory you embrace?
   2. What is the good, or right, thing to do?
   3. Is individual freedom/autonomy a concern?
C. Consequences of the alternatives
   1. What are the short- and long-term benefits (or costs) of all involved for each alternative?
   2. Will there be a big difference in the final outcome based on the alternative selected?
   3. How will the consequences impact you, others, the environment, and the organization?
D. Nature of the alternatives
   1. Do any of the alternatives violate certain human ideals or intrinsic moral rules or values?
   2. Would you be acting immorally?

    E. Reflection on yourself
        1. Would you be enhancing your moral standing?
        2. Can you accept (live with) your own action?
    F. Reflection on society and the environment
        1. What impact will your decision have on society? The environment? In other words, how will others be impacted? Other workers? Members of this person's family?
        2. Is your decision consistent with the way society in general would deal with this?
        3. Is there a norm? Is it ethical?
    G. Categorical imperative
        1. Have you acted as a role model?
        2. Is this how you hope others would act in the same situation?

How will you handle the situation with the alcohol-abusing employee? Do you even have a responsibility to act? If so, who do you talk with first? The employee? The supervisor? Do you go above the supervisor and share the information with those at the next level? Do you do nothing? What is the morally right thing to do? What if the employee is punished or even fired for the behavior? What if the employee hurts someone else at home or on the job because of the alcohol use? What if the newspaper gets ahold of this information and shares it with the whole community? As you can see, moral decisions are not easy to make. They are not to be taken lightly. Responsible action is important. And, remember, this decision will not occur in a vacuum. The "ideal" decision may not be the best decision.

Ethical Issues and Health Education

As noted at the beginning of this chapter, ethical concerns interface with all aspects of our lives. That includes our professional lives too. "Professional ethics seeks to determine what the role of professions is and what the conduct of professionals should be" (Bayles, 1989, p. 13). "Health educators face a complex array of ethical dilemmas in professional practice" (Iammarino et al., 1989, p. 104). While some of the ethical issues faced by health educators are very specific to the profession, such as the ethical issues surrounding getting clients to begin a health-enhancing behavior, the majority of concerns affecting most professions are similar (Hiller, 1987).

    Bayles (1989) has organized the substantive obligations of professions and professionals, regardless of the profession, from which most professional ethical dilemmas arise. The following is a list of these obligations, with several questions that relate the obligations to the practice of health education.

    1. Obligations and availability of services. The primary issue related to this obligation is the equality of opportunity for making professional services available to all citizens. Examples of ethical issues associated with this obligation

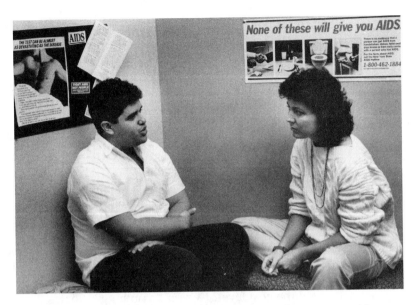

Client–professional relationship is an obligation that is often encountered by health educators. (Rhoda Sidney/Stock, Boston)

include the right to legal counsel, access to health care, and refusal to accept clients for lack of ability to pay. (Who should receive health education? What about clients who are hard to reach? In what settings should it be offered? Should clients have to pay for health education, or should health education be denied if a person cannot pay?)

2. Obligations between professionals and clients. Once the services of a professional have been secured, a number of ethical issues can arise from the professional-client relationship. "The fiduciary model presents the best ethical ideal for the professional-client relationship" (Bayles, 1989, p. 100). In such a model, the professional is honest, candid, competent, loyal, fair, and discrete. At the same time, the client keeps commitments to the professional, is truthful to the professional, and does not request unethical acts from the professional. (Is there ever a time when health educators should not be candid or honest with their clients? How should health educators respond when their clients ask them about their personal behavior?)

3. Obligations to third parties. This obligation revolves around what others need to know about the professional-client relationship. Often professionals are confronted with the issue of whether or not to share client information with family members of the client, people in a supervisory capacity (e.g., teachers, employers), legal authorities (e.g., police, lawyers), or peers (e.g., professional colleagues). (What duty does a health educator have to share information with a student's parents when the student has shared the information with the health educator in confidence? What duty does a health educator have to report the inappropriate behavior of a colleague?)

4. Obligations between professionals and employers. Employed professionals have obligations to employers that are similar to the obligation they have to their clients (see #2 above). "However, the obligation to obey employers is stronger than an obligation to clients. It includes acting as, and only as, authorized" (Bayles, 1989, p. 158). On the other hand, "employers' obligations to professional employees are universal, role related, and contractual" (Bayles, 1989, p. 159). Ethical issues related to this obligation often involve due process, confidentiality, and professional support. (Should health educators always implement "company" policy when they know it is wrong or could bring harm to a client? Is there ever a time when health educators should publicly speak against their employers?)

5. Obligations to the profession. "These obligations rest on the responsibilities of a profession as a whole to further social values" (Bayles, 1989, p. 179). Issues associated with this obligation include conducting research, reforming the profession, and maintaining respect for the profession. (Is there ever a reason health educators should not behave in a professional manner?)

Having identified problems that may cut across all professions, let us examine those that are more specific to health education. First, Penland and Beyrer (1981) state that ethical issues are defined by two criteria. "First they must be 'issues'; that is, there must be controversy related to the problem or topic. There must be 'two sides,' supported by people with two different viewpoints" (p. 6). Issues, by definition, are controversial. For example, the need for youth to know sexual information is not an issue; however, who should provide such information is an issue.

"The second criterion for an ethical issue in health education is that it must involve a question of right and wrong" (Penland & Beyrer, 1981, p. 6). "Can health education programs in the worksite change health behavior?" may be a controversial issue, but it does not deal with rightness and wrongness. Thus, it is not an ethical issue, but "does an employer have the right to make all employees attend the health education program?" is an ethical issue.

Now that we know what comprises an ethical issue, let us look at some of the ethical issues health educators are likely to face. The literature is abundant with examples of ethical issues in health education (see Box 5.1). Issues cited include curriculum development (Barnes, Fors, & Decker, 1980; Penland & Beyrer, 1981; Richardson & Jose, 1983), health behavior change (Hochbaum, 1980; O'Connell & Price, 1983; Read & Russell, 1985; Wikler, 1978), the mission of health education (Penland & Beyrer, 1981), research/scientific inquiry/publishing (Barnes, Fors, & Decker, 1980; Breckon, Harvey, & Lancaster, 1994; Iammarino et al., 1989; Pigg, 1994; Vitello, 1986), the selection of health educators (Barnes, Fors, & Decker, 1980; Penland & Beyrer, 1981), issues and special settings (Pigg, 1994; Roman & Blum, 1987) topical areas (Breckon, Harvey, & Lancaster, 1994;

BOX **5.1**
Practitioner's Perspective

Name:	John Jeffrey Barber
Current Position/Title:	Community HIV/AIDS Consultant
Employer:	Indiana Department of Education
Degree:	Bachelor of Science
Major:	Health Science, Community Health Education
Minor:	History

Please describe an ethical issue which you have had to deal with as a health educator: As a health educator, I have had the opportunity to work with tobacco users through programs designed to help them quit. Within these experiences, I have come across people whose habits, as might be expected, are tied into personal/emotional issues. Some of these clients turned to me as a service provider to help them deal with issues beyond tobacco use. Although their tobacco use may be a symptom of emotional issues, there is a fine line that divides a health educator trained to help people change health behaviors from a professional trained to provide clinical counseling. From a health educator's perspective, I think it is important to recognize and understand the limits of professional training and not step over that line.

How did you handle the issue? The work situations in which these instances have occurred had professional counseling available, so I referred the individuals to the counselors. I was also very up front with the clients, letting them know what my training involved and what was beyond my professional capacity. With some of these clients, it was appropriate to continue tobacco cessation sessions. With others it was apparent that dealing with the deeper issues was best before the tobacco addiction could be addressed.

Looking back on the issue, what might you have done differently? I believe that I would have worked to strengthen my ties with the counselors. This would have provided a bridge back to the tobacco cessation program if the clients so desired and found themselves in a better position to deal with their tobacco problems.

How frequently do you encounter ethical issues in your work? I encounter ethical issues on a regular basis. These situations occur more often than might be expected and at times I believe I address them without consciously thinking about them as issues of ethics.

Have you had any training on how to deal with ethical issues? If yes, please describe it. If no, do you think it should be included in the preparation of health educators? I have not had any formal training specifically regarding ethical issues within health education. I have received training related to confidentiality within a medical setting. I have learned much through professional experiences. This can be risky, however, because this type of learning can be a result of mistakes made from lack of knowledge or training. I definitely think that health educators would benefit from formal ethics training within a health education program. This would help health educators avoid some of the trappings of learning on the job through trial and error.

What recommendations would you give to health education students to help them prepare for ethical issues like the one you described? Health education students would be well-advised to begin thinking about situations that may involve professional ethics and how they handle those situations based on their current training. If they are not receiving training on ethics through their health education program, they must take it upon themselves to be prepared. They should use the library, an organization such as SOPHE, or a professor as a resource to learn before they begin their career. Also, students should use any contact with professionals to gain information. This could be through organizations that provide networking opportunities or through an internship. Specifically, regarding the issue I have described, it is vital for health educators—or any professional, for that matter— to recognize the boundaries of their training. It is almost always possible to find other ways to meet a client's needs without total dependence on oneself— BE CREATIVE!

Fennell & Beyrer, 1989), and the teaching of ethics (Odom, 1988; Patterson & Vitello, 1993). McLeroy, Bibeau, and McConnell (1993) have identified other areas of ethical concern, which reflect the inclusion of health education as a component of health promotion. The major categories of issues raised by McLeroy, Bibeau, and McConnell (1993) include

1. "Assigning individual responsibility to the victim for becoming ill due to personal failures" (p. 314)—for example, becoming ill because one does not exercise, or continues to use tobacco products
2. "Attempting to change individuals and their subsequent behaviors rather than the social environment that supports and maintains unhealthy lifestyles" (p. 314)
3. Using "system interventions to promote health behaviors" (p. 315)—for example, public policy strategies or coercive strategies to modify unhealthy actions
4. Overemphasizing behavior change as a program outcome instead of focusing more on changes in the social and physical environment
5. Overemphasizing the importance of health, forgetting that health is a means to an end, not an end in itself
6. Educating the public on the concept of risk and how to properly use risk factor information
7. Underemphasizing professional behavior, regardless of the health education setting—for example, keeping up-to-date, serving as a role model, and providing ethics education for the next generation of health educators

Ensuring Ethical Behavior

The majority of this chapter has been used to identify and deal with ethical issues and discuss why it is important to act ethically. What we have yet to discuss is how the profession can ensure that professionals will behave ethically. It cannot. Professionals who act unethically usually do so (1) for personal financial gain and reputation and (2) for the benefit of clients or employers without considering the effects on others (Bayles, 1989). However, a profession, and an emerging profession, can put procedures into place to work toward ethical behavior by all.

Some procedures put in place by professions are limited, in some form, to those who are in professional preparation programs and those who have already been admitted to the profession. Traditional ways of doing this have been through (1) selective admissions into academic programs, (2) retention standards to remain in academic programs, (3) graduation from academic programs, (4) completion of internships, (5) the process of becoming credentialed (i.e., certified or licensed to practice), and (6) continual updating to retain the credential. While proceeding through these steps, individuals may have to provide evidence of good moral character.

Once in the profession, professionals are expected to behave according to a system of norms. This system of norms (or professional moral consensus, as some refer to it) is often placed in writing and referred to as a **code of ethics.** A code of ethics is usually not only useful for the professional but also for those who use the services of the professional. An ethical code's principal function is to ensure minimal standards of practice for those for whom it was written (Thomasma, 1979). In other words, an ethical code sets standards "for honor, virtue, and dignity" (Iammarino et al., 1989, p. 101) and "helps professionals become aware of what is generally considered right or wrong professionally" (Richardson & Jose, 1983, p. 5). It also provides the consumers of health education services with an understanding of what they should expect from the provider.

Further, a profession should also have a means by which to deal with (discipline) professionals who violate the code of ethics. Disciplinary measures usually are prescribed by an ethics committee of the profession and often are progressive in nature. First and/or minor violations of ethical behavior often carry disciplinary measures of "warnings." Repeated and/or major violations can lead to loss of ability to practice one's profession.

How does health education stack up to these procedures for ensuring ethical behavior? Currently, the admission procedure into the profession of health education is not clear. Some colleges and universities preparing health educators have selective admission standards, but most have open admissions, meaning that students can enter the health education program if admitted to the institution. Once in the program, all academic institutions have retention standards and graduation requirements, however minimal they may be—minimum grades in certain courses or a grade point average of 2.0 on a 4-point scale. With regard to the amount of education required in the profession, a bachelor's degree is required to sit for the credentialing examination (CHES) (see Chapter 6); however, there is no consensus in the profession that a bachelor's degree should be the standard. Many feel a master's degree is more appropriate. Regardless of whether a bachelor's or master's degree is required to take the credentialing examination, the earned credential (CHES) is not universally accepted, either in or out of the profession, as necessary to practice health education.

The profession of health education has had a code of ethics for a number of years. The first was created in 1976 by the Society for Public Health Education (SOPHE). That code was later revised in 1983 (see Appendix A) and abridged in 1993 (see Appendix B). Though that code was developed more than twenty years ago, it was not universally adopted by the profession. In 1984, SOPHE and the Association for the Advancement of Health Education (AAHE) (now known as American Association for Health Education) appointed a joint committee to develop a professionwide code of ethics. That committee has not been able to create a professionwide code of ethics. Further, in April 1994, AAHE developed another code, the "Code of Ethics for Health Educators" (see Appendix C). Thus, the profession of health education currently has two codes. However, at this writing, the Coalition of National Health Education Organizations, USA (CNHEO) (see Chapter 8) was in the process of trying to blend these codes into a single, professionwide code. Time will tell if the two can be blended and will include a formal procedure for enforcement. At the present time, neither includes such a procedure. At best, the profession has informal enforcement via "the subtle influences colleagues exert on one another" (Iammarino et al., 1989, p. 104).

As can be seen from this analysis, the health education profession is moving in the right direction but still has much room to grow regarding its ethical foundations.

Summary

Ethical questions impact all aspects of life. Individuals on both a personal and professional level are constantly being confronted with ethical dilemmas. To deal with these situations, people must have a basic understanding of how to make an ethical decision. To prepare readers for this task, this chapter presented key terms, such as *philosophy, ethics,* and *morals;* the philosophical, practical, and professional viewpoints of why people and professionals should work from an ethical base; the two major categories of theories (formalism and consequentialism) used to create ethical "yardsticks" for making ethical decisions; a set of principles and a guide for ethical decision making; a sampling of the ethical issues facing health educators today; and a discussion about how a profession, or an emerging profession, can ensure that its professionals will act ethically.

REVIEW QUESTIONS

1. What are the three major areas of philosophy? What does each of them mean?

2. In your own words, how do you define *ethics?*

3. What do the definitions of *ethics* and *moral* share? How are they different?

4. Why is it important to act ethically?

5. How would you summarize the difference between the two major categories of ethical theories?

6. What are Thiroux's five principles that create a common ground for all ethical theories?

7. What should be included in a guide for making ethical decisions?

8. Name five ethical issues currently facing the profession of health education.

9. What can a profession do to ensure that its professionals will act ethically?

10. Define *code of ethics.* Name two sources of codes available to health educators.

ACTIVITIES

Directions for activities 1–4. You will find four scenarios that include an ethical dilemma. Using the guide put forth by Mellert in this chapter, write a response to one of the scenarios. Include in your response a paragraph for each of the components of Mellert's guide. Your eight paragraphs should state your course of action.

1. You have been hired to work for the city health department to complete a project that was begun by your predecessor and funded with money from the National Institutes of Health (NIH). The grant requires the health department to develop X number of programs on the topic of hepatitis and then to present these programs to X number of people representing very specific target groups in the community. After being hired, you discover that the administrator of the grant, your supervisor, has not adhered to the grant guidelines. Only half the number of programs have been developed as the grant required. Further, the number of presentations is less than required, and presentations have been given to people not in the identified target groups. In addition, your supervisor has taken some of the travel funds allocated to pay for your travel to and from presentations and has diverted them into his personal travel fund to attend a national conference in Las Vegas. It is now time for you to develop your year-end report, which will be sent directly to NIH. Your supervisor has provided you with a copy of the original grant proposal and says to make sure your figures agree with those in the proposal. In other words, he expects you to "fudge" the data. What will you do?

2. As the health and fitness director of a large corporate wellness program, you have been asked to provide data to your supervisor that supports the effectiveness of your program. The trend in the company has been to cut programs that

do not "carry their weight." The "bottom line" is important. In your review of the data related to your program, it is obvious that the data are not very strong. However, in fairness to you, the program has been in operation for only two years, and it is too early to see the type of results management is looking for. You are the only one who has access to the data, and no one will know if the data you submit are accurate. How will you handle this situation?

3. You are a high school health teacher. The board of education has just adopted a policy that prohibits the teaching or discussing of any contraceptives or abortion in the district. The only approach that can be mentioned in the classroom is abstinence. As a professional health educator, you have read that the abstinence approach is ineffective with a significant number of students. After class one day, one of your students approaches you and informs you that she is pregnant. She requests your help and asks for the name and location of an abortion clinic. She also asks that you not tell anyone else about this. What will you do?

4. You are the health educator for a large city hospital. Your supervisor has asked you to develop a program on "safer sex" practices for the gay and lesbian population. The program is to be provided to each HIV-positive person who enters the hospital, and it is to be made available to lesbian and gay groups in the community. Because of your strong religious convictions, your personal values and beliefs are opposed to the gay/lesbian lifestyle and the "safer sex" approach. In addition, you feel very uncomfortable dealing with homosexuals in general and especially with anyone who is HIV-positive. How will you handle this situation?

5. Select the code of ethics from either SOPHE (unabridged) (see Appendix A) or AAHE (see Appendix C) and read it thoroughly. Then provide written answers to these question:

   ■ What is your overall opinion of the code? Does it include everything you thought it would? Were there any surprises?

   ■ Is there anything in the code you feel should not be there? If so, what?

   ■ If you could add something else to the code, what would it be?

   ■ Do you think the profession should strive for a single code of ethics? Why or why not?

6. Select one of the ethical theories presented in Table 5.1 to study further. Find and read from other sources explaining the theory. Then write a three-page paper on the theory's application to the practice of health education. Mellert (1995) provides a good overview of the theories.

REFERENCES

Balog, J. E., Shirreffs, J. H., Gutierrez, R. D., & Balog, L. F. (1985). Ethics and the field of health education. *The Eta Sigma Gamma Monograph Series, 4* (1), 65–110.

Barnes, S., Fors, S., & Decker, W. (1980). Ethical issues in health education. *Health Education, 11* (2), 7–9.

Bayles, M. D. (1989). *Professional ethics* (2nd ed.). Belmont, CA: Wadsworth.

Beauchamp, T. L., & Childress, J. F. (1989). *Principles of bioethical ethics* (3rd ed.). New York: Oxford University Press.

Breckon, D. J., Harvey, J. R., & Lancaster, R. B. (1994). *Community health education: Settings, roles, and skills for the 21st century* (3rd ed.). Gaithersburg, MD: Aspen.

Callahan, J. C. (Ed.). (1988). *Ethical issues in professional life.* New York: Oxford University Press.

Dorman, S. M. (1994). The imperative for ethical conduct in scientific inquiry. In R. M. Pigg, (Ed.), Ethical issues of scientific inquiry in health science education. *The Eta Sigma Gamma Monograph Series, 12*(2), 1–5.

Fennell, R., & Beyrer, M. K. (1989). AIDS: Some ethical considerations for the health educators. *Journal of American College Health, 38,* 145–147.

Fox, R. C., & Swazey, J. P. (1997). Medical morality is not bioethics: Medical ethics in China and the United States. In N. S. Jecker, A. R. Jonsen, & R. A. Pearlman (Eds.), *Bioethics: An introduction to history, methods and practice* (pp. 237–251). Sudbury, MA: Jones and Bartlett.

Hiller, M.D. (1987). Ethics and health education: Issues in theory and practice. In P. M. Lazes, L. Kaplan, & G.A. Gordon (Eds.), *The handbook of health education* (pp. 87–108). Rockville, MD: Aspen.

Hochbaum, G. M. (1980). Ethical dilemmas in health education. *Health Education, 11*(2), 4–6.

Iammarino, N. K., O'Rourke, T. W., Pigg, R. M., & Weinberg, A. D. (1989). Ethical issues in research and publication. *Journal of School Health, 59*(3), 101–104.

Jecker, N. S. (1997). Introduction to the methods of bioethics. In N. S. Jecker, A. R. Jonsen, & R. A. Pearlman (Eds.), *Bioethics: An introduction to history, methods and practice* (pp. 113–125). Sudbury, MA: Jones and Bartlett.

McGrath, E. Z. (1994). *The art of ethics: A psychology of ethical beliefs.* Chicago: Loyola University Press.

McLeroy, K. R., Bibeau, D. L., & McConnell, T. C. (1993). Ethical issues in health education and health promotion: Challenges for the profession. *Journal of Health Education, 24*(5), 313–318.

Mellert, R. B. (1995). *Seven ethical theories.* Dubuque, IA: Kendall/Hunt.

O'Connell, J. K., & Price, J. H. (1983). Ethical theories for promoting health through behavioral change. *Journal of School Health, 53*(8), 476–479.

Odom, J. G. (1988). The status of ethics instruction in the health education curriculum. *Health Education, 19*(4) 9–12.

Patterson, S. M., & Vitello, E. M. (1993). Ethics in health education. The need to include a model course in professional preparation programs. *Journal of Health Education, 24*(4), 239–244.

Penland, L. R., & Beyrer, M. K. (1981). Ethics and health education: Issues and implications. *Health Education, 12*(4), 6–7.

Pigg, R. M. (Ed.). (1994). Ethical issues of scientific inquiry in health science education. *The Eta Sigma Gamma Monograph Series, 12*(2).

Read, D., & Russell, R. (1985). Is behavioral change an acceptable objective for health educators? *The Eta Sigma Gamma Monograph Series, 4*(1), 9–61.

Richardson, G., & Jose, N. (1983). Ethical issues in school health: A survey. *Health Education, 14* (2), 5–9.

Roman, P., & Blum, T. (1987). Ethics in worksite health programming: Who is served? *Health Education Quarterly, 14,* 57–70.

Thiroux, J. P. (1995). *Ethics: Theory and practice* (5th ed.). Englewood Cliffs, NJ: Prentice Hall.

Thomasma, D. (1979). Human values and ethics: Professional responsibility. *The Journal of the American Dietetic Association, 75*(5), 533–536.

Vitello, E. M. (1986). Ethical issues: Questions in search of answers. *Health Education, 17*(5), 39–42.

White, T. I. (1988). *Right and wrong: A brief guide to understanding ethics.* Englewood Cliffs, NJ: Prentice Hall.

Wikler, D. I. (1978). Coercive measures in health promotion: Can they be justified? *Health Education Monographs, 6*(2), 223–241.

6 The Health Educator: Roles, Responsibilities, Certifications, Advanced Study

CHAPTER OBJECTIVES

After reading this chapter and answering the questions at the end, you shoud be able to

1. Define *credentialing*.
2. Discuss the history of role delineation and certification.
3. Explain the differences among certification, registration, licensure and accreditation.
4. List and describe the seven major responsibilities of a health educator.
5. Discuss the need for advanced study in health education.
6. Outline factors to consider in applying for master's degree programs.

KEY TERMS

accreditation
certification
Certified Health Education
   Specialist (CHES)
competencies
credentialing
graduate research
   assistantship
graduate teaching
   assistantship

licensure
M.P.H., M.Ed., M.S.
National Commission for
   Health Education
   Credentialing, Inc.
National Task Force on the
   Preparation and Practice of
   Health Educators

objective
primary data
responsibilities
role delineation
secondary data
sub-competencies

Introduction

While education about health has been around since the beginning of human intelligence, health education as a profession is, relatively speaking, an infant. When any infant begins to mature, it takes on its own identity. This chapter is about the emerging identity of health education. It chronicles major historical events that have helped shape the identity of health education since the 1970s. The current identity of health education is also presented in terms of roles, responsibilities, certification, and accreditation. Because the identity of health and health education is a work in progress and constantly changing, this chapter also discusses the importance of advanced study and continuing education in the health education profession.

Credentialing

Credentialing is a process whereby an individual or a professional preparation program meets the specified standards established by the credentialing body and is thus recognized for having done so. Credentialing can take the form of accreditation, licensure, or certification. It is important to be familiar with these terms to understand credentialing as it applies to health education.

Accreditation "is the process by which a recognized professional body evaluates an entire college or university professional preparation program" (Cleary, 1995, p. 39). Thus, the health education program at any particular institution may be accredited by one of several outside agencies to be discussed later in this chapter. For example, the health education program at Alpha University could be accredited by Beta Accrediting Group. Such a process takes place after the program at Alpha University creates a self-study document that shows how it meets the Beta Accrediting Group's standards and after an on-campus visit by representatives from Beta. Throughout the accrediting process, factors such as student-teacher ratio, curriculum, and faculty qualifications would be closely examined.

Licensure is "the process by which an agency or government [usually a state] grants permission to individuals to practice a given profession by certifying that those licensed have attained specific standards of competence" (Cleary, 1995, p. 39). Licensure applies to most medical professionals, such as doctors, nurses, dentists, and physical therapists. The only health educators who are licensed in the United States at the present time are school health educators.

Certification "is a process by which a professional organization grants recognition to an individual who, upon completion of a competency-based curriculum, can demonstrate a predetermined standard of performance" (Cleary, 1995, p. 39). Note that certification is granted to an individual, not a program, and it is given by the profession, not by a governmental body. Certification is available for all health educators, regardless of specialty area. One who is certified is recognized as a **certified health education specialist** and may use the initials **CHES** behind one's name and academic degree.

History of Role Delineation and Certification

The evolution of certification in health education got its formal start about 1978. At that time, individual certification for health educators was not available, except for school health educators, who had to be licensed. Accreditation was available only for school health and public health professional preparation programs. Many public health programs outside schools of public health and all community health programs were not accredited, nor was accreditation available for these programs. This gave rise to a situation in which there were great discrepancies in professional preparation. One program might look very different from another program. To say that an individual was a health educator had little meaning. In describing the situation, Helen Cleary, who was president of the Society for Public Health Education (SOPHE) in 1974, wrote the following:

> What I found in my travels [as SOPHE president] was a profession in disarray. Many, many health educators could neither define themselves nor their role. It was clear that the preparation of most was so varied that there was no common core. There was no professional identity, no sense of a profession. Numbers of competent, bright, young professionals were leaving health education for greener pastures. (Cleary, 1995, p. 2)

As a result of this situation, Cleary began to pursue the idea of credentialing health educators and/or health education programs. She soon discovered that, to undertake such a project, outside expertise and funding would be needed. Thomas Hatch, director of the Division of Associated Health Professions in the

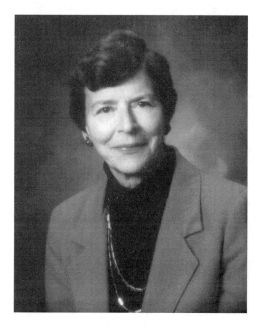

Helen P. Cleary—Person most responsible for establishing certification for health education specialists. (Courtesy of Dr. Helen P. Cleary.)

Bureau of Health Manpower of the Department of Health, Education and Welfare, expressed an interest in the project. Prior to funding the project, however, he needed assurances that members of the profession would work together to create a credentialing system. Hatch wanted to be certain that those who practiced health education in different settings felt enough in common with each other to develop one set of standards.

In response to Hatch's concern, a conference was scheduled. The planning committee for the conference consisted of the presidents/chairpersons and/or their representatives of the eight organizations comprising the Coalition of Health Education Organizations, all of which had an interest in this project. The planning committee formulated two questions to be answered at the conference: (1) what are the commonalities and differences in the function of health educators practicing in different settings? and (2) what are the commonalities and differences in the preparation of health educators? (Cleary, 1995, p. 3). The conference, which has become known as the Bethesda Conference on Commonalities and Differences, was held in February 1978, in Bethesda, Maryland. After much discussion, those attending this conference concluded that health education was one profession and that a credentialing system was necessary. "It was the consensus of the participants that standards were essential if they were to provide quality service to the public and if they were to survive as a viable profession" (Cleary, 1986, p. 130). Further, those who had been on the planning committee for the conference were asked to continue as a task force to develop the credentialing system; thus, the **National Task Force on the Preparation and Practice of Health Educators** was born (see Table 6.1).

In January 1979, funding became available to embark on the project, and **role delineation** for health educators was underway. Alan Henderson was hired as the project director, and under his leadership a working committee of the task force began the difficult task of defining the role of the health education specialist. In describing this process, Cleary (1995) notes, "For the first time in the profession's history, specialists in school health education and in community health education faced each other across the table and learned that each was dealing with similar

TABLE 6.1 **Organizations Represented on the National Task Force on the Preparation and Practice of Health Educators, 1978**

American College Health Association
American Public Health Association, Public Health Education Section
American Public Health Association, School Health Education and Services Section
American School Health Association
Association for the Advancement of Health Education
Conference of State and Territorial Directors of Public Health Education
Society for Public Health Education, Inc.
Society of State Directors of Health, Physical Education and Recreation

concepts, but using different terminology and, as well, applying them in different settings" (p. 5).

Once the initial phase of role delineation was completed, the next step was to verify and refine the role of a health educator. Funding for this became available in March 1980. A survey to verify the role was conducted of health education specialists working in all areas of health education. The results of this survey were very positive. There were no significant differences among practitioners in different settings.

In addition to the survey, a conference for college and university health education faculty members was held in Birmingham, Alabama, in February 1981. The conference provided the opportunity for academics to review the initial role delineation work and discuss its potential impact on the field. The planning committee for this conference was chaired by Warren E. Schaller from Ball State University. Two hundred thirty-eight academics from 125 institutions attended. While many present were happy with the work and direction of the task force, others were not. The polar extremes of these differences centered around the health educator as an expert in content versus the health educator as an expert in process. This difference of opinion probably reflected the different types of professional preparation programs the faculty represented. While these differences were very real, they were not strong enough to alter the work of the task force.

The third step in the process was the development of a curriculum framework based on the verified role of a health educator. Initially, the task force decided to develop a curriculum guide. A curriculum guide is a fairly specific set of guidelines from which a curriculum is developed. Little room is left for interpretation, as the curriculum must meet the standards established in the guide. Betty Mathews from the University of Washington and Herb L. Jones from Ball State University were recruited to do the actual writing.

Once a draft copy of the guide was developed, it had to be pretested. Eleven regional workshops were held around the country to obtain feedback on the guide. Again, differences surfaced regarding whether health educators were specialists in content or process. Further, some felt entry-level preparation should be at the bachelor's degree level, while others believed it should be at the master's degree level. Feedback was also obtained from the professional associations and practitioners in the field.

To deal with some of the criticisms and to make the curriculum guide less prescriptive, it was ultimately transformed into a curriculum framework. A framework merely provides a frame of reference around which a curriculum can be developed. As Cleary (1995) notes, "It does not tell a faculty what to teach or how to teach it. It simply tells them what the students should know when they have completed the program of studies" (p. 9). Marion Pollock was the individual responsible for transforming the curriculum guide into a curriculum framework.

At this juncture, it was important to check with those in the profession to determine if they wanted to continue with the development of a credentialing system and, if so, what kind of a system they wanted. The Second Bethesda Conference was held in February 1986. Ninety-nine individuals attended the conference. Participants were divided into five groups and asked to respond to several predetermined questions. When reports from the groups were analyzed, four of the five were in favor of a certification system for individuals and some form of credentialing for professional preparation programs. They recommended that the task force continue to develop the credentialing system.

Over the next two years, the task force continued to work toward the development of a certification system for individual health educators. The Professional Examination Service (PES), which developed certification and licensure exams for many other professions, was contracted to assist with this process. Not only was its experience in test development vital to the process, but it was also willing to provide start-up funds to get the process off the ground.

By June 1988, the National Task Force on the Preparation and Practice of Health Education had been functioning for ten years. Much had been accomplished, yet there was still much to do. With the certification of individual health educators about to become a reality, it was time to establish a more permanent structure to coordinate and oversee the certification process. As a result, the **National Commission for Health Education Credentialing, Inc.,** was formed to replace the national task force. It is this new organization that oversees the certification process today.

With the PES in place to develop the certification exam and the National Commission for Health Education Credentialing in place to oversee the process, it was time to certify the first health educators.

Individual Certification

In October 1988, the charter certification period began. Charter certification allowed qualified individuals to be certified based on their academic training, work experience, and references without taking the certification exam. When a new certification program is initiated, charter certification is usually available for a limited period of time, after which anyone seeking certification must meet all criteria for certification and pass the examination. The initial requirements for charter certification in health education, through which 1,558 individuals obtained certification, were as follows:

Degree	Experience	References
Graduate degree with health education emphasis (or)	At least four years' experience	Three references
Bachelor's degree with health education emphasis (or)	At least seven years' experience	Three references
Bachelor's degree with other than health education emphasis	At least twenty-five years' experience	Three references

In 1990, the charter certification period ended, and the first examination was held. Six hundred forty-four candidates passed the first exam and became Certified Health Education Specialists.

Currently, eligibility to sit for the CHES exam is based exclusively on academic qualifications. To sit for the exam, one must "possess a bachelor's, master's or doctoral degree from an accredited institution of higher education; *AND* have an official transcript that clearly shows a major in health education, e.g. Health Education, Community Health Education, Public Health Education, School Health Education, etc., *OR* have an official transcript that reflects 25 semester hours (37 quarter hours) of course work with specific preparation addressing the seven responsibilities delineated in the FRAMEWORK" (The National Commission for Health Education Credentialing, 1998).

Graduate Health Education Standards

The roles and responsibilities document, *A Competency-Based Framework for Professional Development of Certified Health Education Specialists* (The National Commission for Health Education Credentialing, 1996), defined the skills needed for the entry-level health education professional. While many health educators with advanced degrees had obtained certification, it attested only to the fact that they had entry-level skills. The document provided guidance for professional preparation programs at the bachelor's degree level, but there was no such guidance available for professional preparation programs at the graduate level.

In June 1992, the Joint Committee for Graduate Standards was established by the Association for the Advancement of Health Education (now called American Association of Health Educators [AAHE]) Board of Directors. Committee membership was initially comprised of Society of Public Health Education (SOPHE) and AAHE members serving on their respective accreditation bodies. To obtain a broader perspective, committee membership was expanded to include members from the Council on Education for Public Health (CEPH) and the National Commission for Health Education Credentialing, Inc. (NCHEC). After much work, discussion, and review, the Joint Committee for Graduate Standards developed a draft document which contains additional responsibilities, competencies, and **sub-competencies** specific to graduate-level preparation.

In February 1996, the draft document was presented to a large group of college-level health educators at the National Congress for Institutions Preparing Graduate Health Educators, which was held in Dallas, Texas. The national congress was convened to "engage professional preparation programs in a review and dialogue about advanced competency-based preparation" (Joint Committee for Graduate Standards, 1996). One hundred thirty-four individuals representing more than one hundred colleges and universities attended the meeting. Throughout the three-day meeting, the graduate competencies were thoroughly discussed and debated. Recommendations for improving the graduate competencies were presented to the planning committee. Despite some dissension, the

BOX **6.1**

New Graduate Standards Released for Health Education

Washington, DC—Marking another milestone for the health education profession, the American Association for Health Education (AAHE) and the Society for Public Health Education (SOPHE) released today new competency-based standards for graduate preparation in health education. The competencies contained in the report *Standards for the Preparation of Graduate-Level Health Educators* outline knowledge and skills all students should be expected to demonstrate on receiving an advanced degree in health education.

"These new standards will help improve the consistency of graduate training programs in health education for the benefit of students and academicians alike," said Randy Schwartz, MSPH, SOPHE president. "Furthermore the standards will delineate for employers the unique role and services of graduate-prepared health educators, and assist practitioners to identify their continuing education needs in this changing health care environment."

The graduate-level competencies are built on a set of entry-level competencies for practicing in the profession, known as "The Framework." These standards have been used by the National Commission for Health Education Credentialing, Inc., to certify Health Education Specialists since 1988. Expanding on the original framework, the new standards include three new major responsibilities for graduate-prepared health educators: applying appropriate research principles and techniques in health education, administering health education programs, and advancing the profession. In addition, they identify forty-six new competencies and sub-competencies related to social marketing, community organization, cultural sensitivity, coalition building, advanced communication techniques, and other areas.

"These graduate standards in health education represent four years of extensive work, validation and consensus development across the profession," said AAHE President Darwin Dennison, Ph.D., CHES (Certified Health Education Specialist). "Health education is one of the few professions to develop measurable educational outcomes, as recommended by the 1993 PEW Report on the health professions."

Health educators plan, implement, and evaluate the effects of educational programs and strategies designed to improve the health of individuals, families, and communities. Health educators work in schools and universities; federal, state, and local public health departments; hospitals and managed care settings; voluntary groups; businesses; international organizations; and other settings. Currently, 134 academic institutions provide graduate training in health education throughout the United States.

"These standards will help ensure health educators are effectively prepared to promote the health of the public, regardless of the institution or its faculty," said Noreen Clark, Ph.D., dean of the University of Michigan School of Public Health. "All graduate professional preparation programs in health education should examine their curricula and ensure students 'make the grade' in these areas."

"The health education profession is at a juncture of unprecedented opportunity," said John Seffrin, executive vice president, American Cancer Society. "Armed with these skills, health educators will be at the forefront in dealing with changes in U.S. demographics, public health infrastructure, health care payment, and other areas to improve individual and community health."

general mood was in favor of the competencies, and the planning committee was urged to move on with the approval process.

Following this meeting, revisions were made to the draft document, and the final version was presented to the AAHE and SOPHE boards of directors for approval. Approval was granted in March, 1997. (See Press Release–Box 6.1.)

Program Accreditation

"Accreditation is a process by which a recognized professional body evaluates an entire program against predetermined criteria or standards" (Cleary, 1995). In most professions, colleges and universities that train students to enter a given profession are accredited by a recognized professional body that operates independent of the college or university. If a program does not meet the standards of the recognized professional body, it can lose its accreditation. A non-accredited program might have difficulty recruiting new students and may be restricted in its participation in the profession. Therefore, accreditation helps ensure that all students entering the profession have similar training and preparation.

In health education, accreditation is available through three accrediting bodies. Health education programs that are affiliated with a college of education and train students for positions in school health may be accredited through the National Commission for the Accreditation of Teacher Education (NCATE). The Council on Education for Public Health (CEPH) accredits schools of public health, public health programs in non-schools of public health, and master's degree programs in community health education. Undergraduate programs in school or community health may elect to obtain accreditation/approval through the Society of Public Health Education/Association for the Advancement of Health Education (SOPHE/AAHE) process.

Having three accreditations available is considered by many to be a weakness in the profession. As Cleary (1995) notes, "There were (and are) huge gaps and great discrepancies in the accreditation/approval process" (p.16). Professional preparation is not at all uniform in the profession (Cleary, 1986). Some programs focus more on content, such as drugs, sexuality, stress, and physical fitness, while other programs emphasize process courses, such as planning, implementing, and evaluating. Some programs stress individual behavior change, while others stress a social ecological approach to change. In 1987, the National Task Force on the Preparation and Practice of Health Educators attempted to develop a registry of health education programs. This effort, however, had to be abandoned. There was too much variety in faculty, administrative arrangements, courses, and philosophies of the various professional preparation programs to agree on criteria for inclusion in the registry (Cleary, 1995).

At the current time, there are 215 programs listed in the 1997 AAHE *Directory of Institutions That Prepare Health Educators.* Many of these programs are not accredited, and there is no professional body monitoring their efforts. At present, there is no concerted effort to improve the accreditation situation in health education. The only hope for improvement at this time rests with the individual certification process. If CHES becomes a recognized and desirable credential to the point that it is required for most health education positions, then it will become important for all professional preparation programs to prepare their students so they can pass the exam and obtain the CHES credential. In other words, professional preparation programs will be forced to conform to minimal standards, or their students will not be able to pass the exam.

Responsibilities and Competencies of Health Educators

The "Responsibilities and Competencies for Entry-Level Health Educators" (see Appendix D) was developed from the *Framework for the Development of Competency-Based Curricula for Entry Level Health Educators* (National Task Force on the Preparation and Practice of Health Educators, 1985). The Responsibilities and Competencies document lists the seven major **responsibilities** of health educators. In essence, these seven responsibilities specify the scope of practice for health educators. Under each of these responsibilities are three or four **competencies.** A competency "reflects the ability of the student to understand, know, etc." (The National Commission for Health Education Credentialing, 1996, p. 12). Each competency is further specified in two to four **sub-competencies.** A sub-competency "reflects the ability of the student to list, describe, etc." (The National Commission for Health Education Credentialing, 1996, p. 12). Although not part of the original document, The National Commission for Health Education Credentialing has recently published a book that identifies several objectives for each sub-competency (The National Commission for Health Education Credentialing, 1996). An **objective** "reflects the ability of the student to perform" (The National Commission for Health Education Credentialing, 1996, p. 12). All prospective health educators, whether focusing their professional preparation on school, community, clinical or worksite settings, should be able to demonstrate the various competencies, sub-competencies, and objectives on completion of their academic program of study.

The "Responsibilities and Competencies for Entry-Level Health Educators" document should be used by health education students on a regular basis during their professional preparation program. The National Commission for Health Education Credentialing (1996) suggests that the competencies be used "as a personal inventory to assess progress toward becoming a health educator; that is to determine which competencies and sub-competencies have been mastered. It is suggested that the student assess his or her progress at intervals during the student's course of study and do a final review at the completion of the health education program" (p. 7). Students who have been diligent in monitoring their progress and who can perform the competencies, sub-competencies, and objectives as indicated will have a much greater chance of passing the credentialing exam to become a Certified Health Education Specialist.

Because the seven major responsibilities identified in the "Responsibilities and Competencies for Entry-Level Health Educators" are the core of what a health educator does, it is important to have a basic understanding of what each responsibility means. The following is a brief description of each responsibility.

Responsibility I: Assessing Individual and Community Needs for Health Education

All health educators, regardless of the setting in which they are employed, must have the skills to assess the needs of those groups or individuals for whom their programs are targeted. Therefore, a school health educator needs to base curriculum on the needs of the students, a health educator in the corporate setting needs to plan programs based on the needs of the company's employees, and public health educators should base their health education efforts on the needs of the community they serve. Health education programs should not be based on the whim of the health educator or any small group of decision makers. Resources are too valuable to waste on programs that do not address the needs of the population being served. As Gilmore and Campbell (1996) noted, "A needs assessment provides a logical starting point for individual action and program development,

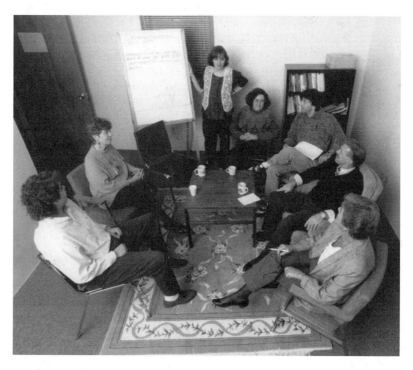

Health educators often need to hold focus groups to learn more about the needs of their target population. (Frank Siteman/Stock, Boston)

as well as a continuing process for keeping activities on track" (p. 5). It is the needs assessment that determines if a health education program is justified and that defines its nature and scope.

To conduct a needs assessment, health educators should know how to locate and obtain valid sources of information that pertain to their specific population or populations with similar characteristics. For example, this may entail a literature review or the accessing of information from local, county, or state health departments. In addition to examining such pre-existing information, which is called **secondary data,** it may be necessary for health educators to gather data of their own, known as **primary data.** They may have to conduct mail or telephone surveys, hold focus group meetings, or use a nominal group process. Once all of this information has been collected, the health educator must be able to analyze the data and determine priority areas for health education programming.

Responsibility II: Planning Effective Health Education Programs

Planning involves more than just determining a location and time for a health education program. Planning begins by assessing the health needs, problems, and concerns of the target population. Early in the planning process, it is important to recruit interested stakeholders, such as community leaders, representatives from community organizations, resource people, and representatives of the target population, to support and help develop the program. Without the help of these stakeholders, it may be impossible to develop effective programs. To be effective in the planning process, the health educator should have strong written and oral communication skills, leadership ability, and the expertise to facilitate diverse groups of people to reach concensus around issues of interest.

As part of the planning process, health educators must be competent to develop goals and objectives specific to the proposed health education program. These goals and objectives establish the foundation on which the program may be evaluated. The health educator must then have the expertise to develop appropriate interventions which will meet these goals and objectives.

Responsibility III: Implementing Health Education Programs

After the initial planning, including the needs assessment, goal and objective setting, and intervention development, it is time to implement the programs. For many health educators, implementation is the most enjoyable of the responsibilities, for it entails the actual presentation of the program.

To successfully implement a program, the health educator must have a thorough understanding of the people in the target population. What is their current level of understanding regarding the issue at hand? What will it take to get the people to participate? Do they need financial assistance or childcare? What time of the day should the program be offered? What location or locations would be most convenient? While some of these questions can be answered from the initial needs assessment, it may also be necessary to obtain additional information about the target population before proceeding with implementation.

In conducting various health promotion and education programs, it is important that the health educator be comfortable using a wide range of educational methods or techniques. In school health, for example, it is not enough to simply lecture to students about "proper" health behaviors. A good health educator includes many teaching strategies such as brainstorming, debate, daily logs, position papers, guest speakers, problem solving, decision making, demonstrations, role playing, drama, music, and current events. In community health, most programs require going beyond developing and distributing a simple pamphlet on a given health topic. Again, a wide variety of strategies should be used, including television, radio, newspapers, billboards, celebrity spokespersons, behavioral contracting, community events, contests, incentives, support groups, and many more. As a general rule, health educators should always use multiple intervention activities when planning and implementing programs.

Once a program is in place and operating, the role of the health educator is not over. The health educator should continue to monitor the program to make certain everything is going as planned. If problems are noted, it may be necessary, even while the program is in progress, to revise the objectives or the intervention activities.

Responsibility IV: Evaluating the Effectiveness of Health Education Programs

In health education, it is critical that accurate evaluation be conducted to measure the success of programs. Without good evaluation, one does not know if the programs being implemented are meeting the specified goals and objectives. Programs that are not properly evaluated may be wasting valuable time, money, and other resources. Further, a program that is not evaluated, and thus cannot "prove its worth," may risk being cut back or even eliminated when resources are short and downsizing occurs.

To conduct an effective evaluation, the health educator must first establish realistic, measurable program objectives. As has already been mentioned, this is an important part of the planning process. Once objectives are in place, the health educator must develop a plan that will accurately assess if the program objectives have been met. Depending on the setting, this may involve developing and administering tests, conducting surveys, observing behavior, or other methods of data collection. Evaluation plans can be very simple or extremely sophisticated, depending on the program being evaluated, the expectations of the program planners, and the requirements of the funding agents.

After data have been collected, they must then be analyzed and interpreted. Reports need to be developed and distributed to the appropriate parties.

Ultimately, the results of the evaluation should be used to modify and improve current or future program efforts.

Responsibility V: Coordinating Provision of Health Education Services

Considering the previous responsibilities, it should be obvious that a great deal of coordination is needed to bring a health education program to fruition. Therefore, coordination is another skill that is critical for health educators to possess. As a first step, health educators need to be aware of related programs to make sure there is not significant overlap in services. By knowing what others are doing, it is also possible to identify gaps in services where important needs may be unmet.

Health educators must facilitate cooperation among personnel, both within programs and between programs. Many public school systems, for example, have initiated coordinated school health programs. This involves coordinating the activities and services of school nurses, counselors, psychologists, food service personnel, physical educators, health educators, teachers, administrators, support staff, parents, and community health agencies. The ultimate goal is to develop both curricular and extracurricular programs to improve the health status of students, faculty, staff, and the community as a whole.

Similar examples can be seen in the community setting. For example, a health department decides to apply for grant funds to reduce the incidence of tobacco use in its community. The health educator may bring together individuals and/or groups with a vested interest in reducing tobacco use to form a coalition. Membership in the coalition might include representatives from the American Cancer Society, American Lung Association, American Heart Association, local medical society, local dental association, public health department, public school system, and YMCA/YWCA. Coordination and integration of the services offered by these various groups would be critical to the successful development of a grant proposal and ultimately to the success of the funded program. It may even be necessary for the health educator to conduct or coordinate in-service training programs to make sure all coalition members have similar levels of knowledge and sophistication related to tobacco prevention programs.

Responsibility VI: Acting as a Resource Person in Health Education

Health educators are often called on to serve as resource persons. It is not unusual for a student to seek out the health teacher for assistance when having a health-related problem. In the corporate setting, health educators get questions about topics ranging from nutritional supplements to cancer signs and symptoms, to the best type of shoe to wear for jogging. Because it is impossible for health educators to know all of the information that could be called for in a given position, they must have the skill to access resources they need. It may be necessary to visit the library; use computerized health retrieval systems; access health databases; find information on specific diseases, obtain local, regional, state and national epidemiological data; and much more. As part of this process, it may be necessary for health educators to select or develop effective educational resources for dissemination.

Being able to retrieve information, however, is not enough. Health educators must establish effective consultive relationships with those seeking assistance, whether they be students, clients, employees, or other health educators. They must instill confidence in those seeking information and develop effective means to communicate the information in a nonthreatening manner. In some situations, health educators may decide to market their skills, via consultation, to individuals or groups and may make serving as a resource person the primary focus of their career.

Responsibility VII: Communicating Health and Health Education Needs, Concerns, and Resources

Health educators must interact with various groups of people, including other health professionals, consumers, students, employers, employees, and fellow health educators. Obviously, health educators must be good communicators. They must be skilled in written communication, oral communication, and mass media use. Health educators need to feel comfortable working with individuals, small groups, and large groups, as the situation warrants. In esssence, communication is the primary tool of the health educator.

It is often necessary for health educators to serve as filters between scientific information and their students or clients. The health educator must have the skill to translate difficult to understand scientific concepts, so that their constituents understand information necessary to improve and protect their health. For example, health educators may be called on to help HMO patients incorporate the recommendations of their physicians. A physician may tell a patient to start an exercise program, reduce fat in the diet, or manage stress better; while many patients have a general idea what these recommendations mean, they do not have the knowledge or skills to implement the recommendations. Most physicians cannot take the time to explain in detail what these recommendations entail. It is often health educators who communicate the detailed information on exercising safely, teach the client to recognize high-fat foods by reading food labels, and instruct the patient how to do progressive neuromotor relaxation. This may involve conducting one-on-one instruction, developing a videotape for patients to watch, developing brochures for distribution to patients, teaching classes, or coordinating support groups—in other words, communicating with the clients.

Summary of Responsibilities and Competencies

The responsibilities, competencies, and sub-competencies required for entry-level health educators do not function independently but are highly interrelated. In conducting all of the responsibilities, one needs to be a good communicator. Conducting a good needs assessment requires the skills to identify and gather appropriate resources. Planning should be based on a valid and reliable needs assessment. When implementing programs, one needs to have good communication skills and serve as a resource person when asked to do so. Evaluation relies on goals and objectives established during the planning process. Coordinating people and programs is necessary in planning, implementing, and evaluating programs.

It is not sufficient to be proficient at one, two, or even six of the responsibility areas. All seven responsibilities are critical for effective health education to take place. It is beyond the scope of this book to provide the level of information necessary to teach the reader how to do these tasks. Rather, it is the intent of this text that the readers become familiar with the responsibilities, competencies, and skills they will be taught in later classes and ultimately practice in their employment settings.

Advanced Study in Health Education

After receiving a bachelor's degree in health education, the student should not stop the educational process. At the very least, health educators should continue to learn on their own. One way of doing so is to belong to and be active in a professional association (see Chapter 8). Such a membership allows for the opportunity to read the professional publications from the association and to attend state, regional, and national meetings of that association. If one is a Certified Health Education Specialist, an average of fifteen continuing education contact hours are required each year (75 over five years) to maintain certification. These may be obtained by reading professional journals and submitting responses to questions on selected articles, by attending various professional meetings and workshops, by taking additional coursework, or by participating in other professional development activities.

At some point, most bachelor's degree-level health educators should consider going on for a master's degree. In some areas of the country and in some health education settings, such as medical care and worksite health education, the master's degree is almost considered the entry-level degree. In other words, to be considered for employment in these settings, the health educator must hold an appropriate master's degree.

In school settings, the master's degree brings additional financial rewards and, in some states, progress toward more permanent teaching certificates. It is usually advised, however, not to complete a master's degree in teaching prior to obtaining one's first teaching position. The additional money it would cost a school district to hire a new teacher with a master's degree versus a new teacher with a bachelor's degree may put the person with the master's degree at a disadvantage in the hiring process.

In community or public health settings, the master's degree may bring additional financial rewards, as well as promotions within the agency. It may also open the door to higher-level positions with other community health agencies or public health departments.

Master's Degree Options

When considering a master's degree, one should first consider the type of degree one wishes to pursue. Typical choices include a Master's of Education **(M.Ed.),** Master's of Science **(M.S.),** Master's of Arts (M.A.), Master's of Public Health **(M.P.H.),** and Master's of Science in Public Health (M.S.P.H.) (Bensley & Pope, 1994). Some colleges and universities may offer only one degree option, while others may offer more than one, giving students the decision of degree choice.

The M.Ed. degree is typically found in institutions where the health education program is located in a College of Education or Teacher's College. While many of the students in such programs may be focusing on school health, this does not mean that all persons with this degree designation have the public schools as their career goal. Some colleges and universities offer the M.Ed. degree with such emphasis areas as community health and corporate health promotion.

The M.S. and M.A. degrees are usually found in universities where the health education program is located in colleges other than education. Because there is no accepted accreditation for these programs, they have much flexibility

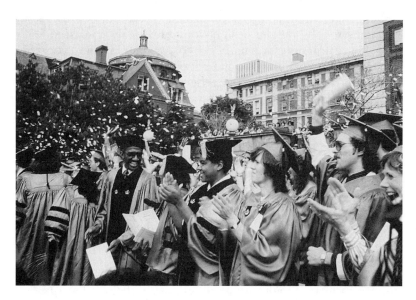

More health education positions require a master's degree either for initial employment or after one is employed. (Van Bucher/Stock, Boston)

to develop programs that meet the needs of the local job market. They offer a variety of emphasis areas, including public health, community health education, and corporate health promotion. When considering differences between the M.S., M.A., and M.Ed. degrees, remember that the M.S. may be the more scientific or research-oriented degree, while the M.A. and M.Ed. may be more practitioner-oriented.

As the name implies, the M.P.H. and M.S.P.H. are the degree choices for many wishing to work in the field of public health. The M.S.P.H. degree is typically more research-oriented than the M.P.H. degree; otherwise, the degrees are similar. The M.P.H. can be awarded in a variety of specialty areas such as an M.P.H. in nursing, M.P.H. in dietetics, or M.P.H. in epidemiology. It is the M.P.H. in health education that is of most interest to health educators. Most M.P.H. degree-granting colleges and universities are accredited by the Council on Education for the Public Health (CEPH). As such, the requirements to obtain an M.P.H. are more standardized than are the requirements to obtain the M.S., M.A., or M.Ed. degrees, which are typically not accredited by any professional body. To obtain accreditation, the curriculum must contain specific core courses. These include biostatistics, epidemiology, health planning, and environmental health. The M.P.H. has the reputation of being a more prestigious degree than the M.S., M.A., or M.Ed. There are, however, many more health educators with M.S., M.A., or M.Ed. degrees than with the M.P.H. degree. The latest AAHE directory lists 126 institutions that prepare health educators at the master's degree level (AAHE, 1997). There currently are twenty-two accredited schools of public health and ten public health programs in community health in the United States (APHA, 1996).

There are great variations between colleges and universities in the program requirements for the degree designations previously discussed. As bachelor's-level health education students begin to consider master's degree options, it would be wise to carefully examine program requirements and degree designation within the context of future career goals.

Selecting a Graduate School

Determining which college or university to attend is a decision that goes hand-in-hand with deciding which degree to pursue. In terms of practicality, factors such as cost, location, and size must be considered. Reputation is also extremely important. Begin by considering the reputation of the college or university. There is a definite hierarchy among colleges and universities in the United States, and graduating from one of the more prestigious institutions may lend instant credibility to the graduate degree and enhance job opportunities.

Next, consider the reputation of the health education program at a given institution. To learn about various programs, bachelor's-level health educators can talk to other professionals in the field whom they admire and trust. A visit or call to their former college professors may also be a good source of information. After narrowing the list to several programs, it is wise to contact each program.

Ask if they can provide written materials describing the program, application forms, admission requirements, a copy of the graduate catalog, and a list of recent graduates and where they have been employed. Contacting recent graduates is also a good way to learn about a particular program.

Finally, do not overlook the college/university library as a resource. Most university libraries subscribe to a microfiche service that provides university catalogs. An overview of graduate health education programs can be obtained from this resource. In addition, many colleges and universities now have home pages on the World Wide Web which provide information about graduate programs and in some cases allow students to complete the application process electronically.

Admission Requirements

As an undergraduate health education student, it is not too early to be concerned about admission requirements to graduate school. While admission requirements vary greatly from one university to another, one factor that has traditionally been important is the undergraduate grade point average (GPA). In general, a student should strive to achieve an overall undergraduate GPA of at least a 3.0 on a 4.0 scale to be sure of consideration by most graduate programs. Some institutions do not specify a minimum GPA (Bensley & Pope, 1994). Instead, they tend to use more individual and subjective criteria in their admission process. In either case, it is important for new health education students to begin with the first term of their freshman year to achieve the best grades possible. Too often, low grades in the first two years of college prevent otherwise good students from being accepted into the master's degree program of their choice.

In addition to GPA requirements, most graduate programs require a completed application form, a letter of application, and several letters of reference. To be considered for admission, some programs also require students to submit scores from a standardized performance test such as The Graduate Record Exam or Miller Analogy Test. These scores may be a major component in the decision-making process, or they may simply be used in conjunction with other applicant information to provide a more well-rounded view of the prospective student.

Financing Graduate Study

Funding the graduate degree may not be as burdensome as funding undergraduate education. Many colleges and universities award assistantships or fellowships to graduate students on a competitive basis. Typically, these graduate awards pay all or part of the graduate tuition and provide students with a monthly stipend to cover living expenses during their graduate studies. In return, students agree to work for the health education program. If the award is a **Graduate teaching assistantship** (or fellowship), the student teaches a specified number of undergraduate courses each term. These are usually introductory health education courses that meet general university requirements or are the first courses for health education majors. If the award is a **graduate research assistantship** (or fellowship), the student usually works closely with one or more faculty members on a particular research project. Students might be assigned to do library research, assist with data collection, enter data into the computer, or a host of other research-related activities.

Graduate assistantships and fellowships not only provide an excellent alternative for funding graduate education but also provide valuable health education work experience for the student.

Summary

Since the late 1970s, many people have worked very hard and dedicated much time to defining and developing the roles and responsibilities of a health educator. The initial stages of this work has become known as the Role Delineation Project. As a result of this work, there is now an agreed-on set of responsibilities, competencies, and sub-competencies for health educators, regardless of whether they ultimately wish to work in schools, communities, clinics, or corporate settings. These responsibilities, competencies, and sub-competencies encourage college and university professional preparation programs to develop their curricula so that a standardized set of skills is taught to all health education students. Further, the responsibilities, competencies, and sub-competencies are the basis for establishing individual certification within the profession. Currently, this certification is available only for entry-level skills. Work is in progress to develop additional responsibilities, competencies, and sub-competencies for graduate-level work, which may lead to advanced levels of certification in the future.

Advanced study in health education is necessary to stay current with health information and new techniques for conducting health education programs. All health educators should read professional journals, join one or more professional associations, and take an active role in their functioning. Certified Health Education Specialists (CHESs) must obtain continuing education credits to maintain their certification. For most bachelor's-level health educators, it would be advisable to consider a master's degree at some point in their career. Decisions concerning graduate study should not be taken lightly. Undergraduate health education students need to be aware of the admission requirements for graduate school and work to make sure they meet these requirements. Graduate assistantships or fellowships provide an excellent alternative to fund graduate education.

REVIEW QUESTIONS

1. Define *credentialing* and explain the differences among certification, registration, licensure, and accreditation.

2. Outline the major events of the Role Delineation Project.

3. Review the "Roles and Responsibilities of a Health Educator" (Appendix D). Do you think they are more focused on health content or the process skills needed to be a health educator? Defend your position and explain why you believe the health education profession has moved in this direction.

4. Identify two ways health educators can stay up-to-date in the field.

5. What is the difference among the following academic degrees: M.A., M.Ed., M.S., M.P.H., M.S.P.H.?

6. Briefly describe the process for applying to graduate school.

ACTIVITIES

1. Read each competency and sub-competency of a health educator. Score each competency and sub-competency using the following scale:
   A. I currently have the skill to meet this competency/sub-competency.
   B. I am uncertain if I have the skill to meet this competency/sub-competency.
   C. I do not have the skill to meet this competency/sub-competency.
   After rating each competency and sub-competency, make a list of things you can do to enhance your skills. Keep this table, and periodically reevaluate your skills throughout your program of study.

2. Write to one or more universities you may wish to attend and request information on their graduate health education programs. Try to learn about their admission requirements, degree options, and financial aid opportunities.

3. Make an appointment with a professor at your school to talk about graduate school. Ask about the schools the professor attended and the degree earned. Finally, ask for advice on what degree to earn and what school to attend.

REFERENCES

American Public Health Association (APHA). (1996). US schools of public health and graduate public health programs accredited by the Council on Education for Public Health. *American Journal of Public Health, 86*(3), 428–429.

Association for the Advancement of Health Education (AAHE). (1997). Directory of institutions offering undergraduate and graduate degree programs in health education. *Journal of Health Education, 26*(2), 107–118.

Bensley, L. B., Jr., & Pope, A. J. (1994). A study of graduate bulletins to determine general information and graduation requirements for master's degree programs in health education. *Journal of Health Education, 25*(3), 165–171.

Cleary, H. P. (1986). Issues in the credentialing of health education specialists: A review of the state of the art. In William B. Ward (Ed.), *Advances in health education and promotion* (pp. 129–154). Greenwich, CT: Jai Press.

Cleary, H. P. (1995). *The credentialing of health educators: An historical account 1970–1990.* New York: The National Commission for Health Education Credentialing, Inc.

Gilmore, G. D., & Campbell, M. D. (1996). *Needs assessment strategies.* (2nd ed.). Madison, WI: Brown & Benchmark.

Joint Committee for Graduate Standards. (1996). National Congress for Institutions Preparing Graduate Health Educators. Program Booklet, 1.

National Task Force on the Preparation and Practice of Health Educators. (1985). *Framework for the development of competency-based curricula for entry level health educators.* New York: The National Commission for Health Education Credentialing, Inc.

The National Commission for Health Education Credentialing. (1996). *A competency-based framework for professional development of Certified Health Education Specialists.* New York: The National Commission for Health Education Credentialing, Inc.

The National Commission for Health Education Credentialing. (1998). *Spring, 1998 Certified Health Education Specialist examination brochure.*

7 The Settings for Health Education

CHAPTER OBJECTIVES

After reading this chapter and answering the questions at the end, you should be able to

1. Identify the four major settings in which health educators are employed.
2. Describe the major responsibilities for health educators in the four major settings.
3. Discuss the advantages and disadvantages of the four major settings.
4. Explain the qualifications and major responsibilities of health educators working in colleges and universities.
5. Identify a variety of "nontraditional" settings in which health educators may be employed.
6. State several action steps that can be taken to help one land one's first job in health education.

KEY TERMS

community/public health
    education
coordinated school health
    program

hard money
health care settings
networking
public health agencies

school health education
soft money
voluntary health agencies
worksite health promotion

Today, most Americans live a healthier and longer life than ever before. Despite this fact, however, it is clear that many, if not most, Americans are not living at their optimal level of health. Hereditary, environmental and behavioral factors predispose too many U.S. citizens to disease, suffering, disability, and premature death. The challenge for health educators is to help these people reduce their risk and increase the probability of a long, happy, and productive life.

To meet this challenge, health educators conduct programs in a variety of settings (Breckon, Harvey, & Lancaster, 1994). The use of multiple settings is important, as it allows health educators to reach the greatest number of people in the most convenient, efficient, and effective ways possible. While the goals of health education and the skills needed to carry out the responsibilities are nearly the same in all settings (English & Videto, 1997), the actual duties of a job may differ greatly from setting to setting.

Professional preparation programs in health education typically prepare students for employment in one or more of four major settings. These settings are schools, hospitals/clinics, community/public health agencies, and business/industry. On obtaining advanced degrees, students from any of these settings may seek employment as college or university health educators. In addition, there are a variety of nontraditional employment areas where health educators can work.

Within this chapter, each of the four major settings for health education will be discussed. After a short introduction to the setting, a description of one day in the career of a health educator from that particular setting is presented. This is designed to give the reader a general idea of what a workday is like. Because of the great diversity in duties from health educator to health educator even within the same setting, it is impossible to say that this is a typical day. For most health educators, there is no such thing as a typical day. Following this is a section that describes additional responsibilities that might be assigned to health educators in the setting. Again, this is not intended to be an exhaustive list but is intended to further the reader's understanding of job responsibilities in that setting. Finally, each section will end with a listing of some advantages and disadvantages for that setting.

School Health Education

Health education, as an area of employment, has been around for more than one hundred years, with some components dating back even further in history (Breckon, Harvey, & Lancaster, 1994). **School health education,** as the name implies, primarily involves instructing school-age children about health and health-related behaviors. The initial impetus for school health stemmed from the terrible epidemics of the 1800s and the efforts of the Women's Christian Temperance Movement to promote abstinence from alcohol in the early 1900s. Many states mandated school health education to inform students about these health hazards. Unfortunately, these mandates have seldom been strictly enforced. Further, teachers have often been underqualified, with only an academic minor or a few elective courses to prepare them for the health classroom. As a result the quality of school health programs has often been compromised (Breckon, Harvey, & Lancaster, 1994).

Despite these limitations, the potential for school districts and the health instruction program in particular to impact students is tremendous. A 1994 study found that nearly 84 percent of Americans appear to support the concept of comprehensive school health education (Seffrin, 1994). Such programs have demonstrated effectiveness when they are well planned, sequential, provided significant

TABLE 7.1 Rules of Good Health—1922

1. Take a full bath more than once a week.
2. Brush teeth at least once a day.
3. Sleep long hours with window open.
4. Drink as much milk as possible, but no coffee or tea.
5. Eat some vegetables or fruit everyday.
6. Drink at least four glasses of water a day.
7. Play part of everyday outdoors.
8. Have a bowel movement every morning.

Source: Data from Bernice C. Regney, "Rules of the Health Game" in *Milk and Our School Children,* U.S. Dept. of the Interior, Bureau of Education, Health Education, No. 11, 1922.

TABLE 7.2 National Health Education Standards

1. Students will comprehend concepts related to health promotion and disease prevention.
2. Students will demonstrate the ability to access valid health information and health-promoting products and services.
3. Students will demonstrate the ability to practice health-enhancing behaviors and reduce health risks.
4. Students will analyze the influence of culture, media, technology, and other factors on health.
5. Students will demonstrate the ability to use interpersonal communication skills to enhance health.
6. Students will demonstrate the ability to use goal-setting and decision-making skills to enhance health.
7. Students will demonstrate the ability to advocate for personal, family, and community health.

Source: A work of the Joint Committee on National Health Education Standards. Reprinted by permission of the American Cancer Society, Inc.

time in the curriculum, and taught by a trained health educator (AAHE, 1990; Green et al., 1985).

The sophistication of school health education programs has increased drastically over the years. Today's school health educator needs to be well trained and prepared to deliver a comprehensive and demanding curriculum. Comparing the 1922 "Rules of Good Health" with the 1995 National Health Education Standards (Joint Committee on Health Education Standards, 1995) clearly illustrates this point (see Tables 7.1 and 7.2).

When the school health education component is made a part of a broader, districtwide approach known as a **coordinated school health program,** the potential to impact students in a positive way is even greater. Allensworth and Kolbe (1987) have defined the comprehensive school health program as follows:

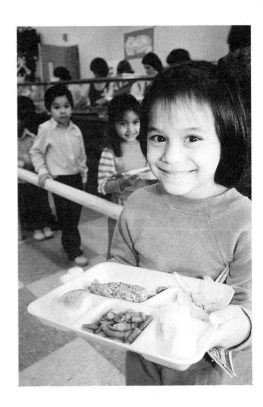

Food service is one component of a coordinated school health program. (Bob Daemmrich/Stock, Boston)

> A comprehensive [coordinated] school health program is an integrated set of planned, sequential, school-affiliated strategies, activities, and services designed to promote the optimal physical, emotional, social, and educational development of students. The program involves and is supportive of families and is determined by the local community based on community needs, resources, standards and requirements. It is coordinated by a multidisciplinary team and accountable to the community for program quality and effectiveness. (p. 60)

In other words, a coordinated school health program coordinates and integrates various aspects of a school district to best impact the health of the students, faculty, staff, administration, and community as a whole. This includes food services, nursing services, school counseling and psychology, health instruction, physical education, administration, school environment, community involvement, and faculty/staff wellness (Allensworth & Kolbe, 1987).

A health educator choosing to work in the school setting will find a challenging and rewarding career. When considering the number of school districts in the United States, it is obvious there is a large number of people teaching health education in the schools. Unfortunately, many of these people are not health education specialists. Some school districts have used biology, physical education, home economics or family life, and consumer science teachers to teach health. Even when certified health education teachers are employed, they

BOX **7.1**

Practitioner's Perspective

Name:	Gretchen L. Anderson
Current Position/Title:	Elementary Teacher
Employer:	Pocatello, ID, School District #25
Degree(s):	Bachelor of Arts, Idaho State University Master of Health Education, Idaho State University
Major:	Elementary Education for the B.A. Health Education for the master's degree
Minor:	Reading and Social Science for B.A.

Primary job responsibilities: I have taught in a sixth grade self-contained classroom and I now teach first and second graders in reading and writing skills through small group instruction in a Title I program.

How did you obtain your position? I obtained my sixth-grade teaching position by applying and then interviewing with the personnel director in our school district. I was officially hired by the building principal. In my current position in Title I, I was interviewed by the Title I director and hired by my principal.

What do you most like about your position? My job is extremely rewarding. I get to work with young people and watch their excitement as they learn to read and write and as they learn about themselves and discover their place in the world around them. I get to use health education nearly every day in my classroom. For example, I use books with health themes to teach reading, and I integrate health into reading, math, and science. Health is a very high interest area for grade-school students. In addition, I create many of my own health lessons, as our district has no health texts for elementary school. With my graduate degree in health education, I can better create age-appropriate lessons and share them with other teachers in our school.

What do you like the least about your position? I dislike the paperwork that is required by the school district, the state, and the federal government.

What recommendations do you have for health education students who would someday like a position like yours? I recommend that they enjoy children and are the type of person who can accept each child for the unique being that she/he is. I also recommend that they diligently study health education methods; health curriculum development; child development; and health topical areas such as diseases, nutrition, fitness, drug abuse, sexuality, mental health, environmental health, and safety. The prospective teacher should also be flexible enough to develop an educational program that fits the needs of the child. Finally, learn the art of including parents as partners in the education of their children.

may have only a minor in health education and are not fully prepared. A further problem confounding the employment situation in the schools is that the requirement for health education is usually less than for other academic subjects. Students typically need only one or two semesters of health education to graduate from high school, while they probably are required to complete four years of English. Thus, with such a minimal requirement, the number of health teachers needed and the resulting demand for health teachers are low. The bottom line is that, in many parts of the country, it is difficult to obtain a job in school health.

Those students who are really committed to being outstanding health teachers, however, should not be deterred from this career path. With time, dedication, and perseverance, those who really want to teach health in the schools can usually find employment. Substitute teaching, coaching, and volunteering are good ways to make oneself known in a school district and increase the likelihood of eventual employment. Students are encouraged to talk to their own professors to determine the job market for school health education in their area.

A Day in the Career of a School Health Educator

At 5:45 A.M. the alarm goes off and Ms. Bell's day is started. Ms. Bell teaches 7th- and 8th-grade health at a junior high school in a suburban school district. After going through the normal morning routine, she arrives at the school building around 7:00 A.M. There is a half hour before homeroom, so she picks up her mail and duplicates a test that she prepared the night before for her 8th-grade health class. In homeroom she takes attendance, gets a lunch count, listens to announcements over the loud speaker, and collects money from a fruit sale fund raiser. The fruit sale is being conducted by the PTA to raise money for new computers in the school. Essentially, homeroom involves administrative responsibilities and a considerable amount of paperwork.

At 7:45 the first period starts. This school has eight fifty-minute periods, with only four minutes between periods. The first three periods, Ms. Bell teaches 7th-grade health. Today's lesson is on refusal skills related to alcohol and drug use. Ms. Bell has written three scenarios students could find themselves in. The scenarios are open-ended, so after each one Ms. Bell leads a discussion on how to use refusal skills to get out of a bad situation. She then asks students to role-play the situations to gain further practice in using refusal skills. Unfortunately, only two of her three classes will get this lesson today. The second-period class is one day behind due to an assembly that was held a week ago. Ms. Bell has to find a way to catch up this group with the rest of the classes.

Ms. Bell's fourth period is divided in half. The first half, she has study hall duty. It is her responsibility to take attendance and monitor the study hall. In today's study hall, two boys become unruly and nearly get in a fight. She sends them to the office for discipline, but the situation is quite upsetting.

The second half of fourth period is Ms. Bell's lunch time. She usually has twenty-five minutes to relax and eat lunch before fifth period begins. Today, however, she must use part of that time to drop by the office for a follow-up discussion with the assistant principal concerning the incident in study hall.

Fifth period, Ms. Bell teaches 8th-grade health. Today is a test day. While the students are taking their test, Ms. Bell works on a future lesson plan for the class.

Sixth period is Ms. Bell's planning period. Today she tries to make a phone call to the parents of one of her students who is having problems in health class, but no one is home. She then grades the test papers from her previous class and records the grades. She averages the grades and starts to develop interim reports for the fifth-period class, but she runs out of time. Seventh and eighth periods are also 8th-grade health classes. While students take their tests, Ms. Bell works on grading papers from the previous classes and writing her interim reports.

School ends for the students at 2:57 P.M. After monitoring the hall while students leave the building, Ms. Bell hurries to the cafeteria for the monthly teacher's meeting. General information and announcements are presented by the principal. The meeting ends at 4:00 P.M.

In addition to her teaching responsibilities, Ms. Bell coaches the junior high girls' volleyball team. Practice goes from 3:15 to 5:00 P.M. After practice, Ms. Bell waits until the last girl leaves the locker room, then returns to her classroom to prepare for the next day's classes. She leaves the school at around 5:30 P.M.

After dinner and her family responsibilities, Ms. Bell spends twenty minutes on the phone with the student's parents who were not at home earlier in the day. She then finishes grading the tests she gave in class and continues working on interim reports. It will take her at least one more evening to finish the interims. At 11:00 P.M. she turns off the light and goes to bed.

Additional Responsibilities

In addition to the lesson planning, grading, parent meetings, disciplining, coaching, and the various administrative duties, teachers may have additional responsibilities. They may be involved in curriculum development, the review of materials for classroom use, the chaperoning of dances or other after-school activities, fund-raising, and the advising of student groups such as yearbook, debate, or student council. School health educators should also be active members of their professional organizations. This allows them to network with other health educators and to stay up-to-date in the field. Finally, school health educators should be strong advocates for school health (Utah State University, 1996). They must make certain that fellow faculty, administrators, school boards, and the community as a whole are aware of the unique contributions of a school health program. (See Table 7.3.)

Community/Public Health Education

Community health education, as defined by the Joint Committee on Health Education Terminology (1991), is

. . .the application of a variety of methods that result in the education and mobilization of community members in actions for resolving health issues and problems which affect the community. These methods include, but are not limited to, group process, mass media, communication, community organization, organization development, strategic planning, skills training, legislation, policy making and advocacy. (p. 105)

The most likely sources of employment for community health educators are voluntary health agencies and public health agencies. **Voluntary health agencies** are created by concerned citizens to deal with health needs not met by governmental agencies (McKenzie & Pinger, 1997, p. 684). As the name implies, they rely heavily on volunteer help and donations to keep them functioning. There are usually paid staff members who are responsible for administration, volunteer recruitment and coordination, program development, and fund-raising. Health educators are hired to plan, implement, and evaluate the education component of the agency's programs. They often, however, are involved in other aspects of the

TABLE 7.3   Advantages and Disadvantages of Working in School Health Education

Advantages
- Health educators have the ability to work with young people during their developmental years.
- Health educators have the potential to prevent harmful health behaviors from forming instead of working with older people after such behaviors have been formed.
- Health educators have the opportunity to impact all students, because health education is usually a required course.
- A graduate degree is not needed for entry-level employment.
- There is good job security.
- Summer months are free and there are nice vacation periods in December and in spring
- Benefits are good.

Disadvantages
- Good health educators usually spend many long hours at their job, including weekends and evenings that may compensate for the long vacation periods.
- Health educators may have relatively low status in a school district when compared with teachers of more traditional subjects such as math, science, and English.
- Pay is low when compared with professionals in other fields, but comparable when compared with that of other health educators.
- Discipline problems are often seen as a major disadvantage.
- Summer "free time" may be consumed with summer employment and/or returning to college for additional required coursework.
- It is difficult dealing with conservative school boards, parents, and community groups when teaching controversial issues such as sex education and drug education.

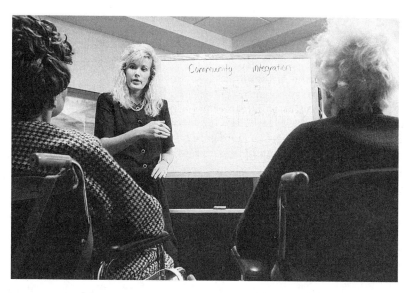

Community health educators work in a variety of voluntary and public health agencies. (Charles Gupton/Tony Stone Images)

agency as well. Voluntary health agencies are usually funded by such means as private donations, grants, fund-raisers, and possibly United Way contributions. Examples of voluntary health agencies include the American Cancer Society, American Heart Association, and American Lung Association. Most of these large, well-known voluntary agencies have national, state, and local divisions.

Public health agencies, or official governmental health agencies, are usually financed through public tax monies. Government has long been responsible for doing for the people as a whole what individuals could not do for themselves. Thus, governments provide police protection, educational systems, clean air and water, and many other important services. Departments of public health, thus, are formed to coordinate and provide health services to a community. Health departments may be organized by the city, county, state, or federal government. They operate primarily with paid staff and typically provide health education services as part of their total program. Table 7.4 contains a list of agencies that have programs for which community/public health educators may be employed.

More diversity in terms of job responsibilities exists in the community/public health education setting than in the other major settings in which health educators are employed. This is due to the large number of community and public health agencies that exist and the vast differences in their missions, goals, and objectives. In some community/public agencies, health educators serve administrative functions such as coordinating volunteers, budgeting, fund-raising, program planning, and serving as liaison to other agencies and groups. In other community/public agencies, the health educator may be more involved in direct program delivery to the clientele of that agency and/or the community at large.

TABLE 7.4   **Possible Sources of Employment in Community/Public Health Education**

State, local, city health departments
U.S. Public Health Service
U.S. Food & Drug Administration
U.S. or state departments of agriculture
U.S. or state departments of transportation
County extension services
U.S. Department of Health and Human Services
U.S. Centers for Disease Control
National Institutes of Health
U.S. or state penal institutions

Most frequently, however, health educators are involved in a little bit of everything.

A Day in the Career of a Community Health Educator

Mr. Fischer is the health educator for a local division of the American Cancer Society (ACS). In that role, he has the responsibility of conducting health education programs in a four-county area of the state. Mr. Fischer usually arrives at the office between 8:30 and 9:00 in the morning. This morning, however, he had an 8:00 meeting with a local coalition that is trying to encourage school districts to implement comprehensive school health education into their curricula. This is an important issue, as the ACS has made comprehensive school health education one of its major priority areas at the national level. Mr. Fischer has been responsible for forming this coalition and was recently elected to serve as its chairperson. As such, he sets the agenda, runs the meetings, takes minutes, and always plans for juice and bagels to be served.

It is 9:30 when Mr. Fischer finally arrives at his office. He spends the next half hour opening his mail and answering telephone calls. From 10:00 to 11:00 is the bi-weekly staff meeting, which is run by Mr. Fischer's supervisor, who is director of the local ACS unit. In these meetings, staff members provide updates on projects for which they are responsible. Issues and problems facing the local unit are discussed, with the intent of involving the group in identifying potential solutions. Information from the state and national levels is also provided.

From 11:00 to 12:00, Mr. Fischer has time to sit at his desk and work on the Great American Smokeout. This is a yearly campaign to help smokers quit smoking for at least one day and hopefully for the rest of their lives. Mr. Fischer is responsible for this event. He has to recruit local sponsors to donate money or prizes for the event, plan a variety of activities to promote the event, contact local media to cover the various events, distribute materials to numerous participating groups, coordinate volunteers to assist with or run various events, develop letters of understanding with each group assisting with the event, and provide letters of

BOX **7.2**

Practitioner's Perspective

Name:	Lisa Koslovsky
Title:	Youth Specialist
	Community Health and Education Services
Employer:	American Red Cross
Degree:	B.S., University of Cincinnati
Major:	Health Promotion & Education
Emphasis:	Community Health

Job responsibilities: My major job responsibility is to market and facilitate delivery of all Red Cross health and safety programs (CPR/First Aid, HIV/AIDS, youth programs) to schools and other youth-serving agencies. As part of this responsibility, I must recruit, train, and place volunteer instructors. In addition, I assist in the preparation of objectives, budgets, statistical reports, and evaluations for all youth and HIV/AIDS program areas.

What do you like most about your job? I like the variety of working with a large number of varied programs on a day-to-day basis. I especially enjoy the daily interaction with volunteers and actually providing services and programs to youth. Most of all, I enjoy working for a national organization that is so highly respected as a community service agency.

What do you like least about your job? I would have to say the salary. By working for a voluntary agency, my salary is at the lower end of the scale for persons with a bachelor's degree. Had I chosen to work in a for-profit organization, I could probably have made more money.

How did you obtain your current position? I began at the Red Cross as an intern during the final quarter of my senior year. On completing my internship, a job was created in Community Health and Education Services to improve Red Cross visibility in the schools. I applied for the job and was hired. I don't believe I would have gotten the job had it not been for the internship experience.

What recommendations would you give to a health education student who would some day like to obtain a position similar to yours? Gain as much field experience as early in the program as possible. This can be done through either employment or volunteer work. As an employee of a voluntary agency, it was amazing for me to learn how many of my colleagues began their careers as volunteers. Volunteering is a win-win situation. Based on the commitment you make, you can establish relationships with influential people and gain the knowledge necessary to make important career decisions. The voluntary agency wins by gaining your valuable time and talents.

thanks to all groups and individual volunteers who assist with the event after it is over. Twice during this hour, Mr. Fischer is interrupted by phone calls from individuals needing information on various cancers. Mr. Fischer writes down their request on a referral slip, along with their name and address. Twice a week he has a volunteer that comes in and mails all of the information that has been requested.

At 12:00 Mr. Fischer heads out for lunch. He usually eats lunch at his desk while working, but today he is speaking to the local Rotary Club about the Great American Smokeout. Although Mr. Fischer enjoys public speaking, he does not have enough time to handle all of the requests and frequently coordinates volunteers to speak on behalf of the ACS.

Mr. Fischer returns to his office shortly before 2:00. He takes another hour to answer phone calls that have come in since the morning and writes some correspondence related to the Great American Smokeout and the Coordinated School Health Coalition. From 3:00 to 5:00, Mr. Fischer is on the phone, calling volunteers to participate in a fund-raiser called Jail and Bail. With this fund-raiser, volunteers are notified in advance that they will be picked up and escorted to "jail," where they will have to stay behind bars until they can raise bail. The jail is actually a temporary structure located at the local mall. Bail is raised by calling friends and acquaintances, requesting donations to the ACS. This is a good fund-raiser and a lot of fun, but it takes considerable staff time to prepare for the event.

Mr. Fischer leaves the office at 5:00 to have dinner with his family. Tonight, however, he has to be back at the office at 7:30 for a meeting of the Youth Education Committee. As the name implies, this committee of volunteers is responsible for all local ACS programs dealing with youth. As the health educator, Mr. Fischer has to be present for all of their monthly meetings. In addition to the Youth Education Committee, there are also board meetings, volunteer recognition nights, Adult Education Committee meetings, and numerous other speaking engagements and responsibilities that require Mr. Fischer to work in the evenings. He averages one or two nights a week on the job. In addition, he occasionally has to work on weekends during special ACS events.

Additional Responsibilities

As can be seen from the Mr. Fischer example, community/public health educators are involved in numerous and varied activities. Planning, implementing, and evaluating programs and events are major tasks, but, in conducting these tasks, health educators get involved in fund-raising, coalition building, committee work, budgeting, general administration, public speaking, volunteer recruitment, grant writing, and media advocacy. (See Table 7.5.)

Worksite Health Education

Since the mid-1970s, business and industry in the United States have been offering **worksite health promotion** programs for their employees. These on-site programs offer a new setting for health educators and allow them to reach segments of the population that had not been easily accessible in the past.

Health promotion programs at worksites differ greatly from site to site. Some are very extensive, include elaborate facilities, and are conducted by full-time staff members hired by the company; others are minimal programs that may include only a brown-bag lunch speaker's program or a discount at the YMCA or health club. Breckon, Harvey, and Lancaster (1994) categorized worksite programs into three groups: (1) educational activities, (2) organizational activities, and (3) environmental activities (Table 7.6).

TABLE 7.5   Advantages and Disadvantages of Working in Community/Public Health Education

Advantages
- Job responsibilities are highly varied and changing.
- There is a strong emphasis on prevention.
- There is usually a high community profile.
- Health educators work with multiple groups of people.
- There is high degree of self-satisfaction.

Disadvantages
- Pay may be low, particularly in voluntary agencies.
- When hired directly by a community or public health agency, job security tends to be good. In such situations, the health educator is said to be employed on **hard money.** Sometimes, however, these agencies hire health educators on money secured through grants, which is known as **soft money.** In these situations, positions are terminated when grant funding is discontinued; so, job security can be a concern.
- Relying heavily on volunteers can be frustrating. While most volunteers are great, some do not demonstrate the same level of commitment as might a paid employee.
- There never seems to be enough money to run all the programs that need to be offered in the way they should be offered.

TABLE 7.6   Worksite Health Promotion Activities

Educational Activities	Organizational Activities	Environmental Activities
- Self-care, first aid, CPR - Nutrition, weight control - Smoking cessation - Stress management - Cancer risk awareness - AIDS prevention - Fitness	- Risk assessment - Smoke-free areas - Screening program - Physical examinations - Newsletter - Support groups - Lending libraries - Counseling hotlines	- Jogging trails - Nutritional items in vending machines - Low-salt/low-calorie foods in cafeteria - Displays, posters - Health fairs

Source: From J. Breckon, J. R. Harvey, and R. B. Lancaster, *Community health education: Settings, roles, and skills for the 21st century,* 3rd edition, 1994. Reprinted by permission.

BOX 7.3
Practitioner's Perspective

Name:	Kimberly A. Jones
Current Position/Title:	Health Educator
Employer:	Delaware County Health Department, Muncie, Indiana
Degrees:	B.S., Penn State University M.S., Ball State University
Major(s):	Exercise Science/Athletic Training Community Health Education
Minor(s):	Health Education

What are your job responsibilities? The responsibilities as a health educator for the county consist of many things. I supervise two additional health educators, who each work approximately twenty hours per week with me. I work very closely with other community social service agencies to address public health issues (teen pregnancy, smoking cessation, minority health, childhood injuries) for all residents of the county. I serve on task forces, coalitions, and executive comittees to develop the framework for programs, health fairs, workshops, and conferences. Needs assessment, program planning, implementation, public relations, and evaluation are many of the areas my job responsibilities fall under.

What do you like most about your job? The most rewarding part of my job is seeing the people to whom I provide educational opportunities make a positive behavioral change (smoking cessation, weight management, etc.). In some situations, a behavioral change cannot immediately be made, but knowing I provided them with the information and skills needed to take control of a situation when it arises is also rewarding.

Providing services for the entire county provides great diversity to the job. I am constantly working with different age groups, different educational backgrounds, and different cultures. Working with other community agencies provides the opportunity to address many health issues. Having a close relationship with other agencies provides me with a great opportunity to network and obtain the newest health information.

What do you like least about your job? Working in an office with a small staff means covering for other people in divisions you aren't familiar with. Answering phones and serving as an information resource for the entire office can get you quickly off focus on the task at hand.

The goal of the County Health Department is to reach people in the entire county and be of easy access to them. I work an 8:30-to-4:30 day, with several evening presentations and classes. There is some flexibility in the schedule, but days and nights are often long.

How did you obtain your current job? Professors from Ball State were very helpful in informing me of position openings in the surrounding area. In addition, the department had an employment bulletin board in the hall. They listed all jobs that came through the office, by word of mouth and the media. My current job was posted in the classified section of the paper.

What recommendations would you give to a health education student who would someday like to obtain a position similar to yours? I would first recommend being active inside and outside of the classroom with the department you are in. Get to know your professors. This will allow them to speak more accurately about you when you use them as references. Volunteer for health education projects. Job shadowing various settings will allow you to explore all the opportunities health educators have. Work hard and be aggressive in your internship. Keep in contact with the company or individuals you did your internship with. They have many connections and may have positions open. Finally, learn from your interviews so you can strengthen the next one. Good luck.

The number of worksite health promotion programs has been growing rapidly. One survey of worksites with fifty or more employees found that two-thirds offered some type of health promotion program or fitness facility (Fielding & Piserchia, 1989). From 1985 to 1992, the percentage of worksites offering at least one health promotion activity increased from 66 to 81 percent (National Coordinating Committee on Worksite Health Promotion, 1993).

There appear to be three main reasons for companies to invest in health promotion programs (Breckon, Harvey, & Lancaster, 1994). First, and foremost, is the economic incentive. Companies initiating health promotion programs hope to decrease absenteeism, increase productivity, reduce turnover, decrease health insurance costs, and decrease disability payments. Second, companies believe worksite health promotion programs may increase employee morale. When employees view health promotion programs as an added benefit and convenience provided by their employers, it may translate into a more positive attitude toward the employer and the job itself. The third reason to become involved in worksite health promotion programs is to improve company image. When companies involve themselves in the health of their employees and the broader health issues of a community, the general public's image of the company may be enhanced. While positions exist in the worksite health promotion setting that are strictly health promotion/education, more frequently expertise in exercise testing and prescription is required. This is because many worksite health promotion programs are based in a fitness center. It is often the fitness center that is the most visible aspect of a worksite health promotion program and attracts many employees to health promotion programs. Therefore, skills related to exercise are important, and these skills are not part of the competencies required by a health educator. As a result, health educators preparing for employment in worksite health promotion

BOX **7.4**

Practitioner's Perspective

Name:	Robert Pabst
Title:	Health/Fitness Technician
Employer:	Tri-Health, Preventive Health Systems
Degree:	B.S. University of Cincinnati
Major:	Health Promotion & Education
Emphasis:	Exercise Leadership

Job responsibilities: I conduct consultations with current as well as new members on their exercise programs. Consultations may include an overview of what the fitness center has to offer, equipment orientations, and exercise recommendations. As a fitness technician, I also conduct general fitness assessments, which include body fat analysis, cardiovascular endurance testing, flexibility testing, and muscular strength testing. I also share responsibility with other fitness center employees for equipment maintenance and cleaning.

What do you like most about your job? I enjoy getting to know the people I work with and especially the members who use our services. It keeps the work interesting and informative. I also enjoy doing fitness assessments/prescriptions and watching people progress through the different levels of fitness. Keeping an eye on the members' progress is especially exciting, because I can see the members improving their health and feeling better about themselves in the process.

What do you like least about your job? Mostly, I do not like the tedious, repetitive aspects of the work. The towels always need to be washed and folded, and exercise machines always need to be cleaned. Fortunately, the staff all pitch in to accomplish these tasks, and the teamwork shows. I also get tired of all the paperwork we have to do, but I guess it all comes with the territory.

How did you obtain your current position? Early in my senior year, I looked at several internship opportunities. Tri-Health is the largest corporate health contractor in the area, and I felt it provided me with the best opportunity to receive a job after the internship, so I applied. I was placed at Proctor and Gamble's Health Care Research Center in Mason, Ohio. At the conclusion of the internship, I applied for several positions within the company. It took about a month before it found a position where I could fit in, and it turned out to be at the General Electric Aircraft Engine's Fitness Center, which is only five miles from where I live.

What recommendations would you give to a health education student who would someday like to obtain a position similar to yours? The best recommendation that I can give is to get as much practical experience in as many places as possible. Volunteering is a great option, but just anything that leads to a related learning experience is important. Another thing I recommend is to start planning early for your internship. In Cincinnati, there were plenty of internship opportunities, but the best ones go early, so do not waste your time. Start planning and making contacts at the beginning of your senior year.

should strongly consider a minor or second major in exercise science. Beyond exercise expertise, a master's degree is also required for many entry-level health promotion/education positions in business and industry. In addition to the Certified Health Education Specialist (CHES) credential, certifications more specific to exercise are available from the American College of Sports Medicine and may be required at some worksite settings. The Association for Worksite Health Promotion is in the process of developing an additional certification for worksite health promotion providers and directors. Certifications for specific aspects of worksite health promotion, such as aerobic dance, first aid, and CPR, and for smoking cessation instructors are also available and encouraged. In general, the more degrees, certifications, and credentials one has, the better one will compete in the job market.

A Day in the Career of a Worksite Health Educator

The day begins early for Alisa. The fitness center opens promptly at 5:00 A.M. so that those employees who start to work at 6:00 A.M. can have time to work out prior to beginning their shift. Alisa has to be there at 4:45 A.M. to open the doors, turn on the lights, and greet the first members. The first two hours of her day are spent working the floor. This means she greets members as they enter the facility; walks around the machines, providing instruction where needed; chats with the members; answers health-related questions; and basically makes everyone feel important and welcome. By 7:00, all of the shift workers have left the fitness facility and, by 8:00, most of the managerial employees have cleared out.

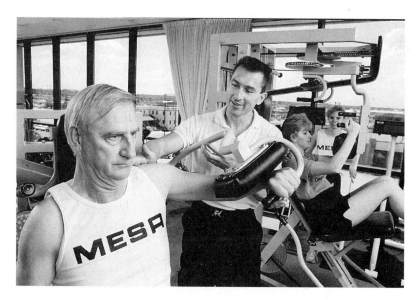

Health educators are employed by business and industry to provide programs to improve the health of employees. (Charles Thatcher/Tony Stone Images)

From 9:00 to 11:00 is a slow time in the center. A few retired employees and a couple spouses use the machines, but this is basically the time for Alisa to get other tasks done. She begins by laundering the dirty towels and folding those that come out of the dryer. Next she provides the routine maintenance to the machines. This involves cleaning them with disinfectant and applying a lubricant to the moving parts. Once this is completed, Alisa has about an hour to work at her desk. Today she is writing an article on the different types of dietary fats to be included in the Wellness Center newsletter she publishes each month. The newsletter is distributed to all active employees and retirees of the company. Alisa is always amazed at how important writing skills are to her position in worksite health promotion.

Between 11:00 and 12:15, Alisa teaches two aerobics classes for the employees. The first is a beginners' class for new members. The second is supposed to be a more advanced class. Unfortunately, many of the shift employees have no choice in their lunch time, so Alisa ends up with some very advanced members in the beginners' class and some beginners in the advanced class. This is frustrating and could be avoided if there were another fitness center employee. There are, however, only two employees in the center, and Rob, the other health educator, must work the floor with the lunch crowd while Alisa teaches. Alisa is going to pursue the possibility of hiring a part-time aerobics instructor just for the lunch hours. This would allow her to offer a beginning and an advanced class at each time slot.

From 12:15 to 1:00, Alisa runs an ongoing support group for employees trying to lose weight. All participants bring a brown bag lunch that is supposed to contain food appropriate for a weight-loss diet. They weigh in weekly, and Alisa provides each participant with a voluntary body composition (fat vs. lean) analysis every three months. At least twice a week, Alisa prepares a twenty-minute lecture on a weight-loss topic or invites a guest speaker from the community.

At 1:00 the employees are back at their work stations, and there is again a quiet time in the health promotion center. Alisa spends the next hour eating lunch at her desk and working on a new incentive program for employees to join the health promotion center that will be offered next month. She has to develop all of the brochures, promotional material, and registration forms and arrange for the purchase of incentive items.

At 2:00 she has a meeting with upper management of the company. She has been encouraging the company to establish a no-smoking policy for the past five years. Two years ago, the company did restrict smoking to specified smoking areas, which was a major accomplishment. Today she will present a proposal to phase out all smoking over a one-year period. Alisa would be responsible for offering several smoking cessation classes over the twelve month period prior to the no-smoking policy taking effect.

By 2:30 she is back in the health promotion center. The second shift employees are in the center now ahead of their shifts, so Alisa is again working the floor. Today she has to do initial fitness assessments on three new employees. This involves running the employees through a standardized series of tests. Based on the results of these tests, she prescribes an individualized exercise program for each employee. She then takes the employees through the fitness center and teaches them how to use the equipment and maintain a record of their progress.

By 3:30 Alisa is finished with the assessments. Since she had the early shift, opening the facility, she is finished for the day. Rob, who came in later, will stay and close the facility at 7:00.

Additional Responsibilities

The responsibilities involved in working in a corporate health promotion center are many and varied. In some facilities, maintaining records such as who is using the center, which programs are most popular, fitness assessment results, and health profiles is a major task. There are always many little things that need to be done, such as the creation and updating of bulletin boards, equipment maintenance, and towel distribution and laundering. Many times, annual health fairs and company-wide health screenings are the responsibility of the health promotion staff.

In addition to being employed in the corporate world, health educators with an exercise background can also seek employment in a host of other settings. See Table 7.7 for a partial listing of opportunities and Table 7.8.

Health Education in Health Care Settings

Positions are available for health educators in a variety of **health care settings,** including public and for-profit hospitals, free-standing medical care clinics that provide both routine and emergency services, home health agencies that provide

TABLE 7.7   Employment Opportunities in Health Education with an Emphasis in Exercise and Fitness

Corporations, business, and industry
Corporate/industrial parks
YMCAs/YWCAs
Private health and fitness clubs
Special population clubs (women, elderly, etc.)
Community parks & recreation programs
Colleges/universities
Hospitals
Sports medicine centers
Entrepreneurial enterprises (aerobics studios, consulting, club owner)
Fitness product/service companies (sales and marketing)
Condos and apartment complexes
Hotels
Spas
Resorts and cruise lines

TABLE 7.8   Advantages and Disadvantages of Worksite Health Education

Advantages

■ It affords excellent opportunities for prevention. It provides access to individuals who may not participate in community programs.

■ Health educators work with multiple and diverse groups of people, including everyone from upper management to shift workers.

■ Most health educators in the corporate setting enjoy their positions and report a high degree of job satisfaction.

■ Pay is usually higher than in other health education settings. Benefits are usually good, but they vary considerably from employer to employer.

■ Health educators have access to fitness facilities for personal use.

Disadvantages

■ Hours are long and irregular. To cover employees on all shifts in a company may necessitate health educators' working hours very early in the morning or late in the evening. It is not unusual to work more than eight hours a day.

■ Upward mobility may be a problem. Typically, there is only one or two managerial positions in health promotion at any given worksite. This makes it difficult for health educators to move up. In addition, those holding managerial positions as directors of health and fitness have nowhere to move up in a company unless they are willing to get out of the health promotion field.

■ Health promotion programs and fitness centers often seem to be low on a company's priority list. Such programs are often the first to receive budget cuts in difficult times and often seem to be short the staff necessary to run optimal programs.

■ Some companies subcontract their health promotion and fitness programs to outside vendors. Some of these outside vendors hire part-time employees, pay lower wages, and provide few or no benefits.

■ Health educators have strong pressure to be extremely fit and healthy role models for other employees.

in-home care designed to replace or reduce the need for more expensive hospitalization, and physician organizations such as health maintenance organizations (HMOs) and preferred provider organizations (PPOs) (Breckon, Harvey, & Lancaster, 1994).

In hospitals and other health care settings, health educators have been hired to direct health and fitness programs for company employees, much the same as in other worksite settings (Breckon, Harvey, & Lancaster, 1994). Sometimes these programs are also open as an outreach service to community members. Other times, health educators are responsible for developing and conducting health and fitness programs specifically designed for community members.

Health educators have also been used in health care settings to provide patient education. For example, a patient is diagnosed with heart disease. That patient is then referred to the health educator for information about exercise, nutrition, weight control, stress management, smoking cessation, and so on. This could involve one-on-one education or counseling sessions with the patient, or it

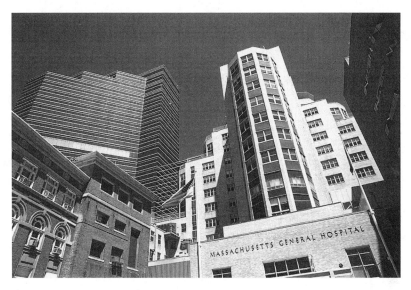

Hospitals employ health educators to provide programs for employees, patients, or the community at large. (Michael A. Dwyer, Stock, Boston)

might involve group programs in which multiple patients receive the same program at the same time.

Unfortunately, patient education has not emerged as a major source of employment for health educators. Although it seems like an ideal activity for health educators, health insurance companies do not typically reimburse for the services of a health educator. Thus, many patient education positions have gone to nurses who can also serve other functions in the health care setting. While health insurance companies are certainly concerned about reducing health care costs, their strategies to date have been more short-term. The impact of health promotion and education programs may not be seen for years, and cause and effect relationships are difficult to establish. Therefore, without the availability of third-party payment, there is a major disincentive for hospitals, clinics, and private practice physicians to offer health promotion and education services to their patients (Hale & Greenberg, 1989).

Of all health care settings, HMOs have been most receptive to hiring health educators. The first HMOs were established in the 1970s as a result of federal money that was made available to help with start-up costs and to study the effectiveness of this health care delivery mechanism. In essence, patients belonging to an HMO pay one set fee for all their medical services in a given year. It therefore benefits the HMO to provide preventive health services and health education programs to keep their patients healthy. The fewer services a patient uses, the greater the cost benefit to the HMO. In the initial HMO legislation, one of the criteria for establishing an HMO was providing health education. Unfortunately, there were no stipulations on the professional preparation of the health education provider.

Often, nurses or other individuals with no health education preparation or experience were given the responsibility of providing health education programs. As a result, some HMOs have developed outstanding health education programs with health educators, while others do very little.

There is, however, reason to be optimistic about future employment opportunities in health care settings for health educators. With changes in the medical care system rapidly occurring, the increased emphasis on cost-cutting measures, and movement toward more managed care, it is likely that prevention will take a higher profile in the future. As these changes occur, health educators will be the best-prepared professionals to assume responsibility for helping individuals adopt healthy lifestyles.

A Day in the Career of a Health Care Setting Health Educator

Mary's day begins at 8:30, when she arrives at the hospital, picks up her mail, and proceeds to her office. She is the only health educator employed by this large metropolitan hospital, but she does have a secretary/assistant who works closely with her to carry out the duties of the position.

At 9:00 Mary has to attend the weekly staff meeting. This is a meeting with all department heads at the hospital. Much of the agenda does not concern Mary directly, but it is important for her to know what is going on in all departments. At today's meeting, it was decided to have an open house for the public to see the newly renovated obstetrics wing of the hospital. Mary is given the responsibility of planning and advertising this event.

At 10:00 Mary has an appointment with the administrative head of the Cardiac Rehabilitation Program at the hospital. The purpose of the meeting is to begin planning the development of two brochures that will eventually be distributed to all cardiac rehabilitation patients. One brochure will be on stress-management strategies, and the other on different types of dietary fat. They brainstorm ideas, and Mary agrees to develop a rough draft of the content of the brochures for the administrative head to review prior to their next meeting. They will also discuss graphics, layout, and production at the next meeting.

At 11:00 Mary leaves the hospital to drive to one of the local malls. The mall has decided to conduct a three-day health fair, and the hospital has agreed to be a cosponsor of the event. Today is a planning meeting for all of the agencies and businesses that will participate. In addition to serving on the planning committee, Mary is responsible for setting up the hospital's display and coordinating nurses and physicians to work in several screening stations. During the health fair, Mary will be at the hospital's booth all day, handing out materials, answering questions, and promoting the hospital's community outreach health promotion programs.

After lunch, Mary returns to the hospital around 1:00 and spends the next two hours working on the hospital's health and wellness newsletter. As a public service and to promote the hospital, Mary is responsible for developing a

BOX **7.5**

Practitioner's Perspective

Name:	Jill Sinclair Hopkins
Title:	Health Educator
Employer:	Franciscan Health System of the Ohio Valley, Inc.
Degree:	B.S., University of Cincinnati
Major:	Health Promotion & Education
Emphasis:	Community Health

Job responsibilities: I am responsible for coordinating all internal wellness programs for hospital employees. In addition, I help plan, design, implement, teach, and evaluate health education programs offered by the hospital for the community at large. I am certified to teach CPR, first aid, Smoke Stoppers, I Can Cope Cancer Support, and the ACS Fresh Start programs. I sit on various community action committees, write articles, develop ad layouts, and conduct promotional campaigns for health education programs.

What do you like most about your job? There is always something different to do in my job. No two days are ever the same, and I never get bored. The people I work with have a positive energy, and I enjoy being around them. I feel good about the type of work I do and how it impacts people's lives.

What do you like least about your job? I really do not like the long hours, which includes many nights and some weekends. To be successful, we must offer programs when people are available to attend them. There is also a side to my job that is unpredictable—some programs are successful; others are not. This can be very stressful. I often feel I have to explain my job, as many people do not understand what I do. People in the hospital often assume I have a nursing background. While we are not a revenue-generating program, we must justify that we save the hospital money.

How did you obtain your current position? I obtained my job directly through my internship. I did my internship in another department of the hospital, which does prenatal and lactation education. While in the internship, I met the director of the community health education program. When the internship was completed, a position opened up in the community health education program. I applied for the position and was hired.

What recommendations would you give to a health education student who would some day like to obtain a position similar to yours? Take your internship seriously, and get as many certifications as possible. While in school, get involved in school-related activities. I was president of our Eta Sigma Gamma chapter while in school, and this allowed me to practice some of the skills that were being taught in our program and helped me to get to know the faculty on a more personal level. Take advantage of independent studies and/or electives related to topics that interest you and relate to your field.

newsletter every other month that is mailed to all households in the hospital's immediate service area. Each edition of the newsletter features one department in the hospital and contains several additional articles about health and wellness. Mary writes much of each newsletter, using information she obtains from the Internet as well as a variety of health journals and newsletters she subscribes to regularly. She designs and formats the newsletter with a desktop publishing program she has on her computer. She marvels at how important the computer is to her everyday functioning.

At 3:00 Mary leads a weight-loss support group for hospital employees. Most of the participants are nurses and housekeeping staff from either the first or second shift. At each session, participants weigh in, share their experiences over the previous week, and listen to a thirty-minute presentation designed to enhance their weight-loss program. Mary is responsible for each week's presentation. In addition, she provides participants with healthy recipes, exercise tips, motivational incentives, and recognition awards.

After class, Mary answers phone calls and ties up loose ends until it is time for her to go home at 5:00. It is not unusual for Mary to take some work home in the evenings or on weekends. Tonight, however, Mary must return to the hospital at 7:30 to teach a stress-management class for the community. The stress class is part of the hospital's ongoing community outreach program. Each month a different health topic is taught, and Mary is responsible for either teaching the class or lining up the instructor for the class.

Additional Responsibilities

Health educators working in health care settings are involved in numerous and varied activities. The actual responsibilities can vary greatly from one health care setting to another. Planning, implementing, and evaluating programs and events are certainly major tasks. Health educators may also be involved in grant writing, one-on-one or group patient education services, publicity, public relations, employee wellness activities, and various collaborative efforts with other hospital staff, community agencies, or departments of public health.

Administration is a major responsibility of many health educators working in hospitals. They are often hired as managers, directors, or coordinators of programs. Hospitals often adopt a "team" approach to health education, in which doctors, nurses, physical therapists, and other health specialists are all part of the team. Health educators plan and coordinate the programs and serve as resources for the other team members, who actually present the programs. In this type of position, the health educator provides little direct client service (Breckon, Harvey, & Lancaster, 1994). (See Table 7.9.)

Health Education in Colleges and Universities

Colleges and universities have been another source of employment for health educators. Within the college setting, there are typically two types of positions

TABLE 7.9   Advantages and Disadvantages of Health Care Setting

Advantages
- Job responsibilities are highly varied and changing.
- There is increased credibility due to health care connection.
- There is usually a high community profile.
- Health educators work with multiple groups of people.
- Wages and benefits are good.
- There is a high degree of self-satisfaction.

Disadvantages
- Health education may have low status and low priority within health care settings.
- Jobs are difficult to obtain.
- Turf issues over educational responsibilities can develop.
- Hours may be long and irregular.
- Some medical doctors may be difficult to work with.

health educators hold. The first is an academic, or faculty, position and the second is a health educator in a health service or wellness center.

As a faculty member, the health educator typically has three major responsibilities: teaching, community and professional service, and scholarly research. The amount of emphasis on each of these major responsibilities is dependent on the institution. In very large research institutions, faculty may spend most of their time writing grants and conducting research. In smaller four-year colleges, teaching may be the major responsibility. In addition to the major responsibilities, faculty may be asked to advise students, serve on committees, coordinate or lead student groups, attend professional conferences, and accept administrative duties.

The minimum qualifications for working as a faculty member in the college/university setting is usually a doctoral degree in health education. While some junior colleges and small four-year schools may hire faculty with only a master's degree, most faculty positions require the doctorate for tenure track positions. In addition, depending on the position for which one is applying, it may be necessary to have had prior experience or training in school health, community/public health, or worksite health promotion. Holding or being eligible for a Certified Health Education Specialist (CHES) credential is often listed as a preference or requirement for faculty positions.

As a health educator in a university health service or wellness center, the major responsibility is to plan, implement, and evaluate health promotion and education programs for the target population. In some universities, the target population is the students, while in others it is the faculty and staff. Many times programming responsibility is for both groups. In addition to program planning, the health educator may be responsible for maintaining a resource library; counseling one-on-one with students; developing and coordinating a peer education program; speaking to residence hall, fraternity, and sorority groups; conducting incentive programs, and planning special events.

The minimum qualifications for working in a university health service or wellness center typically includes a bachelor's or master's degree in health education. Students interested in working in this setting are advised to work as a volunteer or consider completing a practicum or internship in the campus wellness center while an undergraduate. Many universities have peer education programs in which undergraduate students are trained by the professional health educator to conduct programs for their peers. This type of experience is invaluable, whether or not a student ends up employed in a university health service or wellness center. It would also be a good idea to obtain the CHES credential for work in this area.

International Opportunities

Health education professionals may wish to consider working in foreign countries for all or a portion of their careers. There is great need for professionals with health education skills in many developing countries. These positions often require special dedication, as the living and working conditions may be more challenging than those experienced in the United States. For those so inclined, however, the rewards in terms of personal satisfaction and accomplishment can be tremendous. Further, the experience gained by planning, implementing, and evaluating health promotion and education programs in foreign countries can be invaluable to one's professional development.

Working in developing countries many times requires the health educator to examine different health problems and to try different approaches. For example, instead of helping people reduce high-fat and cholesterol diets, as in the United States, the health educator may be helping people deal with problems of starvation, malnutrition, and parasitic and bacterial infections. Instead of dealing with heart disease and lung cancer, the health educator in a developing country may be facing schistosomiasis, diarrhea, and ascaris and tapeworm infections.

Consider the case of Sofia. Sofia was working as a community health educator for the health department in a rural community of about two thousand people in a developing country. The water source for this community consisted of several large ponds. These ponds were the only source of drinking water and were also used for bathing, clothes washing, and care of animals. Many people were getting sick with severe diarrhea, and there had been several deaths among the elderly and very young. To alleviate this problem, it was decided to develop an educational campaign to get people to boil their water prior to consumption. Sofia was given the responsibility for developing this campaign. There was no local newspaper or radio stations and, no billboards, and many of the people could not read. After consulting with local leaders, it was decided that the best way to get out the information would be to use a "mobile communication system." This was accomplished by hooking up an old stereo system to a car battery and driving around the community, broadcasting information about the importance of boiling water. In addition, Sofia set up several demonstrations around the community about

TABLE 7.10   International Health Organizations

National Council for International Health
American Association for World Health
World Health Organization (WHO)
Pan American Health Organization
U.S. Agency for International Development (A.I.D.)

how to boil water effectively. These sessions were also advertised via the "mobile communication system."

As can be seen from Sofia's experience, health educators working in foreign countries must be able to develop creative, innovative programs to solve identified health problems. Most often, these programs must be low-cost, easily developed and implemented, acceptable to the social norms of the community, and available to all aspects of the public. It is imperative that these programs be developed in conjunction with the local people being served. It is also helpful when programs are sponsored by organizations seen as credible by the target population.

One of the best ways to begin a career in international health is to volunteer with the Peace Corps. Health education professionals are in demand by the Peace Corps, and students should begin the application process during their senior year. Many colleges and universities are visited by Peace Corps recruiters every year, and talking to one of these Peace Corps volunteers is a good place to start. There may also be faculty members on your campus that were former Peace Corps volunteers, and talking to these individuals can provide valuable insight into the Peace Corps experience.

There are many advantages to volunteering with the Peace Corps. The Peace Corps provides volunteers with some of the best language and technical training in the world. Each Peace Corps volunteer is granted a monthly allowance for housing, food, clothing, and miscellaneous expenses. Free dental and medical care are provided, as well as free transportation to the placement setting and twenty-four vacation days per year. After completing the two-year experience, volunteers are given a postservice readjustment allowance of $5,400. They are also given preference for federal jobs and have enhanced scholarship and assistantship opportunities at more than fifty major colleges and universities. In addition, successful Peace Corps experience may serve as a stepping-stone to paid positions in other international health organizations (see Table 7.10).

Nontraditional Health Education Positions

In addition to the traditional settings for health education that have been described in this chapter, there are also a variety of nontraditional jobs health educators may wish to consider. These positions may or may not carry the title of health educator. In some cases, they require the health educator to use the skills and competencies in different or unique ways. Further, it is often necessary for health educators to sell themselves to get these positions, as the persons doing the hiring may be unfamiliar with the skills and training of a health educator.

Given health educators' knowledge of health and fitness, sales positions related to health are a real possibility. Pharmacy sales, fitness equipment sales, and the sales of health-related textbooks are all areas in which health educators have found employment. Life and health insurance are two additional options to consider in the area of sales.

By emphasizing the communication competencies that are part of the professional training in health education, the health educator may seek employment in journalism, TV, or radio. Many television stations have a regular health or medical reporter who does feature stories on health-related issues. Newspapers may have a health column that could and should be written by a health educator. Again, it is necessary for health educators to sell themselves to obtain these positions. Taking elective classes in media, communications, and journalism and doing one's internship in these settings may also assist those interested in this career field.

Health educators should always be alert to unique job opportunities, many of which may not even carry the title of health educator. One health educator, for example, was hired by a state mental hospital as a "Teacher II." His job was to teach drug education to patients who had a history of drug problems and sex education to patients who had a history of sex problems. The remainder of his work schedule involved tutoring patients in math and science who were studying to obtain their high school general equivalency diploma.

Landing That First Job

At first, it may seem unusual to discuss landing one's first job while still an undergraduate in an introductory course, but this is the best time to consider the issue of future employment. There are several actions students can take during their undergraduate years to enhance their chances of obtaining employment. By following the suggestions made in this section, a student will be far ahead of those who wait until the end of their bachelor's degree program to address these issues.

No matter in what setting a health educator hopes to eventually work, landing the first job can be a frustrating experience. Students often find themselves in a dilemma. Employers want their new employees to have had "experience," but where are students supposed to get experience if they can't get hired? There are several possible answers to this question. One way to gain experience is to obtain part-time or summer employment in one's preferred health education setting. Typically, there are many more students looking for this type of employment than there are employment situations. Should such an opportunity be available, however, it is an excellent way to get experience prior to graduation. Another way to obtain experience is to volunteer time in the chosen health education setting. Most professional health educators working in the field are more than willing to accept and use the volunteer time of health education students. In addition to experience, volunteering also begins the important process of **networking.** Networking involves establishing and maintaining a wide range of contacts in the field that may be of help when looking for a job and in carrying out one's job responsibilities once hired.

Carefully planning internships and practicums can help students obtain their first professional position. Required field experiences are often the best way to obtain practical experience in one's chosen setting. Students should consider what they would like to be doing five years after graduation and select an experience that closely matches that goal. Often students are hired by the agency after completing their practicum or internship experience.

In addition to obtaining experience, students should strive to obtain an excellent academic record. When there is heavy competition for an open position, one of the first strategies in making hiring decisions is to examine grade point average. This is not to say that the person with the highest grade point average is always the best person or that the person with the highest grade point average will always get the job. But, when there are fifty applications for one job, grade point average is an easy way to begin limiting the field.

Consider what certifications are going to be important in landing your first job and carefully plan to make sure they are awarded either prior to graduation or as soon after graduation as possible. All professional health educators should pursue the CHES credential. In the future, this may be a prerequisite for many health promotion and education positions. Depending on one's work setting and job responsibilities, other certifications should be obtained as needed.

Get to know your faculty. They are a great source of information about jobs and how to compete for them successfully. Often employers contact faculty directly, asking for the names of students who might be interested in a particular position. Unless a faculty member knows a student by name and knows that the student is in the job market, there is little the faculty member can do.

Most colleges and universities have placement centers that provide a variety of services to students. They may assist with developing the resume, maintain a list of job openings, provide workshops or handouts on interviewing skills, and establish reference files for students. It would be a good idea to contact the placement center well before graduation to determine when and how to access its services.

A final suggestion is to join one or more of the professional associations (see Chapter 8). Employers are typically impressed when they see that a young professional has been a member of the professional organization and perhaps has attended several professional meetings. If your campus has a chapter of Eta Sigma Gamma, the professional health education honorary, try to get involved. Eta Sigma Gamma recognizes high academic achievement, provides opportunities to obtain valuable leadership experience, and allows students to plan, implement, and evaluate various service projects and social activities.

Summary

There are many settings in which a health educator can seek employment. In this chapter, we have discussed in detail health education positions in schools, community/public health agencies, worksites, health care facilities, colleges and universities, and international settings. In addition, we have examined the potential for employment in nontraditional settings and have considered what introductory-level undergraduate students can do to help themselves land that first job.

REVIEW QUESTIONS

1. Identify four major settings and two non-traditional settings in which health educators are employed.

2. Compare and contrast the roles and responsibilities of health educators working in schools, community/public health agencies, worksites, and health care facilities. How are all of these settings similar? How are they different?

3. What is the difference between a position funded with hard money and a position funded with soft money? Which position is preferable and why?

4. Explain why it might be said that health education has never reached its real potential in the health care setting. What factors have kept health education positions at a minimal level in this setting?

5. What is networking and why is it important in health education?

6. What can introductory-level health education students do now that might help them land their first job after graduation?

ACTIVITIES

1. Select the one setting you think you would most like to work in. Develop a short essay describing why you prefer this setting to other health education settings.

2. Visit a health education professional who works in the setting in which you would most like to be employed. Develop a job description for this person's position that explains the qualifications and responsibilities needed for the job.

3. Examine the classified ads of a major city Sunday newspaper. Circle in red those jobs you find that specifically ask for a health educator. Next look through the same classified ads and circle in blue those that do not ask for a health educator but that require the same competencies and skills of a health educator.

4. Interview someone who is responsible for hiring health educators. Find out what that person looks for in a letter of application, a vita, and a personal interview.

5. Contact the placement office at your institution. Determine what services it offers and when these services should accessed.

REFERENCES

Allensworth, D., & Kolbe, L. (1987). The comprehensive school health program: Exploring an expanded concept. *Journal of School Health, 57,* 409–412.

Allensworth, D., Lawson, E., Nicholson, L., & Wyche, J., (Eds.). (1997). *Schools & health: Our nation's investment.* Washington, DC: National Academy Press.

Association for the Advancement of Health Education (AAHE). (1990). *Health education works!* (Video), Reston, VA.

Breckon, J., Harvey, J.R., & Lancaster, R.B. (1994). *Community health education: Settings, roles, and skills for the 21st century.* Gaithersburg, MD: Aspen Publishers.

English, G.M., & Videto, D.M. (1997). The future of health education: The knowledge to practice paradox. *Journal of Health Education, 28(1),* 4–7.

Fielding, J. & Piserchia, P.V. (1989). Frequency of worksite health promotion activities. *American Journal of Public Health, 79,* 16–20.

Green, L.W., Cook, T.D., Doster, M.E., Fors, S.W., Hambleton, R., Smith, A., & Walberg, H.J. (1985). Thoughts from the School Health Education Advisory Panel. *Journal of School Health, 55(8),* 300.

Hale, J.F., & Greenberg, J.S. (1989). Patient education in primary care settings: A review of the literature. In J.H. Humphrey (Ed.), *Advances in health education* (pp. 195–234). New York: AMS Press.

Joint Committee on Health Education Standards. (1995). *National health education standards: Achieving health literacy.* Atlanta, GA: American Cancer Society.

Joint Committee on Health Education Terminology. (1991). Report of the 1990 Joint Committee on Health Education Terminology. *Journal of Health Education, 22(2),* 97–108.

McKenzie, J.F., & Pinger, R.R. (1997). *An introduction to community health.* Sudbury, MA: Jones and Bartlett.

National Coordinating Committee on Worksite Health Promotion. (1993). *Health promotion goes to work: Programs with an impact.* Washington, DC: U.S. Department of Health and Human Services.

Seffrin, J.A. (1994). Americans' interest in comprehensive school health education. *Journal of School Health, 64(10),* 397–399.

Utah State University. (March 16, 1996). *Careers in health education.* Available: http://www.ed.usu.edu/coe/hper/advising/careers.html

CHAPTER

8 Agencies/Associations/ Organizations Associated with Health Education

CHAPTER OBJECTIVES

After reading this chapter and answering the questions at the end, you should be able to

1. Define each of the following terms and give several examples of each: governmental health agency, quasi-governmental health agency, nongovernmental health agencies.
2. Briefly describe the levels of governmental agencies and provide several examples of each.
3. List and explain the three primary activities of most voluntary health agencies.
4. Explain the purpose of a professional association/organization.
5. Identify the benefits derived from membership in a professional organization.
6. Identify the primary professional associations/organizations and coalitions associated with health education.
7. Describe the process by which a person can become a member of a professional association/organization.

KEY TERMS

American Alliance for Health, Physical Education, Recreation and Dance (AAHPERD)
American Association for Health Education (AAHE)
American College Health Association (ACHA)
American Public Health Association (APHA)
American Red Cross (ARC)
American School Health Association (ASHA)

Association for Worksite Health Promotion (AWHP)
Association of State and Territorial Directors of Health Promotion and Public Health Education (ASTDHPPHE)
Coalition of National Health Education Organizations, USA (CNHEO)
Eta Sigma Gamma (ESG)
governmental health agencies

International Union for Health Promotion and Education (IUHPE)
local health department
National School Health Education Coalition (NaSHEC)
nongovernmental health agencies
philanthropic foundations
professional health associations/organizations

190

| quasi-governmental health agencies | Society of State Directors of Health, Physical Education, and Recreation (SSDHPER) | voluntary health agencies |
| Society for Public Health Education, Inc. (SOPHE) | | |

There are many health agencies, associations, and organizations with which health educators interact. Most of these agencies/associations/organizations were created to help promote, protect, and maintain the health of individuals, families, and communities. For many health educators, these agencies/associations/organizations will be places of employment. These groups regularly hire health educators to plan, implement, evaluate, and coordinate their educational efforts. Health educators not employed by these groups will find them to be valuable sources of up-to-date information and materials. This chapter classifies the agencies/associations/organizations into three major categories: governmental, quasi-governmental, and nongovernmental. Because information on most of these agencies/associations/organizations that support the efforts of health education/promotion is available elsewhere (Green & Ottoson, 1999; McKenzie, Pinger & Kotecki, 1999; Miller & Price, 1998; & Reagan & Brookins-Fisher, 1997) and because this text was written primarily as an introduction to the profession, the primary emphasis of this chapter is on the professional health education associations/organizations.

Governmental Health Agencies

Governmental health agencies, are health agencies that are designated as having authority for certain duties or tasks outlined by the governmental bodies that oversee them. For example, a **local health department** has the authority to protect, promote, and enhance the health of people living in a specific geographical area. It is given this authority by the county or city government that oversees it. Governmental agencies, which are primarily funded by tax dollars (they may also charge fees for services rendered) and managed by government employees, exist at four governmental levels: international, national, state, and local (city and county). Table 8.1 provides examples of governmental agencies and their governing bodies.

Quasi-Governmental Health Agencies

Quasi-governmental health agencies are so named because they possess some of the characteristics of a governmental health agency, but they also possess some of

TABLE 8.1   Governmental Agencies and Their Governing Bodies

Level/Agency	Governing Body
International Level	
World Health Organization (WHO)	United Nations
Pan American Health Organization (PAHO)	An independent agency
National Level	
Department of Health and Human Services (DHHS)*	U.S. government
Environmental Protection Agency (EPA)	U.S. government
State Level	
State health department	Individual state governments
State environmental protection agency	Individual state governments
Local Level	
Local health department (LHD)	City or county governments
Local school districts	Local school boards

*On October 31, 1995, this agency was reorganized (see *Federal Register* of November 9, 1995). Within the department are a number of smaller (sub-) agencies (e.g., Centers for Disease Control and Prevention, Food and Drug Administration, etc.) that may be of particular interest to health education students.

the characteristics of nongovernmental agencies. They obtain their funding from a variety of sources, including community fund-raising efforts such as the United Way, charges for services rendered, donations, and governmental bodies. They carry out tasks that are often thought of as services of governmental agencies, yet they operate independently of governmental supervision.

Probably the best-known quasi-governmental health agency is the **American Red Cross (ARC).** It was founded in 1881 by Clara Barton as an outgrowth of her work during the Civil War. Today, the ARC has several official responsibilities given to it by the federal government, such as (1) acting as the official representative of the United States government during natural disasters (Disaster Services) and (2) serving as the liaison between members of the active armed forces and their families during family emergencies (Services to the Armed Forces and Veterans). The ARC also provides many nongovernmental services such as its blood drives and safety services classes such water safety, first aid, and CPR.

Nongovernmental Health Agencies

Nongovernmental health agencies "operate, for the most part, free from governmental interference as long as they meet Internal Revenue Services guidelines

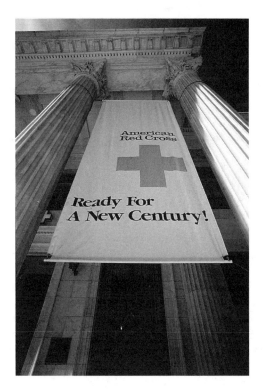

The American Red Cross is one of the best examples of a quasi-governmental agency. (Robert Rathe/Stock, Boston)

with regard to their tax status" (McKenzie & Pinger, 1997, p. 47). They are primarily funded by private donations, or, as in the case with professional and service groups, membership fees. The nongovernmental agencies can be categorized into the following subgroups: voluntary, philanthropic, service, religious, and professional.

Voluntary Health Agencies

Voluntary health agencies are some of the most visible health agencies in a community. Voluntary health agencies are an American creation and grew out of unmet needs in communities. When governmental or quasi-governmental agencies were not in place to meet the needs of communities, interested citizens came together to form voluntary agencies. Such was the case with the American Cancer Society, American Heart Association, American Lung Association, A Better Way, and Mothers Against Drunk Driving (MADD). The number of voluntary agencies seems endless, with agencies for about every disease and part of the body impacted by a disease or an illness. Most voluntary agencies have three primary purposes: (1) raise money to fund research, (2) provide education to both professionals and the public, and (3) provide service to those individuals and families affected by the disease or health problem.

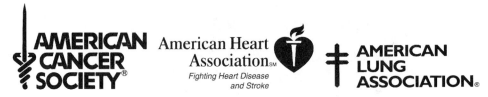

The three largest voluntary health agencies are the American Cancer Society, American Heart Association, and American Lung Association. (Symbols courtesy of organizations shown.)

Philanthropic Foundations

Philanthropic foundations play an important role by funding programs and research on the prevention, control, and treatment of diseases and other health problems. *Philanthropy* means "the effort to promote the happiness or social elevation of mankind, as by making donations" (Landau, 1979, p. 492). Philanthropic foundations differ from voluntary health agencies in two primary ways. First, they were created with an endowment and, thus, do not have to raise money. Second, they are able to finance long-term projects that may be too expensive or risky to be funded by other agencies. Examples of some philanthropic foundations that have supported work by health educators are the Ford Foundation, the Robert Wood Johnson Foundation, and the Rockefeller Foundation.

Service, Fraternal, and Religious Groups

Each of the many different service, fraternal, and religious groups has also been important to health educators. Even though none of these groups has the primary purpose of enhancing the health of a community, they often get involved in health-related projects. Examples of service and fraternal groups (and their health-related projects) include the Kiwanis Club (Quest: Skills for Living), Fraternal Order of the Police (food and clothing donations for the needy), Lions (preservation of sight), Shriners (children's hospitals), and American Legion (community recreation programs).

Religious groups have also contributed to the work of health educators' projects, both on a global level (e.g., the Protestants' One Great Hour of Sharing, the Catholics' Relief Fund, and the United Jewish Appeal) and on a local level (e.g., food pantries, sleeping rooms, soup kitchens).

Professional Health Associations/Organizations

As noted at the beginning of this chapter, the primary focus of this chapter is the professional health associations/organizations. The mission of **professional health associations/organizations** is to promote the high standards of professional practice for their respective profession, thereby improving the health of

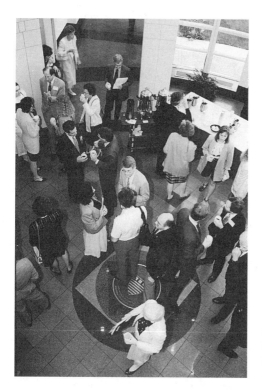

Annual professional conventions are an important benefit of membership in a professional organization. (D. Wells/The Image Works)

society by improving the people in the profession (McKenzie & Pinger, 1997). The mission is carried out by advocating for the profession; keeping the members up-to-date via the publication of professional journals, books, and newsletters; and providing the members with an avenue to come together at professional meetings. At these meetings, members have the opportunity to share and hear the new research findings, network with fellow professionals, and find out more about the latest equipment and published materials in the field. In addition, professional associations/organizations provide their members with "perks" such as reduced rates on insurance (accidental death and dismemberment, auto, cancer, disability, health, hospital, life, long-term care, Medicare Supplement, and professional liability), participation in tax-deferred annuity programs, discounts (annual national conventions, car rental, eye wear, long-distance telephone calls, publications, travel), job placement, and a variety of other associated items.

Professional associations/organizations are comprised, for the most part, of health professionals who have completed specialized education and training and who are eligible for certification/licensure in their respective professions. These associations/organizations are funded primarily by membership dues, but it is becoming more common for these associations/organizations to seek grant funds (soft money) to help promote their missions. Most of these associations/organizations hire staff for day-to-day operations, but the officers of the associations/organizations are usually elected professionals (see Box 8.1).

BOX **8.1**

Practitioner's Perspective

Name:	Cathy Nickels
Current Position/Title:	Cancer Control Manager
Employer:	Marion County (IN) Health Department
Degree:	Bachelor of Science
Major:	Health Science, Community Health emphasis
Minor:	Educational Psychology
Professional association in which you hold an office:	Indiana Association of Health Educators (IAHE)
Office held:	President
Length of term:	One year

Primary responsibilities of the office: Coordinate the functions of the organization: plan and facilitate board meetings, assist in planning of semi-annual meetings, chair nominations committee, assist in maintaining and directing functions of committees and any sub-committees, conduct business meetings associated with semi-annual meetings

How did you get into this office? I was invited to run for the office of president-elect by the nominations committee. The position of president-elect is the first position in a series of three: president-elect, president, and past president, each lasting one year. Once elected president-elect, I then rotated through each of these positions.

Why did you want to hold this office? The profession of health education is currently under-recognized. As a practicing health educator, I feel that membership in professional organizations that support and advance the field are vital to the survival of the profession. I wanted to help motivate professional advancement with my peers. As a member and officer of IAHE, I am able to initiate change and promote efforts that can lead to better opportunities for health educators in Indiana.

What do you like most about holding this office? The most exciting aspect of holding this office was the interaction with peers. Learning more about others' experiences, goals, and aspirations for the health education profession helped revitalize my support of the field. Also, the networking associated with the position provided a number of opportunities for my work and for my personal advancement.

What do you like least about holding this office? Arranging and conducting meetings was the biggest challenge I encountered during my term as president. All of the executive committee members were extremely active in their work, with other professional organizations, and in their personal lives. While their involvement in several different organizations served as a benefit to IAHE, it made planning meetings and getting people to attend meetings a rather complicated challenge.

What recommendations would you give to a health education student who would someday like to hold an office in a professional organization? I consider every bit of the energy and time I have spent as a member and officer in IAHE to have been well spent. Additionally, I strongly encourage all preservice and new professionals to get involved in at least one professional organization. And, if possible, get involved as an officer. However, it is important to keep in mind time commitments and to be aware of how much you can give to an organization. If time restricts your involvement, offer your services in another manner; write letters of support for activities, contribute meeting ideas, participate on a committee, attend at least one membership meeting each year, write for the newsletter, encourage increased membership, and/or assist in implementation of activities. Professional involvement is reciprocal and benefits the individual as much as it benefits others.

In the remaining portions of this chapter, we will present information on the national professional associations/organizations that help promote the health education profession. The reader should also be aware that many of these national associations/organizations have affiliates and other related groups at the regional and/or state level. For example, the American Public Health Association is at the national level, but there are also state associations such as the Ohio Public Health Association. In addition, there are also some state-only organizations that are not affiliated with any national organization. One such example is the Indiana Association of Health Educators. (Ask your instructor if there are any such organizations in your state.) Table 8.2, and Appendix E contain information about the following organizations.

The American Alliance for Health, Physical Education, Recreation, and Dance. The **American Alliance for Health, Physical Education, Recreation, and Dance (AAHPERD)** is an alliance of six national associations (American Association for Active Lifestyles and Fitness, American Association for Health Education, American Association for Leisure and Recreation, National Association for Girls' and Women's Sports, National Association for Sport and Physical Education, National Dance Association) and six district associations (Central, Eastern, Midwest, Northwest, Southern, and Southwest). (Note that the district associations are comprised of AAHPERD members located in the states represented by these parts of the country. Also, states have an affiliate organization of AAHPERD—for example, the Ohio Association of Health, Physical Education, Recreation and Dance. A professional can be a member of both the state and national organizations, or just one or the other.) AAHPERD is several generations of professional organizations removed from its beginning back in 1885, when "Dr. William G. Anderson invited a small group of professionals to meet with him to discuss mutual interests and concerns related to physical training. The purposes of the embryo association, resulting from this meeting, were simply stated: to disseminate knowledge, to improve methods, and to bring those interested in the subject into close relationship with each other" (Anderson, 1985, p. 94). The association continued to grow and turned into the American Physical Education Association (APEA) in 1937. In that year, the APEA "accepted an invitation from the National Education Association (NEA) to merge with its School Health and Physical Education Department to become an NEA Department with three divisions: health, physical education, and recreation" (Anderson, 1985, p. 1). The merger resulted in the formation of the American Association for Health and Physical Education. The word *recreation* was added to the title in 1938, creating AAHPER. In the mid-1960s, the NEA began to feel pressure, because of a challenge from the American Federation of Teachers, to become more active in the welfare movement for teachers. This challenge made the NEA look more closely at its focus. It was supporting thirty departments which had members of their own, most of which were not members of NEA (Anderson, 1985). In 1968, the NEA changed its "bylaws regarding their departments: to remain a department, all its members had to join the NEA: one alternative was to become an affiliated organization, still identified with NEA and paying a small fee for rent and services; another choice was to become an autonomous associated organization paying the full costs of services rendered by NEA" (Anderson, 1985, p. 95). In 1968, AAHPER chose the former. "This status continued until September 1, 1975 when another NEA bylaws change discontinued this affiliated relationship and AAHPER became completely disassociated from NEA" (Anderson, 1985, p. 95). AAHPER added *dance* to its title in 1979 (Anderson, 1985).

Though all the associations in AAHPERD are associated with the promotion of healthy lifestyles, the one most directly related to the discipline of health education is the American Association for Health Education. Therefore, it will be the only one discussed here.

The **American Association for Health Education (AAHE)** is a relatively new name (as of July 1, 1996) for the older organization the Association for the Advancement of Health Education (also AAHE). The Association for the Advancement of Health Education evolved from the School Health Division of AAHPER when the AAHPERD was formed in 1974 (Nolte, 1985). Membership in AAHE is open to current, retired, and student (preparing for careers as) health educators and health promotion specialists regardless of their work setting. Current membership is at approximately 11,000 members. The mission of AAHE "is to advance health by encouraging, supporting, and assisting health professionals concerned with health promotion through education and other systematic strategies" (AAHE, no date-b, p. 1).

The AAHE produces several publications that health educators find very useful. AAHE's peer-reviewed (a journal in which other professionals in the field decide what is published and what is not) "*Journal of Health Education,* published bimonthly, provides penetrating articles on research findings, teaching ideas, community learning strategies, industry trends, and recent resource materials. Many articles are designed as self-study courses, with continuing education questions and response forms built right in" (AAHPERD, no date, p. 2). AAHE's newsletter is called "HE-XTRA." It is published five times per year and updates members on health issues, sample curricula, continuing education programs, association activities, advocacy issues, and career opportunities. In addition, AAHE publishes a bi-annual directory of undergraduate and graduate professional programs in school, community, and public health education (AAHE, 1995).

In recent years, AAHE has been involved in several activities of note:

- AAHE Professional Health Education Network (ProNet). Established in 1990, ProNet "organizes professional development activities in a manner that will make such programs easier to access" (AAHE, no date-a, p. 1). This allows health educators who are Certified Health Education Specialists (CHESs) to obtain needed continuing education contact hours directly from AAHE.
- SOPHE/AAHE Baccalaureate Program Approval Committee (SABPAC). A joint committee of SOPHE and AAHE "responsible for directing and carrying out the undergraduate program approval process for eligible college and university programs preparing undergraduate preservice health education specialists" (AAHE, no date-a, p. 1).
- AAHE/ASHA Committee on Health Education Preparation Responsibilities and Competencies for Elementary Teachers. In January 1990, AAHE and ASHA formed a joint committee to establish guidelines to prepare elementary teachers in health education. The resulting guidelines were titled "Health Instruction Responsibilities and Competencies for Elementary (K–6) Classroom Teachers" (AAHE, no date-a).
- NCATE/AAHE. The National Council for Accreditation of Teacher Education (NCATE) has allowed AAHE to be the professional health education association/organization to be responsible for reviewing folios submitted to NCATE by colleges and universities when they are seeking NCATE accreditation for their teacher education programs.
- The development of the AAHE Code of Ethics, which outlines conduct for ethical health education research and practice. This code was developed in 1994. (See Appendix C for a copy.)

American Public Health Association. The **American Public Health Association (APHA)** is the oldest and largest of the professional associations/organizations discussed in this chapter. The APHA was founded in 1872 "as a result of the public health movement to combat yellow fever and other diseases in the 1870s" (APHA, no date, p. 3). The purposes of the APHA are "to protect and promote personal and environmental health; to exercise leadership with health professionals and the general public in health policy development and action, with particular focus on the interrelationship between health and the quality of life and on developing a national policy for health care and services and on solving technical problems" (Cauffman, 1982, p. 93).

Membership in the APHA is open to professional, student/trainee, and retired health workers, as well as consumers who are interested in supporting the

TABLE 8.2   Information about Key Professional Associations/Organizations

American Alliance for Health, Physical Education, Recreation and Dance (AAHPERD)

Address:
1900 Association Drive
Reston, VA 20191-1599

Telephone:
800/213-7193
703/476-3404

Facsimile:
703/476-9527

Internet:
membrshp@aahperd.org
http://www.aahperd.org

American Association for Health Education (AAHE)

Address:
1900 Association Drive
Reston, VA 20191-1599

Telephone:
703/476-3437

Facsimile:
703/476-6638

Internet:
aahe@aahperd.org
http://www.aahperd.org

American College Health Association (ACHA)

Address:
P.O. Box 28937
Baltimore, MD 21240-8937

Telephone:
410/859-1500

Facsimile:
410/859-1510

Internet:
acha@access.digex.net
http://www.acha.org

American Public Health Association (APHA)

Address:
1015 Fifteenth Street, NW
Washington, DC 20005

Telephone:
202/789-5674
202/789-6573 (TDD)

Facsimile:
202/274-4577

Internet:
comments@msmail.apha.org
http://www.apha.org

American School Health Association (ASHA)

Address:
7263 State Route 43
P.O. Box 708
Kent, OH 44240

Telephone:
330/678-1601

Facsimile:
330/678-4526

Internet:
treed@ashaweb.org
http://www.asha.web.org

Association for Worksite Health Promotion (AWHP)

Address:
60 Revere Drive, Suite 500
Northbrook, IL 60062

Telephone:
847/480-9574

Facsimile:
847/480-9282

Internet:
tsgi@aol.com
http://www.awhp.com

Eta Sigma Gamma (ESG)

Address:
2000 University Avenue
Muncie, IN 47306

Telephone:
800/715-2559
765/285-2258

Facsimile:
765/285-2351

Internet:
etasigmagam@bsu.edu
http://www.cast.ilstu.edu/temple/esg.htm

International Union for Health Promotion and Education (IUHPE)

International Office
Address:
2, Rue Auguste Comte
92170 Vanves (Paris), France

Telephone:
(33) (1) 46 45 00 59

Facsimile:
(33) (1) 46 45 00 45

Internet:
iuhpemcl@worldnet.fr

North American Regional Office
Address:
c/o APHA, 1015 15th Street, NW, Suite 300
Washington, DC 20005

Telephone:
c/o AAHE, 703/476-3437

Facsimile:
c/o AAHE, 703/476-6638

Internet:
c/o AAHE, aahe@aahperd.org

Society for Public Health Education, Inc. (SOPHE)

Address:
1015 Fifteenth Street, NW, Suite 410
Washington, DC 20005

Telephone:
202/408-9804

Facsimile:
202/408-9815

Internet:
sopheauld@aol.com

mission of the association. Currently, the approximately 32,000 members come from seventy-seven disciplines in public health and related fields. Once individuals become members, they have the opportunity to select one or more of the sub-groups of the organization. These sub-groups are referred to as section, or special primary interest, groups. They allow members to pursue specific professional interests and provide the technical and scientific foundations for the association activities. More specifically, these sub-groups propose policy statements, advise on publications, provide testimony and reports, help develop the content and structure of annual meetings, and assist in APHA governence (APHA, no date). The sections most closely related to health education are (1) Public Health Education Section, which formed in 1922 and in 1991 changed its name to Public Health Education and Health Promotion Section, and (2) School Health Education Section, which formed in 1942 and in 1980 changed its name to School Health Education and Services Section. The purpose of the Public Health Education and Health Promotion Section (CNHEO, 1996, p. 15) is

- To provide a unit within the framework of APHA for consideration and inclusion of public health education and promotion in health programs and in the efforts of APHA
- To provide for the coordination of the activities within the section and collaboration with the APHA boards, committees, sections, and affiliates
- To provide APHA with recommendations about public health education and health promotion and serve as a medium through which the section may obtain recommendations about concerns of APHA
- To stimulate thought, discussion, and research concerning health problems in which public health education is involved and to investigate approaches for their solution
- To provide opportunities for improving health education and promotion within the broad perspective of public health
- To promote the recognition of outstanding individuals who have made substantial contributions to, and have demonstrated leadership in, public health education and promotion

The purpose of the School Health Education and Services Section (CNHEO, 1996, p. 11) is

- To provide a section within the association which works independently, with other association substructures, and with external organizations toward the improvement of early childhood, school, and college health programs
- To interpret the functions and responsibilities of health agencies to daycare, preschool, school, and college personnel
- To interpret early childhood, school, and college health education and service objectives to other public health personnel and assist them in integrating the objectives in their community
- To provide a forum for discussion of practices and research in early childhood, school, and college health
- To encourage the provision of health promotion programs within the school and college settings which address the needs of children and school personnel
- To encourage among interested association members the study and discussion of procedures and problems in early childhood, school, and college health services, health education, and environmental health programs

The primary publication of APHA is the *American Journal of Public Health (AJPH)*. This peer-reviewed journal is published monthly. A typical issue of the *AJPH* includes editorials, commentaries, book reviews, job announcements, notification of upcoming meetings, and authoritative articles in both general and specialized areas of research, policy analysis, and program evaluation of public health. Areas covered in the articles include the environment, maternal and child health, health promotion, epidemiology, administration, occupational health, education, international health, statistics, and more (APHA, 1996). The association also publishes *The Nation's Health* eleven times per year. This newspaper includes reporting on current and proposed legislation, policy issues, news of actions within the federal agencies and Congress, and special features. The publication also includes association news, job openings, and information on upcoming conferences. In addition to the *AJPH* and *The Nation's Health,* the APHA also publishes books on a variety of public health topics. Examples include the best-selling titles *Control of Communicable Disease Manual* (Benenson, 1995) and *Healthy Communities 2000: Model Standards* (APHA, 1991).

There are other professional health associations that have a more focused mission. Some of those include the American College Health Association (ACHA), the American School Health Association (ASHA), the Association for Worksite Health Promotion (AWHP), and the Society for Public Health Education, Inc. (SOPHE).

American College Health Association. The **American College Health Association (ACHA)** was founded originally as the American Student Health Association in 1920. In 1948, the name of the association was changed to its current name. "The association's mission is to be the principal advocate and leadership organization for the college health field. It is committed to providing advocacy, education, and service for its members to enhance their ability to improve the health of all students" (ACHA, no date, p. 4). The association has two distinct types of memberships. One is for institutions of higher education. Currently, there are more than 900 such members. ACHA also serves more than three thousand individual members who are interested in college health—that is, the health of college students. Included in the members are physicians, nurses, psychologists, health educators, college and university administrators, student affairs personnel, and students, both as preprofessionals and as consumers (*Scope and Guidelines for Contributors*, 1992). Most of these members are associated with the health service facilities on their respective campuses.

Like some of the other associations/organizations, the ACHA also has subgroups. "On the regional and state level, ACHA recognizes six regions comprised of a total of 11 affiliate organizations. These affiliates play an important role in helping college health providers forge strong links with colleagues in their state or region. For example, each affiliate conducts an annual meeting, which is typically a prime networking opportunity for all levels of staff" (ACHA, no date, p. 5). In addition, ACHA has ten membership sections, which are defined by the disciplines of college health. The Health Education Section was formed in 1958.

"ACHA publishes several newsletters, numerous health information brochures, and other special publications. The cornerstone of ACHA's publishing effort is the membership newsletter 'Action'. This quarterly publication features articles on legislative issues, the latest association offerings, and general news briefs" (ACHA, no date, p. 6). The professional journal of the ACHA is the *Journal of American College Health.* It is published bi-monthly and is the only journal devoted entirely to the health of college students. The journal publishes articles encompassing many areas of college health, "including clinical and preventive medicine, dentistry, environmental health, health promotion and education, management and administration, mental health, nursing, and sports medicine" (*Scope and Guidelines for Contributors,* 1992, p. 308).

American School Health Association. The **American School Health Association (ASHA)** began on October 27, 1927, as the American Association of School Physicians. It began to use its current name in 1936 (ASHA, 1976). The mission of the ASHA

> is to protect and improve the well-being of children and youth by supporting comprehensive school health programs. These programs significantly affect the health of all students, in preschool through grade twelve, and the health of school personnel who serve them. School health programs prevent, detect, address and resolve health problems, increase educational achievement and enhance the quality of life. The Association works to improve school health education, school health services and school health environments. The Association also works to support and integrate school counseling, psychological and social services, food services, physical education programs and the combined efforts of school, other agencies and families to improve the health of school-aged youth and school personnel. (ASHA, no date, p. 1)

The association is open to individuals, both inservice and preservice, who are interested in promoting comprehensive school health. Four primary groups of people comprise the more than eight thousand members of the association: school health educators, school nurses, school physicians, and university faculty members who help prepare school health personnel. With membership in the ASHA comes the opportunity to join sub-groups of the association called sections and councils. These sub-groups allow members to interact with others who have the same school health interests. Examples of a few of the councils are health behaviors, international health, school health instruction and curriculum, nutrition education and school-based food service.

The ASHA has several publications. They include the *Journal of School Health,* which is published ten times per year; "The Pulse," a newsletter that is published four times per year and provides the latest news and analysis of the ASHA; "Healthy Youth: Agenda for Action," a quarterly publication that is topic-specific and includes reproducible fact sheets, policy examples, lesson plans, individualized health plans, and assessment instruments; and "Network News," which is issued twice a year and offers in-depth reviews of priority problems facing youth,

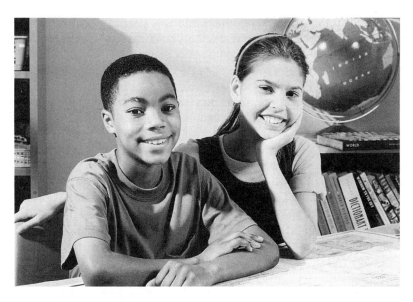

The American School Health Association focuses on the health of the school-aged child.

along with valuable resource lists. *The Journal of School Health* is recognized widely and includes in-depth articles, results of professional research, case studies of successful school health programs and practices, school health service applications, teaching techniques, book reviews, commentaries, and other current information such as job and workshop announcements. The *Journal* "publishes material related to health promotion in school settings. The readership of the *Journal* includes administrators, educators, nurses, physicians, dentists, dental hygienists, counselors, social workers, nutritionists, dietitians, and other health professionals. These individuals work cooperatively with parents and the community to achieve the common goal of providing children and adolescents with the programs, services and environment necessary to promote health and to improve learning" (ASHA, 1996, p. 307).

Association for Worksite Health Promotion. The **Association for Worksite Health Promotion (AWHP)** is the name of a professional association that was originally founded in 1974 as the American Association of Fitness Directors in Business and Industry. The original organization changed its name in 1983 to the Association for Fitness in Business. The current name was adopted in 1993 to better reflect the mission of the association, which is "to advance worksite health promotion throughout the world" (AWHP - b, no date, p. 1). The AWHP "is dedicated to enhancing the the personal and organizational health and well-being of employees and their families" (AWHP - b, no date, p. 1). The Association and its approximately 3,000 members work to achieve their mission by "advocating the value of worksite health promotion to business and government leaders; supporting health promotion professionals through education; providing resources to those who offer health promotion at the worksite; and serving as a catalyst to advance research and learning in the field" (AWHP - b, no date, p. 1). Unlike some of the other associations/organizations mentioned in this chapter, the Association's membership is comprised of many other professionals than just health educators. "Members include human resource directors, health educators, corporate and nonprofit organization wellness directors, government officials, exercise physiologists, dietitians, organizational health consultants, benefits managers, physical and occupational therapists, occupational health; nurses and physicians, fitness instructors, personal trainers, and exercise facility managers/owners" (AWHP, no date-a, p. 1).

AWHP is truly an international association, with eight regional chapters in the United States, two Canadian chapters, and a chapter in the United Kingdom. Like the other associations, the AWHP has a variety of membership services, an annual conference, and several regularly produced publications. The publications of the AWHP include a quarterly journal called *Worksite Health*; a bi-monthly newsletter available only to the members, called "Action"; and an annual AWHP membership directory and buyers' guide. In addition to these regular publications, the association has prepared several other publications that have been very popular with those interested in worksite health promotion:

1. *Guidelines for Employee Health Promotion Programs.* A publication that provides a step-by-step approach to the start-up phases of employee health promotion programs
2. *Economic Impact of Worksite Health Promotion.* A compendium of articles and survey results "of available research on the efficacy of worksite health promotion organized into three parts: economics and worksite Health Promotion, Assessment and Evaluation, and Worksite Health Promotion Profiles" (AWHP, no date-b, p. 2)
3. *Worksite Health Promotion Economics.* An "up-to-date and concise analysis available on the effectiveness of worksite health promotion programs" (AWHP, no date-b, p. 3)
4. *National Compensation and Benefits Survey.* "Defines and reports on the responsibilities, benefits, experience, education, and salary levels of worksite health promotion practitioners" (AWHP, no date-b, p. 3)
5. *Job Opportunity Bureau (JOB)* A listing of job openings that is published twice a month (AWHP, no date-b)
6. *University Internship Services (UIS).* A quarterly international directory of internship opportunities for students (AWHP, no date-b)

Society for Public Health Education, Inc. The **Society of Public Health Educators (SOPHE),** which was founded in 1950, is the only professional organization devoted exclusively to public health education and health promotion. In 1969, the organization changed its name to the **Society for Public Health Education, Inc. (SOPHE).** The purpose of SOPHE is "to promote the health of all people by: stimulating research on the theory and practice of health education;

supporting high quality performance standards for the practice of health education and health promotion; advocating policy and legislation affecting health education and health promotion; developing and promoting standards for professional preparation of health education professionals; promoting networking among health education professionals" (SOPHE, 1996, p. 1). Membership in SOPHE is open to individuals with formal training and/or interest in health education and health promotion. Total national membership is about 1,750 individuals. Another approximately 2,200 individuals belong to one of the seventeen state or regional chapters of SOPHE (SOPHE, 1996). Like several of the other associations/organizations, SOPHE members have the opportunity to associate with one or more of its eight special-interest groups within the larger organization.

SOPHE publishes three primary publications. They include its peer-reviewed journal *Health Education and Behavior,* a newsletter called "News & Views," and a membership directory that is prepared annually to facilitate networking among the members. *Health Education and Behavior* is a well-respected journal that is aimed primarily at the dissemination of research findings, but a typical issue also includes book reviews and SOPHE-related information. "News & Views," like the journal, is published quarterly and includes information, the latest trends, public policies, meetings, and tools of the trade (SOPHE, 1996).

Over the years, SOPHE has had a good working relationship with the APHA. As can be seen in Table 8.2, SOPHE is located in the same building as the APHA in Washington, DC. In addition, SOPHE holds its annual meeting the weekend prior to the APHA annual meeting in the same city as the APHA. Like several of the other associations/organizations, the annual meeting of SOPHE provides opportunities to share and receive the most recent research findings, to earn continuing education contact hours, to participate in its job bank service, and to network with other professionals.

In addition to the above-mentioned items, SOPHE has been involved in some other special projects:

- The development of the SOPHE Code of Ethics, which outlines conduct for ethical health education research and practice. This code was last revised in 1983 (see Appendix A) and abridged in 1993 (see Appendix B).
- The creation of an annual transcript of continuing education contact hours earned at SOPHE events
- An annual mid-year scientific conference each June, which focuses on a topic of special interest to those in the health education and health promotion disciplines
- Partnership in the SOPHE/AAHE Baccalaureate Program Approval Committee (SABPAC) (see p. 199).

International Union for Health Promotion and Education.   Though all of the professional associations/organizations noted already in this chapter have members from countries other than the United States, there is one professional association that is truly worldwide. It is the **International Union for Health Promotion and Education (IUHPE),** with a membership of about two thousand. The IUHPE, which was founded in 1951 in Paris, is a global association of people and organizations from more than ninety nations "working in the fields of health promotion and health education, dedicated to the promotion of world health through education, community action, and the development of healthy public policies" (IUHPE, no date, p. 2).

Among the activities of the IUHPE (IUHPE, no date, p. 2) are

- *Advocacy.* To promote the development of informed public opinion on health matters
- *Liaison.* To maintain constant relations with national and international bodies concerned with the promotion of health
- *Networking.* To stimulate and support effective links with international, national, and regional organizations and people in the fields of health promotion and health education
- *Consultancy.* To provide advice and support to WHO, UNESCO, UNICEF, and other international agencies on health promotion and health education implications of their policies and programs
- *Information.* To facilitate worldwide exchanges of information and experiences on all matters related to health promotion and health education
- *Training.* To promote the improvement of the knowledge, skills, and competencies required to deal effectively with health promotion and health education policy and practice
- *Research.* To promote scientific research, including field studies, related to health promotion and health education
- *Conferences.* To provide opportunities for study and discussion through international conferences, regional seminars and meetings

Because IUHPE is a worldwide organization, it is organized through six regional offices (Europe [IUHP/EUR], Latin America [IUHPE/ORLA], North America [IUHPE/NARO], Northern Part of the Western Pacific [IUHPE/NPWP], South-East Asia [IUHPE/SEARB], and South-West Pacific [IUHPE/SWP]) and has a total international conference only once every three years. The most recent one was in San Juan, Puerto Rico, in June 1998. The peer-reviewed journal of the organization is *Promotion & Education.* A typical issue of the journal, which is published quarterly, includes "articles on the theory and practice of health promotion and health education as well as news about major events throughout the world" (IUHPE, no date, p. 4)

Eta Sigma Gamma.   Founded in 1967, **Eta Sigma Gamma (ESG)** is the national health education honorary. The idea for the organization was born when three professors from Ball State University, Drs. William Bock, Warren E. Schaller, and Robert Synovitz, were on their way to a professional conference and were talking about the need for an honorary for the discipline. Their discussion lead to the formation of the organization, which has had, from its very beginning, the primary purpose of furthering the professional competence and dedication of individual members of the health education profession (ESG, 1991). The ideals of the honorary are symbolized in its seal. The seal (see Figure 8.1) "is divided into four equilateral triangles, each carrying a symbol. A lamp of learning is in the center triangle, surrounded by an open book representing teaching, a microscope signifying research, and an outstretched hand representing service. These three elements form the basic purposes of the organization and profession; teaching, research, and service. The unifying element of these purposes is symbolized by the lamp of learning, since it is through the learning process that each purpose is achieved" (ESG, 1991, p. 2).

As noted in Table 8.2, the national office of Eta Sigma Gamma is located in Muncie, Indiana, on the campus of Ball State University in the Department of Physiology and Health Science. This is also where the the Alpha Chapter (the first chapter of the honorary) is located. As of October 1998, there were one hundred chapters located on university/college campuses throughout the United States (see Appendix E). Chapters are awarded to colleges/universities based on a review and vote by the National Executive Committee of Eta Sigma Gamma on an application prepared by personnel at the petitioning college/university. From its beginnings, Eta Sigma Gamma has focused on the student members. It is while individuals are either undergraduate or graduate students that most people join the honorary. Membership is open to those who have a major or minor in health education and a grade point average equivalent to at least a *B-*. In fact, students can achieve membership only by affiliating through a collegiate chapter. It is through their affiliation with the collegiate chapters that they are eligible to apply for the awards and scholarships of the honorary. Professionals active in the discipline of health education and holding a degree can affiliate through the Chapter-At-Large (ESG, 1991). To obtain more information about joining Eta Sigma Gamma or starting a new chapter contact the national office.

Eta Sigma Gamma regularly produces three publications; its journal, *The Health Educator; The Health Education Monograph Series;* and "The Vision," a newsletter. Each of these publications is distributed twice a year. Like the publications of the other associations/organizations, these publications include the current works of the professionals in the field. However, unlike the others, only individuals who are current members of Eta Sigma Gamma can write articles for *The Health Educator* and *The Health Education Monograph Series.* Another unusual

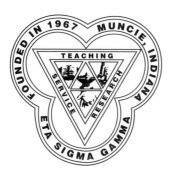

FIGURE 8.1 Seal of Eta Sigma Gamma

Source: National Office of Eta Sigma Gamma, 2000 University Ave., Muncie, IN 47306.

characteristic of the publications of Eta Sigma Gamma is that one entire issue of the *Monograph Series* each year is comprised of articles written only by student members. This is another indication that the honorary is very concerned about the preservice professional.

One final bit of information about Eta Sigma Gamma is that it is the professional health association/organization that is responsible for processing the health education entries for the U.S. Department of Health and Human Service's Secretary's Award for Innovation in Health Promotion. This is an annual competition among students from all health science professions for the top proposals for community-based programs in health promotion. For more information about this competition, contact the national office of Eta Sigma Gamma.

Associations for Directors.   There are two other professional groups that have ties to health education. They are the (1) Association of State and Territorial Directors of Health Promotion and Public Health Education and (2) Society of State Directors of Health, Physical Education, and Recreation. Unlike all the other professional groups discussed, membership in these organizations is determined by the professional position held; not by application for membership. The individuals who belong to these organizations are employees of their respective state/territorial departments of health or education. The primary functions of the **Association of State and Territorial Directors of Health Promotion and Public Health Education (ASTDHPPHE),** which was formed in 1926, are to work to enhance the health education standards in public health agencies and to provide a means by which its members have an opportunity to network with one another. More specifically, ASTDHPPHE has the following purposes (CNHEO, 1996, p. 3):

- To serve as a channel through which directors of public health education programs of states and territories of the United States may exchange and share methods, techniques, and information for the enrichment and improvement of public health education programs
- To establish position statements and make recommendations on legislation and public policy related to and having implications for public health education
- To participate with the Association of State and Territorial Health Officials (ASTHO) in promoting health and preventing disease
- To identify methods of improving the quality and practice of education, public health education, and health promotion
- To elicit the cooperation and coordination with those national, public, private, and voluntary agencies related to public health programs
- To provide a forum for continuing education opportunities in public health education and health promotion

This association is also an affiliate of the Association of State and Territorial Health Officials, which is the association for those who oversee state and territorial health departments. You can obtain more information about ASTDHPPHE by contacting any state or territorial department of health.

The Conference of State Directors of Health, Physical Education, and Recreation, which later changed its name to **Society of State Directors of Health, Physical Education, and Recreation (SSDHPER),** was founded in 1967 and has the primary function of promoting comprehensive health, physical education, and recreation programs in the K–12 schools of the states. The purpose of the society is "to help insure that every student has the opportunity to participate in a broad, constructive, continuing series of educational experiences in health, physical education, and recreation throughout their entire school career" (CNHEO, 1996, p. 7). You can obtain more information about SSDHPER by contacting any state department of education.

Coalitions.   Because of the large number of professional health education associations, there are times when there is a need to have a common voice for the profession. To help provide such a voice, coalitions of health associations/organizations have been created. The two most prominent coalitions are the Coalition of National Health Education Organizations, USA, and the National School Health Education Coalition.

The **Coalition of National Health Education Organizations, USA (CNHEO)** is comprised of representatives (delegates and alternates) from eight national associations/organizations that have identifiable health educator memberships and ongoing health education programs. The associations/organizations included are American College Health Association, Health Education Section; American Public Health Association, Public Health Education and Health Promotion Section; American Public Health Association, School Health Education and Services Section; American School Health Association; American Association for Health Education; Association of State and Territorial Directors of Health Promotion and Public Health Education; Society for Public Health Education, Inc.; and Society of State Directors of Health, Physical Education, and Recreation (CNHEO, 1996).

The CNHEO was formed on March 1, 1972, after a series of three meetings in 1971 and 1972 to determine the feasibility of such an organization. The primary mission of the coalition is "the mobilization of the resources of the Health Education Profession in order to expand and improve health education, regardless of the setting" (CNHEO, 1996, back cover). The work of the CNHEO is financed by funds obtained from coalition member organizations, public and private agencies, and contributions and gifts from individuals. Over the years, the working relationship of the member organizations has been outlined in the *Working Agreement of the CNHEO.* Also, included in this document are the purposes of the coalition (CNHEO, 1996, back cover):

1. Facilitates national level communication, collaboration, and coordination, among the member organizations.
2. Provides a forum for the identification and discussion of health education issues.
3. Formulates recommendations and takes appropriate action on issues affecting member interests.

4. Serve as a communication and advisory resource for agencies, organizations, and persons in the public and private sectors concerning health education issues.
5. Serve as a focus for the exploration and resolution of issues pertinent to professional health educators.

Since its inception, the CNHEO has operationalized its purposes in a number of ways, which has contributed to the growth of the profession. One way has been the creation of position papers on topics of importance to the profession. Two of the most recent statements dealt with the preparation of elementary school teachers in the area of health education and the strengthening of health education in the public health arena. Other issues the coalition has addressed include federal legislation for health education, professional preparation programs, and the credentialing of health educators. With regard to the last issue, coalition co-sponsorship, with the National Commission for Health Education Credentialing, Inc. (NCHEC), held a forum in June 1995 to examine the future of the health education profession (NCHEC & CNHEO, 1996). It brought together twenty-four professionals, representing NCHEC and each of the member associations/organizations of CNHEO. In addition, Eta Sigma Gamma was invited to send a representative to the forum "because of its widespread contact with preservice professionals" (NCHEC & CNHEO, 1996, p. 291). The goal of this forum was four-fold (NCHEC & CNHEO, 1996, p. 292):

- Develop goals which will provide direction for the profession
- Identify actions needed within the profession to move it into a significant role in the United States
- Identify actions needed external to the profession to move it into a significant role in the United States
- Develop an action plan which identifies who will do what when

From this forum came a working document (NCHEC & CNHEO, 1996) that participants were asked to (1) share with their respective association's/organization's officers, executive directors, and board members and (2) respond to collectively to NCHEC and CNHEO. The working document included four major components (NCHEC & CNHEO, 1996):

- Emerging goals for the health education profession
- The question, What do we need to do to achieve the goals of the health education profession?
- The question, How will we implement these actions?
- The question, Where do we go from here?

It was also concluded that another meeting with additional participants was essential. It was decided that the participants from the forum were to serve as the steering committee to bring a larger group of representative professionals together (NCHEC & CNHEO, 1996). At the time of this writing, that second conference had not been held.

The current project of CNHEO has been to develop a unified code of ethics for the profession. More about this project is noted in Chapter 5.

More information about CNHEO can be obtained by contacting the office of any of the member organizations.

The other major coalition associated with the profession of health education is the **National School Health Education Coalition (NaSHEC).** It was established in 1982 and "provides leadership and advocacy to ensure that all children, pre K–12, receive quality comprehensive health education as a cornerstone of a comprehensive health program in the schools and communities" (NaSHEC, 1995, p. 1). Membership in NaSHEC is open to any agency/association/organization that has a "commitment to improving the health and education of children and youth, and an interest in comprehensive school health" (NaSHEC, 1995, p. 1). Today it has more than ninety members, which include national education and health organizations, agencies and corporations, and state and local coalitions. Like any coalition, the strength of NaSHEC lies in its ability to mobilize its members to work together for a focused cause—in this case, comprehensive school health education.

NaSHEC has three primary means of keeping its members and others interested in comprehensive school health education informed: the "NaSHEC Newsline," the "NaSHEC Legislative Status Report," and its annual membership meeting. Both the "Newsline" and the "Report" are quarterly publications. The "Newsline" keeps the members up-to-date on the news of the coalition, plus notices of new resources, upcoming events, new member profiles, other news of interest, and comments from the staff. The *Report* is intended to provide legislative updates (primarily federal legislation) on critical health, education, and social programs that aim to improve the health and well-being of children and youth (NaSHEC, 1996). The annual membership meeting of the coalition is often, but not always, held in conjunction with the annual conference of the American School Health Association. The membership meeting provides an opportunity to "discuss issues critical to improving the health and educational status of children and youth, and in assuring the provision of health programs in schools nationwide; share information about program activities and policies; and conduct business" (NaSHEC, 1995, p. 1).

More information on NaSHEC can be obtained by contacting its office at 1400 I Street, NW, Suite 520, Washington, DC 20005, 202/408-0222 (voice), 202/408-8922 (fax).

Joining a Professional Health Association/Organization

Becoming a member of a professional organization is not difficult. With the exception of a few of the associations/organizations previously noted (the two coalitions, Eta Sigma Gamma, and ASTDHPPHE and SSDHPER), membership in a professional organization can be obtained by completing an application form (available from any of the organizations or included in many of the official publications) and sending the money of the desired length and category of membership (different rates apply to different types of membership—for example, student, professional, retired) to the association/organization of choice. Most individuals join a professional association/organization for a year at a time. Some associations, however, provide multiple-year memberships at a reduced rate or even a lifetime membership. In general, the cost of a membership in a state or regional association/organization is separate from and less than a membership in a national association/organization. If you are interested in joining a state or local association/organization, you can usually contact its national office to find out whom to contact locally.

Summary

This chapter discussed the various health agencies, associations, and organizations with which the profession of health education interacts. The agencies/associations/organizations were presented within three major categories: governmental, quasi-governmental, and nongovernmental. The primary emphasis of the chapter was to present information about a sub-category of the nongovernmental associations/organizations, the professional associations/organizations. Those discussed included the American Alliance for Health, Physical Education, Recreation and Dance; American Association for Health Education; American Public Health Association; American College Health Association; American School Health Association; Association for Worksite Health Promotion; Society for Public Health Education, Inc.; International Union for Health Promotion and Education; Eta Sigma Gamma; and associations for directors (Association of State and Territorial Directors of Health Promotion and Public Health Education and Society of State Directors of Health, Physical Education, and Recreation). Also, information about two coalitions—the Coalition of National Health Education Organizations, USA, and the National School Health Coalition—was presented. The chapter concluded with information on how to become a member of a professional association/organization.

REVIEW QUESTIONS

1. Define and explain the differences among the following types of agencies: governmental health agency, quasi-governmental health agency, nongovernmental health agency.

2. At what levels do governmental agencies exist? Provide an example of an agency at each level.

3. What are the three primary activities of most voluntary health agencies? Give an example of each.

4. What are the purposes of a professional association/organization?

5. What are the benefits derived from membership in a professional association/organization?

6. What is the oldest and largest professional health association in the United States?

7. Name three professional health associations/organizations that focus their efforts on work settings for health educators. Name two other professional health associations/organizations that are not as focused on a work setting.

8. What is the name of the health education honorary? Where was it founded and where is the national office located? In general, where are the chapters of the honorary found?

9. What is a coalition? What are two coalitions that support the profession of health education? What is the primary purpose of each of these coalitions?

10. How does a person become a member of a professional organization?

ACTIVITIES

1. Closely examine one professional health association/organization and write a two-page paper on the history of that association/organization.

2. Interview two health education faculty members at your school and ask them
   - Do they belong to any professional health education associations/organizations?
   - If they belong, why?
   - What benefits do they see in belonging to them?
   - What association/organization would they recommend that you join?

3. Does your school have a chapter of Eta Sigma Gamma? If not, make an appointment with the department head/chairperson to inquire about the possibility of starting one on your campus.

4. Write a one-page paper using the following two sentences to start the paper:

   "If I could join one professional health association/organization, it would be _____. My reasons for choosing that association/organization are _____."

REFERENCES

American Alliance for Health, Physical Education, Recreation and Dance (AAHPERD). (no date). *Give yourself a healthy promotion.* Reston, VA: Author.

American College Health Association (ACHA). (no date). *American College Health Association.* Baltimore, MD: Author.

American Public Health Association (APHA). (no date). *The American Public Health Association: Keeping public health in the public eye for more than a century.* Washington, DC: Author.

American Public Health Association (APHA). (1991). *Healthy Communities 2000: Model standards* (3rd ed.). Washington, DC: Author.

American Public Health Association (APHA). (1996). *Publications catalog 1996*. Washington, DC: Author.

American School Health Association (ASHA). (no date). *American School Health Association*. Kent, OH: Author.

American School Health Association (ASHA). (1976). *History of the American School Health Association, 1926–1976*. Kent, OH: Author.

American School Health Association (ASHA). (1996). Statement of purpose. *Journal of School Health, 66*(8), 307.

Anderson, G. (1985). AAHPERD from the beginning. *Journal of Physical Education, Recreation and Dance, 56*(4), 94–96.

Association for the Advancement of Health Education (AAHE). (no date-a). *The Association for the Advancement of Health Education introduces ProNet*. Reston, VA: Author.

Association for the Advancement of Health Education (AAHE) (no date-b). *Mission statement*. Reston, VA: Author.

Association for the Advancement of Health Education (AAHE). (1995). Directory of institutions offering undergraduate and graduate degree programs in health education. *Journal of Health Education, 26*(2),107–118.

Association for Worksite Health Promotion (AWHP) (no date-a). *Fact sheet*. Northbrook, IL: Author.

Association for Worksite Health Promotion (AWHP). (no date-b). *Give yourself the AWHP advantage*. Northbrook, IL: Author.

Benenson, A. S. (Ed.). (1995). *Control of communicable disease manual*. (16th ed.) Washington, DC: Author.

Cauffman, J. G. (1982). A history of the Coalition of National Education Organization: Its first ten years and future directions. *The Eta Sigma Gamma Monograph Series, 1*(2).

Coalition of National Health Education Organization (CNHEO). (1996). *Directory: Coalition of National Health Education Organization U.S.A.* Columbia, MO: Author .

Eta Sigma Gamma (ESG). (1991, November). *Eta Sigma Gamma*. Muncie, IN: Author.

Green, L. W., & Ottoson, J. M. (1999). *Community and population health* (8th ed.). Boston: WCB McGraw-Hill.

International Union for Health Promotion and Education (IUHPE). (no date). *International Union for Health Promotion and Education* (a pamphlet about membership). Vanves (Paris), France: Author.

Landau, S. I. (Ed.). (1979). *Funk & Wagnalls standard desk dictionary* (Vol. 2, N–Z). New York: Funk & Wagnalls.

McKenzie, J. F., & Pinger, R. R. (1997). *Introduction to community health* (Web-enhanced edition). Sudbury, MA: Jones and Bartlett Publishers.

McKenzie, J. F., Pinger, R. R., & Kotecki, J. E. (1999). *An Introduction to Community Heatlh* (3rd ed.). Sudbury, MA: Jones & Bartlett Publishers.

Miller, D. F. & Price, J. H. (1998). *Dimensions of community health* (5th ed.). Boston, MA: WCB/McGraw-Hill.

National Commission for Health Education Credentialing, Inc., & Coalition of National Health Education Organizations, USA (NCHEC & CNHEO), (1996). The health education profession in the 21st century: Setting the stage. *Journal of School Health, 66*(8), 291–298.

National School Health Education Coalition (NaSHEC). (1995, October). *Resource Guide*. Washington, DC: Author.

National School Health Education Coalition (NaSHEC). (1996). *NaSHEC legislative status report: Spring 1996*. Washington, DC: Author.

Nolte, A. E. (1985). Health education: An alliance commitment. *Journal of Physical Education, Recreation and Dance, 56*(4), 107–108.

Reagan, P. A., & Brookins-Fisher, J. (1997). *Community health in the 21st century*. Boston: Allyn and Bacon.

Scope and guidelines for contributors. (1992). *Journal of American College Health, 40*(6), 308.

Society for Public Health Education, Inc. (SOPHE). (1996). *SOPHE snapshot 1996*. Washington, DC: Author.

9 The Literature of Health Education

CHAPTER OBJECTIVES

After reading this chapter and answering the questions at the end, you should be able to

1. Describe the difference between a primary, a secondary, and a popular press literature source.
2. Write an abstract or a summary of an article from a refereed journal.
3. Use appropriate questions to critique a journal article.
4. Name the most commonly used journals in the field of health education.
5. Locate an article related to some aspect of health education, using an index or an abstract.
6. Identify the most commonly used on-line computerized databases for finding health education information.
7. Conduct an Internet search for information about a health-related topic, using one of the World Wide Web sites listed in the chapter.
8. Critique the validity of the information obtained from searching a site on the Internet.

KEY TERMS

abstracts	hypertext transfer protocol	refereed journal
browser	indexes	search engine
computerized databases	internet	secondary sources
home page	popular press publications	Uniform Resource Locators
hypertext	primary sources	World Wide Web
hypertext markup language		

Introduction

It is no secret that the amount of information about any given topic is growing at almost an exponential rate. Terms such as *information overload* and *information burnout* are being heard more and more. Arguably, the area in which information is growing fastest and in which there is tremendous public interest is health. People today seem almost obsessed with the need to gather information about such health topics as diet, exercise, stress management, vitamins, drugs, sexuality, depression, safety, disease, violence prevention, and the formation of positive personal relationships.

The fact that there is an increasing demand for information, coupled with the fact that information is being produced at an ever greater rate, creates added responsibility for health educators. Two of the major responsibilities of a health educator as discussed in Chapter 6 involve being a resource person for health information (Responsibility 6) and communicating to others health education needs, concerns, and resources (Responsibility 8). In order to perform these tasks, the health educator must have the skills to find information, evaluate the source of the information to determine its credibility, and disseminate the information through the appropriate channels to consumers. This chapter introduces prospective health education students to the most common sources of health-related information used by health educators. It also describes how to access the information from these sources.

Types of Information Sources

When accessing information, it is important to note whether the source is primary or secondary. **Primary sources** of data or information are published studies or eye-

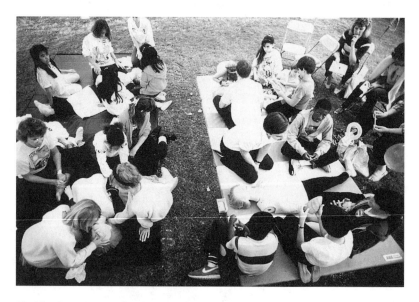

Health educators are often asked to conduct presentations on a variety of health topics to community groups. This photo shows a CPR class for children. (Spencer Grant/Stock, Boston)

witness accounts written by the people who actually conducted the experiments or observed the events in question. A journal that publishes original manuscripts only after they have been read by a panel of experts in the field (referees) and recommended for publication is termed a **refereed journal**. Examples of primary sources are research articles written by the researcher(s), personal records (autobiographies), official records of legislative sessions or minutes of community meetings, newspaper eyewitness accounts, and annual reports.

Secondary sources, on the other hand, are usually written by someone who was not present at the event or did not participate as part of the study team. The value of these sources is that they often provide a summary of several related studies or chronicle a history or sequence of events. The writers of secondary sources may also provide editorial comments or alternative interpretations of the study or event. An additional function served by secondary sources is that they often provide a bibliography of primary sources. Examples of secondary sources are journal review articles, editorials, and noneyewitness accounts of events occurring in the community, region, or nation.

Although refereed journals most often have primary source articles published in them, secondary source articles can sometimes be found as well. The types of secondary source articles most likely to be found in a refereed journal are articles summarizing the results of several studies, editorials, or positions deemed important enough (by the panel of expert reviewers) to be of interest and utility to those who read the journal.

A third type of source of health information, and probably the most difficult to check for credibility, is the **popular press publications**. Popular press publications range from weekly summary-type magazines (e.g., *Time, Newsweek, U.S. News & World Report*) and newspaper supplements (e.g., *Parade*) to monthly magazines (e.g., *Reader's Digest, Better Homes and Gardens, Esquire*) and tabloids (e.g., *The Star*). At times, any of these may be a primary source of information (as in an interview). Most often, however, they are secondary sources at best. Often, articles in the popular press include opinions or editorials that contain the bias of the author or the editor of the publication. Popular press publications should be heavily scrutinized as to the source of the information in the article before being cited as authentic and accurate.

Sorting through the maze of health information can be a daunting task, even for the most skilled health educator. In order to equip the health educator for assuming the responsibilities associated with providing and disseminating information, several tasks need to be mastered. The next several sections of this chapter are designed to provide background for the student in: (1) identifying the components of a research article; (2) critically reading a research article; (3) ascertaining the accuracy of the information in articles that are nonresearch-based or are from secondary or popular press sources; (3) writing an abstract or a summary of a journal article; (4) identifying and locating primary and secondary sources most commonly used by health educators using indexes, abstracts, and computerized databases; and (5) retrieving health-related information on the Internet.

Identifying the Components
of a Research Article

A research article usually begins with an abstract which is a brief description of the study about which the article is reporting the results. The abstract describes the research questions that were tested, outlines the study design, and lists one or two major findings from the study. The abstract is meant to communicate essential information, so that readers will know whether or not the study has information related to the topic they are interested in. An example of an abstract (McKinney et al., 1997) follows:

> The authors analyzed self-reported questionnaire data from the 1987 National Medical Expenditure Survey (NMES) to determine smoking patterns of veterans. Using NMES data, the authors compared veterans versus nonveterans overall, women veterans versus women nonveterans, Vietnam-era veterans versus other veterans, and veterans whose usual source of medical care was the Department of Veterans Affairs system (VA) versus veterans who received care elsewhere. The likelihood of ever having smoked cigarettes was higher for veterans than for nonveterans and for women veterans than for nonwomen veterans. The prevalence of current smoking was higher for veterans than for nonveterans and higher for those seeking care in the VA system. Given the enormous health care costs associated with smoking, health promotion efforts should be developed to reduce the high rate of smoking among veterans—especially those who are consumers of VA health care. (p. 212)

The introduction section follows the abstract. Its purpose is usually three-fold: (1) to give readers a more detailed description of the research question(s) or hypotheses being tested, (2) to review related literature, and (3) to explain the need for or the significance of the study. This section communicates the rationale behind the researchers' decision to conduct the study.

The methodology section comes directly after the introductory material. In this section, there is usually a description of (1) the research design used, (2) the subjects who took part in the research, (3) the instruments used to gather the information necessary to answer the research questions, and (4) any administrative procedures involved in conducting the research, such as methods used to select the subject, gather the data, or protect the rights of the subjects.

Following the methodology section are the results and discussion sections. The results section gives the research findings by describing the results of the statistical procedures used in analyzing the data (in the case of studies involving quantitative methods—methods involving the analyses of numerical data) and provides an overall answer to the research questions or hypotheses that were described in the introductory section. The discussion section provides a forum for the researcher to interpret the conclusions and meanings and to comment on the implications of the data analyses. In addition, the researcher often includes a narrative about the limitations of the study and makes recommendations for further research on the topic.

Critically Reading a Research Article

The volume of articles on any one health topic continues to escalate. It is important to be able to evaluate the information found in any source for accuracy and saliency. Beginning students to the field of health education are not expected to be able to immediately understand every nuance in a research article. It is essential, however, to begin to frequently read scientific reports and journal articles to become familiar with the style in which they are written. Often, preformulating generic questions suitable for critiquing any study can help when evaluating study results. Following is a list of hints that have been found to be of help when such an evaluation is necessary. The list is adapted from information found in *Studying a Study and Testing a Test* (Riegelman & Hirsh, 1989).

1. Were the aims of the study defined in a clear manner?
2. Were the research questions/hypotheses clearly stated?
3. Was the description of the subjects clear? Did the article state how the subjects were recruited?
4. Were the design and location of the study described clearly?
5. Were the data collection instruments described?
6. Did the results directly address the research questions/hypotheses?
7. Were the conclusions logical in terms of the research design and data analyses performed?
8. Were the study implications meaningful to the population you serve?

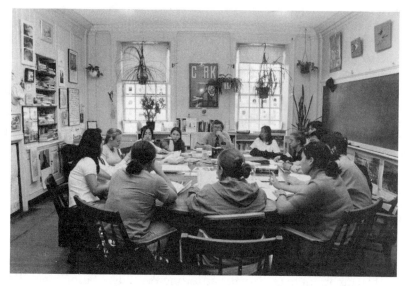

Summarizing research articles in small group settings sharpens the ability to correctly interpret research findings. (Lionel Delevingne/Stock, Boston)

The final test comes when students can read an article and begin to view themselves in the position of a reporter who has the task of describing the study, its findings, and its limitations to an audience with a time allotment of no more than five minutes. People who can restate study findings in their own words have accomplished much in becoming a critical consumer of scientific and nonscientific literature, as well as a better resource for others.

Evaluating the Accuracy of Nonresearch-Based Sources

As with journal articles that are research-based, it is important to be able to evaluate whether or not the information presented is reliable, regardless of the source. McKenzie (1987) published a checklist for helping readers ascertain the accuracy and reliability of information found in almost any type of journal or magazine. It lists 16 questions about the author, the publication source, and the information presented that the reader should consider when evaluating an article for accuracy of information. When using this list with his classes, Cottrell (1997) found that he could shorten it to include the following:

1. What are the author's qualifications? Does the person have an academic degree in the field being written about? A note of caution—a degree does not make someone absolutely qualified, but it provides evidence to suggest that the person is qualified.
2. What is the style of presentation? Look for health information written in a scientific style of writing, not a style that uses generalities or testimonials.
3. Are references included? A well-written article provides references to the primary sources used. Be aware when someone is writing about another person's research, as that individual may be interpreting the results in a different way than the author did.
4. What is the purpose of the publication? Be aware of news publications and publications that contain advertisements designed to sell items being discussed in the articles.
5. What is the reputation of the publication? Is it refereed? Professional journals are good sources of information. Popular press publications can sometimes have poor information related to health issues.
6. Is the information new? When reading for the first time, be skeptical. Information must be validated over time. New information is newsworthy but may not be valid.

It is important to realize that acquiring the skill of becoming a skeptical, critical consumer of printed health information is an important first step in being seen by others as credible. In order for the public to use the expertise and training of health educators to a greater degree, the health educators must develop a reputation for providing accurate and current information.

Writing an Abstract or a Summary

Another valuable skill that is of assistance when reading and interpreting health-related literature of any kind (primary, secondary, or popular press) involves learning to write an abstract or a summary of an article. Although abstracts and summaries are both short forms of describing a research study, the major differences lie in the extent of the content. Abstracts are short (usually 150-250 words). They are written to identify the purpose of the research, the study questions, the methods used by the researcher, and one or two major findings. Summaries, on the other hand, may be two to three pages in length and include all of the elements of the abstract. In addition, summaries are meant to reveal any secondary findings, to describe study limitations, and to provide for a more detailed review of the researcher's conclusions and recommendations from the viewpoint of the summary's author.

It is recommended that beginning health educators practice writing both abstracts and summaries of the articles they read. Using this technique sharpens the ability of the health educator to discriminate between health-related articles that are of substance and meaning for health promotion and those that contain erroneous or misleading claims or information.

Locating Health-Related Information

Health educators serve as major health information resource persons for many constituencies. It does not matter if they are employed in the school, the clinic, the worksite, or the community setting. In all cases, inquiries from a variety of people wanting to know about a health topic or wanting interpretation of the latest research findings are directed to health educators. Therefore, it is essential that they be knowledgeable about how to locate the information requested. The next section identifies resources that health educators can use to locate information on health education and health promotion, and it explains how the information can be accessed.

Journals

As has been previously mentioned, much of the information that health educators use to make decisions when planning, implementing, and evaluating health promotion programs can be found in journals that publish primary research articles and position papers about health topics and health programs. The following are examples of journals commonly used by health professionals. The list is by no means inclusive of all journals of benefit to the health educator.

1. *American Journal of Health Behavior* (formerly *Health Values*). Articles accepted for publication feature research about the impact of personal behavior patterns, practices, and characteristics on health promotion. Examples of successful multi-disciplinary approaches to improving health at the community level are also included.

2. *American Journal of Health Promotion.* Original research articles, the testing of health behavioral theory on selected populations, and program evaluation are prominent. It is an excellent source of articles related to worksite health promotion.

3. *American Journal of Health Studies* (formerly *Wellness Perspectives*). Articles target health promotion and wellness in the broadest sense. Readers will find selections on social and environmental support for health, health program planning strategies and evaluation methods, the testing of health behavioral theory, and opinions on the implications of health policy.

4. *American Journal of Public Health.* Published by the American Public Health Association, this journal features reports related to health research, program evaluations, and health policy analysis, as well as articles on special topics on the health of selected groups and communities.

5. *Evaluation and the Health Professions.* Articles generally focus on research related to the development, implementation, and evaluation of community-based health programs. Philosophical and innovative aspects of evaluation are also covered.

6. *Family and Community Health.* Articles contain information and research on nutrition, exercise, health-risk appraisals, and the physical and emotional development of a variety of age groups. The overall goal of this journal is to publish articles that foster the role of self-care in health promotion.

7. *The Health Educator: The Journal of Eta Sigma Gamma.* Published by Eta Sigma Gamma, the health education honor society, users will find articles related to most health education or health promotion topics in a variety of settings. Many of the studies and commentaries are submitted by undergraduate and graduate students in health education/public health programs.

8. *The Hastings Center Report.* This journal focuses on the ethical, social, legal, moral, economic, and religious tenets of health policy and health decisions.

9. *Health Education Quarterly.* The official publication of the Society for Public Health Education, Inc. (SOPHE), its articles center on health behavior and education, case studies in health, and program evaluation. Each submission includes a commentary on the application of findings to the practice setting.

10. *Health Education Research: Theory and Practice.* It features articles concerning health promotion program planning, implementation, and evaluation. An effort is made to publish articles that provide a mechanism to assist those in the field apply the results of the studies.

11. *Health Promotion International.* The majority of research studies and commentaries are on issues related to health promotion in schools, clinics, worksites, and communities located outside of the United States.

12. *The International Electronic Journal of Health Education.* This journal published its first edition in January 1998. It features articles on nearly every aspect of health education, including school health, community health, worksite health promotion, the ethical implications of health education, and the philosophy of health education.

13. *The Journal of American College Health.* Published by the American College Health Association, its articles are limited to those that relate to health promotion or health service provision in the college or university environment.

14. *Journal of Community Health.* This is an all-inclusive journal, with articles relating to all aspects of community health, preventive medicine, and socio-economic, biocultural, and ethical issues in public health.

15. *Journal of Health Education.* This journal is published by the American Association for Health Education. Most articles have broad application to the field of health education. Readers might find articles concerning opinions, original research on health issues and policies related to schools, communities or worksites, and methods and strategies for health instructional programs.

16. *Journal of Rural Health.* Published by the Rural Health Association, this journal's articles focus on professional practice, research, theory development, and policy issues related to health in the rural setting.

17. *Journal of School Health.* Published by the American School Health Association, all material is related to the public or private school setting at the preschool through 12th-grade levels. Articles generally focus on children's health issues but may include information related to other aspects of coordinated school health programs, such as employee wellness.

18. *Promotion and Education.* This journal is affiliated with the World Health Organization and the International Union for Health Promotion and Education. Most issues are topical in nature (e.g., environmental health, population health, infectious disease prevention) and feature articles related to the application of public health and health promotion in countries around the globe. Articles are published in several languages.

19. *Public Health Reports.* The official publication of the Public Health Service, this journal reports findings from many avenues of research related to health services acquisition, health policy development, and health promotion at the community level.

Indexes

Indexes are books that provide a link to articles from many refereed journals, books, and research reports. Each index references articles from journals, books, and reports pertaining to topics that fall under the subject headings for which the index was created. For example, *Index Medicus* lists articles relating to clinical and preventive medicine and does not include references to articles in the social sciences.

The procedures for locating references in an index and the list of journals that are included in the index are found in the front pages of each volume. Many of the indexes are now also found on CD-ROM, but the method of locating an article or a topic is the same. Generally, there are many similarities in how references can be located from one index to the next. Users begin by looking up the topic of interest in the index (e.g., health behavior). Using a volume of the 1995 *Index Medicus* as an example, two samples of citations from the topic "health behaviors" are listed:

> The transitional model of change and HIV prevention: a review. Prochaska JO, et al. **Health Educ Q** 1995 May; 22(2): 190–200 (48 ref).

> Self-esteem and the value of health as determinants of adolescent health behavior. Torres R, et al. **J Adolesc Health** 1995 Jan; 16(1): 60–63. (43 ref).

When reading the citation, the parts are as follows: the title of the article in the journal, the authors' names, the abbreviated title of the journal, the year and month of publication, the volume number, the page numbers, and the number of references that can be found in the bibliography of the article.

Health educators then need to go to the journal listed and find the article of interest. Indexes that are most used by health educators are

1. *Index Medicus.* This index includes references to more than three thousand biomedical journals. It is updated monthly and cumulated annually.
2. *Cumulative Index to Nursing and Allied Health Literature (CINAHL).* Included are references to more than three hundred nursing, allied health, and health-related journals. It is updated bi-monthly and cumulated annually.
3. *Education Index.* this index references more than four hundred journals on topics related to education. The index is updated monthly and cumulated annually.
4. *Physical Education Index.* This index includes references to more than four hundred periodicals on physical education, health education, dance, physical therapy, and sports medicine. It is published six times a year and cumulated annually.
5. *Current Index to Journals in Education (CIJE). CIJE* includes references to more than 775 journals related to education. The index citations correspond to Educational Resources Information Center (ERIC) reference numbers. (See the "Computerized Databases" section later in this chapter for more information.) It is updated monthly and cumulated annually.

Abstracts

Abstracts are book volumes that include short summaries of research studies that have appeared in other journals. An abstract is usually more valuable than an index in that an abstract provides both a reference and a summary for each article included. This allows the user to decide whether or not the article has information worth pursuing further, whereas, when using an index, the reader has only the title of the article.

To use an abstract, locate the index at the end of each volume. The index is organized so you can search by subject or author. Find the subject or author you are interested in, and look at the titles of the articles listed under that subject/author heading. At the end of each article reference there is a number. Go to the volume of the abstract that includes that number (the numbers included in each volume are listed on the outside binding of the volume), turn to the number of the article you are interested in (the numbers are listed consecutively), and locate the desired article abstract. A sample abstract (number 34782) from *Psychological Abstracts* (1993, p. 4144) under the subject area "cardiovascular disorders" follows:

> 34782. Fleury, Julie. (U of North Carolina, School of Nursing, Chapel Hill) **The application of motivational theory to cardiovascular risk reduction.** *IMAGE: Journal of Nursing Scholarship*, 1992(Fall), Vol 24(3), 229–239. -Examines the primary motivational theories used to explain and predict individual adherence in the initiation and maintenance of cardiovascular risk reduction. Research findings from both nursing and related disciplines are presented within each theoretical framework. The application of the health belief model (I.M. Rosenstock, 1974), health promotion model (N.J. Pender, 1987), theory of reasoned action (I. Ajzen and M. Fishbein, 1980), theory of planned behavior (Ajzen, 1985), and self-efficacy theory (A. Bandura, 1986) to the initiation and maintenance of cardiovascular health behavior is discussed.

The abstracts most commonly used by health educators are

1. *Psychological Abstracts.* This abstract includes abstracts of journal articles and books in psychology and other social and behavioral sciences.
2. *Sociological Abstracts.* It includes a collection of abstracts of the literature in sociology and related disciplines. It is published six times a year and cumulated annually.
3. *Biological Abstracts.* Indexed by author, subject, biosystem, and generic heading, this resource includes articles from more than five hundred biology-related publications. It is published bi-monthly and cumulated annually.
4. *Resources in Education.* It includes abstracts on hundreds of studies and papers related to education and provides information on how a copy of an article or a speech can be obtained (e.g., request from the publisher, microfilm).

Computerized Databases

Computerized databases provide an alternative to searching indexes or abstracts manually, in that they are large compilations of references stored on a computer. Like an index or abstract, each database has a general subject area that it covers (e.g., education, medicine, psychology). However, a database provides access to the cumulative information found in several index or abstract sources. Computer searches using databases are usually faster than manual searches, and they have the advantage of allowing the user to link several concepts together to narrow the search. For example, instead of looking up "health behavior" or "cardiovascular disorders," as demonstrated earlier, the user can enter the terms into the computer and connect them by placing the word *and* between them. The result will be to eliminate any articles that do not have both "health behavior" and "cardiovascular disorders" as key terms. Other terms can be used to further narrow a search to be as specific as needed. The main concern the computer database user faces is to accurately specify the key terms associated with the information desired, so the resulting list of references will be useful. Computerized searches require very little computer knowledge; however, it is advisable to seek the assistance of a librarian when beginning to seek information. The databases most used by health educators are

1. *Educational Resources Information Center (ERIC).* It includes the previously mentioned *Current Index to Journals in Education (CIJE)* and *Resources in*

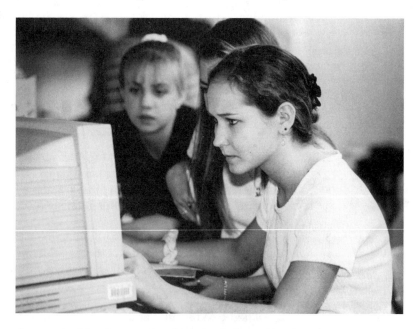

Computerized databases can be a big help when searching for information on a particular topic. (Jeffrey Muir Hamilton/Stock, Boston)

Education (RIE). ERIC is an information clearinghouse that collects, sorts, classifies, and stores thousands of documents on topics pertaining to education and allied fields of study. An advantage to using ERIC is that many types of documents are contained in the database that are not journal articles—for example, proceedings of meetings, teaching strategies, lesson plans, commentaries, and policy documents.

2. *MEDLINE.* This is the premier biomedicine database indexing more than 3,600 journals. It covers the fields of medicine, nursing, dentistry, veterinary medicine, and preclinical sciences.

3. *Cumulative Index to Nursing and Allied Health Literature (CINAHL).* It contains more than 300,000 citations from 1983 until the present. It references journal articles and book chapters, pamphlets, audiovisuals, educational software, and conference proceedings in the areas of nursing, health education, health services, and health care administration.

4. *BIOETHICSLINE.* This database covers ethical, legal, and public policy issues surrounding health care and biomedical research. Citations are derived from the literature of law, religion, ethics, social sciences, philosophy, the popular media, and the health sciences.

5. *Psychological Abstracts (PsychLit).* This database is the analog of *Psychological Abstracts* in computerized form. As with all computer databases, narrowing a search to a specific topic can be accomplished more easily using PsychLit.

6. *Health Services, Technology, Administration, and Research (HealthSTAR).* This is a database formed by merging two former National Library of Medicine databases. It focuses on clinical (patient outcomes and effectiveness of procedures, products, services) and nonclinical (health care administration, planning, policy) aspects of health care.

The Internet and the World Wide Web

Until a few years ago, it was only possible to dream about the day when health information would be readily available at home or at the office at the "touch of a button." Today, of course, that dream is a reality through the use of the Internet and the World Wide Web. The **World Wide Web** is an interactive information delivery service that includes a repository of resources about almost any subject imaginable. In "the web," documents that are related by subject area or place of origin are linked to each other, thus creating a web, or network, of materials. The web relies mainly on **hypertext** as its means of interaction with users. Hypertext is nearly the same as regular text in that it can be searched, edited, and stored, but hypertext contains connections within the text to documents (in the form of printed matter, pictures, graphics, and/or sound) found on computers connected to each other around the globe. This integrated network of computers is known as the **Internet.**

In order to use the web, a person must have access to a **browser.** The browser is a software package that can be installed on any computer with a graphical interface and can greatly simplify the ability to access information on the web. Examples of commonly available browsers include Netscape, Mosaic, and Internet Explorer. Use of the browser involves entering a web address, which usually starts with the characters "http://" (http stands for **hypertext transfer protocol**). Web addresses are known as URLs, or **Uniform Resource Locators,** which are unique identifiers for a location on the global Internet much as the mailing address of your home is unique to where you live. The URL is composed of the Internet access protocol, the location, and the file—for example, http://www.yahoo.com/headlines/Health/ is the URL for the **home page** of the Yahoo Health News Daily. A home page is analogous to a combination of a cover and a table of contents in a book, in that it names the site and directs the user to a list of information options available within the site. In the example, the "http://" is the Internet access protocol; the "www.yahoo.com" is the location; and "headlines/Health/" is the file.

Assume you are looking for information concerning the current population in a region of the United States. In order to obtain the information, you might open Netscape (or any similar browser) by double clicking on its icon. Once Netscape is opened, place the cursor on the "File" column at the top left-hand side of the screen. Click and hold down the mouse to reveal the menu below "File." Move the mouse to "open location" and release. A dialogue box will appear on the screen that asks you to type in the address of the location you are seeking. In this case, enter the address of the U.S. Census Bureau—http://www.census.gov—and the home page of the Census Bureau will appear (as shown in Figure 9.1).

On the home page will be some buttons to click to direct you to find the information you are looking for. In addition, any blue wording on an organization's home page can be double clicked with the mouse, and information that relates to the word or phrase that is clicked will be provided. The blue wording denotes a topic or name that has been linked to another site to help the user access additional information about that topic.

Another method for locating information on the Internet involves using a **search engine.** Various search engines are available (e.g., Yahoo, Alta Vista, Excite, Infoseek, Webcrawler, Lycos, PubMed, Hotbot). The advantage of using a search engine over typing in a URL (which is specific to one site) is that the search engine allows you to type in the name of the topic you want to find information about, and after a few seconds identifies and lists several sites related to that topic. All the user needs to do to access the information from any of the sites listed is to click the pointer on the name of the site and it will appear. The search engines are usually located on the main search page of the browser.

For example, as a health educator, you have been asked to find some information on "sexually transmitted diseases." You can go to the main search page of your browser, Netscape in this case, and click on the button on the toolbar above the screen that is labeled "net search." The button takes you to one of the search engine web pages that has a box in it for typing in the words for a search. Click in the box and type "sexually transmitted diseases." See Figure 9.2 for an example.

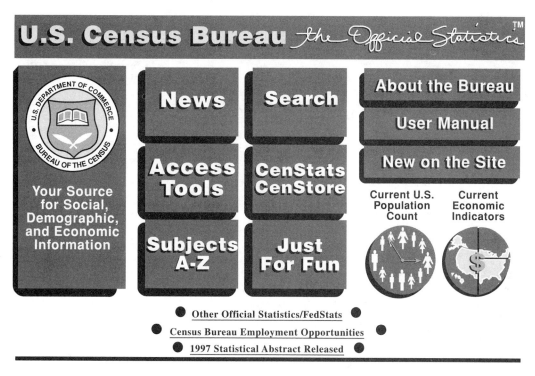

FIGURE 9.1   Home page of the U.S. Census Bureau as found on the Internet.

Then hit "return" or "enter" on your keyboard and wait several seconds. In a short while, you will see a list of sites on your screen related to "sexually transmitted diseases (Figure 9.3)." Click on any one of the sites, and you will be transported to the page and information that correspond to that site.

Sometimes you may want to use a specific search engine. Because all of the search engines have nearly the same URL, the home page for any of the search engines can be readily accessed by typing in the specific web address (URL) from the Netscape 'File" menu, as was demonstrated in the example using the Census Bureau. For example, the URL for Yahoo is http://www.yahoo.com; for Infoseek, it is http://www.infoseek.com; for Alta Vista, it is http://www.altavista.com.

If the term you are searching for has more than one word (such as "sexually transmitted diseases"), it is wise to use quotation marks around the term when it is entered into the box marked "search." This will let the search engine know that all of the words are to be included in the term when the search engine is seeking sites that match. If quotation marks are not used, the search engine may seek sites that match only the first word in the multiword term (in this case, it might search only for the word *sexually*), and the search engine might locate some sites that do not have anything to do with the topic of sexually transmitted diseases.

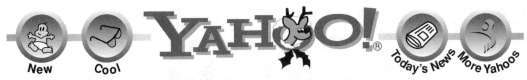

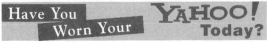

"sexually transmitted diseases"   Search   options

Yellow Pages - People Search - Maps - Classifieds - Personals - Chat - **Email**
Holiday Shopping - My Yahoo! - News - Sports - Weather - Stock Quotes

- **Arts and Humanities**
  Architecture, Photography, Literature...

- **Business and Economy [Xtra!]**
  Companies, Finance, Employment...

- **Computers and Internet [Xtra!]**
  Internet, WWW, Software, Multimedia...

- **Education**
  Universities, K-12, College Entrance...

- **Entertainment [Xtra!]**
  Cool Links, Movies, Music, Humor...

- **Government**
  Military, Politics [**Xtra!**], Law, Taxes...

- **Health [Xtra!]**
  Medicine, Drugs, Diseases, Fitness...

- **News and Media [Xtra!]**
  Current Events, Magazines, TV, Newspapers...

- **Recreation and Sports [Xtra!]**
  Sports, Games, Travel, Autos, Outdoors...

- **Reference**
  Libraries, Dictionaries, Phone Numbers...

- **Regional**
  Countries, Regions, U.S. States...

- **Science**
  CS, Biology, Astronomy, Engineering...

- **Social Science**
  Anthropology, Sociology, Economics...

- **Society and Culture**
  People, Environment, Religion...

Yahooligans! for Kids - Beatrice's Guide - MTV/Yahoo! unfURLed - Yahoo! Internet Life
What's New - Weekly Picks - Today's Web Events
Visa Shopping Guide - Yahoo! Store

World Yahoos Australia & NZ - Canada - Denmark - France - Germany - Japan - Korea
Norway - SE Asia - Sweden - UK & Ireland

Yahoo! Metros Atlanta - Austin - Boston - Chicago - Dallas/Fort Worth - Los Angeles
Get Local Miami - Minneapolis/St. Paul - New York - S.F. Bay - Seattle - Wash D.C.

Smart Shopping with **VISA**

How to Suggest a Site - Company Info - Openings at Yahoo! - Contributors - Yahoo! to Go

FIGURE 9.2   Yahoo Search Engine page with "sexually transmitted diseases" entered in the
"Search" box.

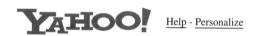

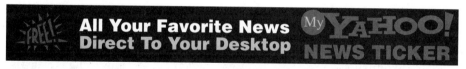

Categories	Web Sites	Alta Vista	News Stories	Net Events
Found **3** categories and **16** sites for **sexually transmitted diseases**				

Yahoo! Category Matches   (1 - 3 of 3)

Health: **Diseases** and Conditions: **Sexually Transmitted Diseases** (STDs)

Regional: Countries: Australia: Health: **Diseases** and Conditions: **Sexually Transmitted Diseases** (STDs)

Regional: Countries: United Kingdom: Health: **Diseases** and Conditions: **Sexually Transmitted Diseases** (STDs)

Yahoo! Site Matches   (1 - 16 of 16)

Health: **Diseases** and Conditions: **Sexually Transmitted Diseases** (STDs)

- **Sexually Transmitted Diseases** Research Group - Johns Hopkins University - info about our research in STDs and links for health care providers in this field.
- my **sexually transmitted** disease - True story of the time I had nonspecific urethritis.
- **Sexually transmitted** disease (STD) (venereal disease) prevention for everyone.
- International Union against the Venereal **Diseases** and the Treponematoses - working to achieve international cooperation in controlling **sexually transmitted diseases**, including HIV infection.
- Communicable **Diseases**
- American Social Health Association - ASHA's mission is to stop **sexually transmitted diseases** (STDs) and their harmful consequences to individuals, families, and communities.
- Clinic 275 - **Sexually Transmitted Diseases** Clinic operated by the South Australian Health Commission's STD Control Branch.

Entertainment: People

- Wright, Michael P. - summarizes my professional activities relating to **sexually transmitted diseases**, American Indians, and coal industry.

Health: **Diseases** and Conditions: AIDS/HIV: Education: Organizations

- American Social Health Association - ASHA's mission is to stop **sexually transmitted diseases** (STDs) and their harmful consequences to individuals, families, and communities.

Health: General Health

- Wellness on the Web Prevention Resource Center - for information about **sexually transmitted diseases**, Medical and natural healing approach to treatment.

FIGURE 9.3   Yahoo page with site matches to the search query for the term "sexually transmitted diseases."

Practitioner's Perspective

Name:	Jenny J. Bair
Current Position/Title:	Peer Education & Healthy Lifestyle Center Coordinator
Employer:	Idaho State University, Department of Health and Nutrition Sciences
Major(s):	B.S. Health Education—Southwest Texas State University
Minor(s):	None

Primary job responsibilities: I coordinate training sessions and retreats, teach the peer education class, and supervise the Healthy Lifestyles Center. I plan, implement, and evaluate all peer education programming initiatives such as Safer Spring Break, Great American Smokeout, Breast Cancer Awareness Month, and World AIDS Day. I also order all educational materials for the Lifestyles Center and market the peer education classes.

How I obtained my position: One of my undergraduate professors put my resume on the Internet, and Idaho State University responded by phone. I expressed interest in their position (which was for a graduate assistantship with the duties described above); I had a phone interview; I came on campus for an interview with departmental faculty and staff in the Student Affairs Office; and I was offered the position.

How I utilize health information resources: Each and everyday I search for pertinent and up-to-date health information on the World Wide Web. In addition, I have become very familiar with most health and wellness pamphlets and posters available that might appeal to a college audience. Finally, I utilize the library extensively, searching CD-ROM databases for articles and studies that might assist me and the other peer educators in obtaining factual, current information that will be of value to students. The database searches have also assisted me in finding approaches to health education that have been used by other institutions.

What I like most about my position: I have a deep passion for the ever-changing field of health promotion. I love helping others lead more positive lifestyles that enable them to better reach goals and life visions. I enjoy working with college students. My job is never dull or boring but always challenging! I have to be creative to reach students of all religious persuasions, ethnic backgrounds, cultures, and sexual orientations. When students share a story of positive transformation, I am renewed and feel most blessed. I also am proud and privileged to coordinate a group of intelligent, unique, creative students (our peer educators) who want to make a positive change in their campus community. These students teach me much about myself and life each and every day.

What I like least about my position: I am frustrated by financial constraints. Programming and education materials can be very expensive. I spend much time prioritizing what to buy and creating many of the materials from scratch.

Recommendations for health education students who want to have positions similar to mine: I think it is highly beneficial to become involved in health-related student organizations and to attend conventions. As overwhelming and as "scary" as it may be to some students, take advantage of public speaking opportunities. Doing these activities will help develop your organization, communication, and leadership skills. You will build self-confidence and continue to be motivated to contribute toward positive changes in your community for a lifetime.

Evaluating Information on the Internet

Earlier in the chapter, directions were given for evaluating the accuracy and validity of information from journal and popular press sources. Because of the massive amount of information available on the Internet and because nearly anyone who has a knowledge of "html" (**hypertext markup language,** the programming language used on the Internet) can publish on the World Wide Web, it is equally imperative that the health educator know how to evaluate information obtained via an Internet search. Jatkevicius (1998), an electronic reference specialist at the Oboler Library at Idaho State University, has published a handout listing several areas to consider in evaluating information retrieved on the Internet:

1. Content. Material included has been verified or has survived a minimal screening or refereeing process. Sources are cited. Frequently, the addresses end in ".edu," ".gov," or ".org" if from a known professional organization.
2. Authority. The credentials of the authors are clearly presented. The authors' e-mail addresses and/or phone numbers are provided for contact.
3. Publisher-source. This information should be unambiguous and clearly identifiable. It should be readily apparent who is sponsoring or otherwise representing the page.
4. References. Have other pages used this site as a link to their own page?
5. Documentation. Documentation is consistently provided. The sources are important, because a source that lacks documentation often falls in the opinion or editorial category.
6. Facts. Are the facts consistent with information obtained from other sources? Be cautious of sites that have an address ending in ".com," as they are commercial sites and may be selling a product.

Selected Health-Related Web Sites

Larsson (1996), Daniel (1997), Kittleson (1997), and Rivard and Olpin (1998) have published lists of sites with information that has proved to be helpful to health educators. The lists given by Kittleson (1997) and Rivard and Olpin (1997) are part of texts providing detailed descriptions on how to use the Internet to retrieve health information. For those students wishing more information on this topic or for identifying the URLs of many more health sites, either of these texts is recommended. The following list of sites is not meant to be exhaustive in scope but representative of the many sites that are available on the World Wide Web. The best way to learn about web sites is to log on to the computer and start experimenting.

Epidemiological and Statistical Information
1. CDC Wonder
   http://cdc.wonder.gov

2. Morbidity and Mortality Weekly Report
   http://www.cdc.gov/epo/mmwr.html
3. U.S. Statistical Data from the U.S. Bureau of the Census
   http://www.census.gov/

Infectious Diseases
4. MMWR Summary of Notifiable Diseases
   http://www.crawford.com/epo/mmwr/mmwr_snd.html
5. National Center for Infectious Disease Statistics
   http://www.cdc.gov/ncidod/ncid.htm

Chronic Diseases
6. Chronic Diseases
   http://www.os.dhhs.gov/progorg/io/chronic/htm
7. National Cancer Institute
   http://www.nci.nih.gov/

Disease Control and Prevention
8. The CDC Prevention Guidelines Database
   http://wonder.cdc.gov/wonder/prevguid/prevguid.html
9. The National Clearinghouse for Alcohol and Drug Information
   http://www.health.org
10. American Diabetes Association
    http://www.diabetes.org/
11. CDC's Division of HIV/AIDS Prevention
    http://www.cdc.gov/nchstp/hiv_aids/dhap.htm
12. Immunization Action Coalition
    http://abdominable.winternet.com/~immunize/
13. Children's Safety Network
    http://www.edc.org/HHD/csn
14. FDA Center for Food Safety and Applied Nutrition
    http://vm.cfsan.fda.gov/list.html
15. Oncolink's Smoking, Tobacco, and Cancer Web Page
    http://oncolink.upenn.edu/topics/smoking_menu.html
16. Travel Medicine
    http://www.hslib.washington.edu/clinical/travel
17. CDC's Division of Tuberculosis Elimination
    http://www.cdc.gov/nchstp/tb/dtbe.html
18. Harvard Women's Health Watch
    http://www.med.harvard.edu/publications/Women/.index.html
19. Environmental Health Center: Radon and Indoor Air Quality
    http://www.nsc.org/nsc/ehc/radon/html

National Agencies
20. CDC—Centers for Disease Control and Prevention
    http://www.cdc.gov

21. DHHS—Department of Health and Human Services
    http://www.os.dhhs.gov/
22. EPA—Environmental Protection Agency
    http://www.epa.gov
23. IHS—Indian Health Service
    http://www.tuscon.ihs.gov/
24. ODPHP—Office of Disease Prevention and Health Promotion
    http://nhic-nt.health.org

International Agencies
25. WHO—World Health Organization
    http://www.who.ch/
26. PAHO—Pan American Health Organization
    http://www.paho.org/english/index.htm

Web-based MEDLINE Search Systems
27. HealthGate (free access to MEDLINE)
    http://www.healthgate.com/
28. MEDLINE Simple Search
    http://healthgate.com/HealthGate/MEDLINE/search.shtml

Public Health Practice
29. Public Health Practice Program Office (CDC)
    http://www.cdc.gov/phppo.htm
30. Public Health Practice Publications
    http://www.hsph.harvard.edu/Organizations/php/publicat.html

State and Local Public Health Departments
31. Local Health Departments (USA and Canada)—by name
    http://weber.u.washington.edu/~larsson/hsic94/resource/phealth/
    lhd/ihddepts.html

General Health Information
32. Alta Vista Health Topics Search
    http://www.altavista.digital.com/
33. Health A to Z
    http://www.HealthAtoZ.com/
34. Yahoo Search/Health
    http://www.yahoo.com/Health/
35. Healthwise's "Go Ask Alice"
    http://columbia.edu/cu/healthwise/alice/html
36. The Virtual Public Health Center
    http://www-sci.lib.uci.edu/~martindale/PHealth.html
37. Cal Berkeley Wellness Letter
    http://www.enews.com/magazines/ucbwl/

38. Healthfinder
http://www.healthfinder.gov
39. Internet Connections/Health
http://www.mcrel.org/connect/health.html
40. Community Health Sites
http://web.indstate.edu/hlthsfty/ch/bookmarks.htm
41. Association for Worksite Health Promotion
http://www.awhp.com/
42. University of Alberta's Health Information Page
http://www.ualberta.ca/~jhancock/HealthEd.html

News Stories
43. Reuters Health Information Service
http://reutershealth.com/
44. USA Today Healthline
http://167.8.29.13/life/health/lhd1.htm

Health Education/Health Promotion Jobs
45. Health Education Professional Resources
http://www.nyu.edu/education/hepr/

Summary

This chapter has presented an overview on accessing and evaluating health-related information. The fact that there is an increasing demand for health information, coupled with the fact that the information is being produced at an ever greater rate, creates added responsibility for health educators. Two of the major roles of health educators as discussed in Chapter 6 involve being resource people for health information and communicating to others health education needs, concerns, and resources. In order to perform these tasks, the health educator must have the skills to find information, must evaluate the source of the information to determine its credibility, and must disseminate the information through the appropriate channels to consumers. Becoming familiar with the tools found in this chapter is a necessity for all students wanting to enter the field of health education.

REVIEW QUESTIONS

1. Describe the difference between a primary, a secondary, and a popular press source.

2. How do an article abstract and an article summary differ in content?

3. What are the questions you should ask yourself when critiquing a journal article? What are the differences between the questions asked when evaluating a primary research article and the questions asked when evaluating a secondary or popular press article?

4. What are five of the most commonly used journals in the field of health education? What types of information would you expect to find in each of the journals you named?

5. What is the difference between using an abstract and using an index to find health-related information?

6. What is the Internet and how does it enable one to access so much information?

7. How does one go about evaluating information retrieved from the Internet?

8. In your own words, describe how to access information concerning "breast cancer" on the World Wide Web.

ACTIVITIES

1. You are employed as a health educator in a district health department and have just received a call from a member of a local coalition wanting to know where to find an article that summarizes the content and effectiveness of available school-based sexuality education curricula. Use an index and find a reference to an article that meets those criteria.

2. Was the article you located in activity #1 a primary or secondary source of information? Provide rationale for your answer.

3. Using a database (CINAHL, MEDLINE, or ERIC), find a primary research article relating to traffic safety (e.g., the use of seatbelts, airbags, road surfaces). Critique the article by applying the questions found in the "critically reading a research article" section of the chapter.

4. As a newly employed health educator in a hospital outpatient clinic, one of your jobs is to provide information to patients after they have seen the physician. Ms. X has just been diagnosed with coronary artery disease, and the physician has sent her to you to discuss the role of lifestyle on her condition. Using the World Wide Web, find several sources of information that you could give her to read that might assist you with the education process. Evaluate the accuracy of the information you retrieve.

5. Make a list of the health education journals described in this chapter that are available at your college/university library. For those journals not in your library's holdings, check with a librarian to determine if they are available through interlibrary loan or another exchange service.

REFERENCES

American Psychological Association. (1993). *Psychological Abstracts, 80,* p. 4144. Washington, DC: American Psychological Association.

Cottrell, R. R. (1997). *A guide to evaluating a journal article.* Unpublished manuscript

Cozby, P.C. (1993). *Methods in behavioral research* (5th ed.). Palo Alto, CA: Mayfield.

Daniel, E.L. (1997). *Jump start with weblinks: A guidebook for fitness/wellness/personal health.* Englewood, CO: Morton.

Jatkevicius, J. (1998). *Internet resource evaluation guidelines.* Pocatello, ID: Eli Oboler Library, Idaho State University.

Kennedy, G.E., & Montgomery, T.T. (1993). *Solving problems through technical and professional writing.* (pp. 1–82). Boston: McGraw-Hill.

Kittleson, M. J. (1997). *Web sites for health professionals.* Sudbury, MA: Jones and Bartlett.

Larsson, L. (1996, November). *Internet demonstration for public health practitioners.* American Public Health Association Convention, New York.

Levene, L. A. (1990). Health educators and library resources. *Health Education, 21*(5), 25–29.

McKenzie, J.F. (1987). A checklist for evaluating health information. *Journal of School Health, 57*(1), 31–32.

McKinney, W.P., et al. (1997). Comparing smoking behavior of veterans and nonveterans. *Public Health Reports, 112*(3), 212–217.

National Commission for Health Education Credentialing. (1996). *A competency-based framework for professional development of Certified Health Education Specialists.* New York: National Commission for Health Education Credentialing.

Riegelman, R.K., & Hirsh, R.P. (1989). *Studying a study and testing a test: How to read medical literature,* (2nd ed., pp. 3–91). Boston: Little, Brown, & Company.

Rivard, J.D., & Olpin, M. (1997). *Quick guide to the Internet for health.* Boston: Allyn and Bacon.

Shi, L. (1996). *Health services research methods* (pp. 61–112). Albany, NY: Delmar.

Thomas, J.R., & Nelson, J.K. (1985). *Introduction to research in health, physical education, and dance* (pp. 31–53). Champaign, IL: Human Kinetics.

10 Future Trends in Health Education

CHAPTER OBJECTIVES

After reading this chapter and answering the questions at the end, you should be able to

1. Identify two settings in which health educators will practice to a greater degree than they do today.
2. Describe four major societal changes that will influence the practice of health education into the next century.
3. Explain how demographic changes will impact health education delivery into the future.
4. Delineate the major implications of credentialing for future health educators.
5. Compare and contrast the roles of health educators in the four practice settings.
6. Identify several reasons that health educators should be optimistic about future employment opportunities.
7. Describe the need for health educators in two alternative settings.

KEY TERMS

conservative	microlevel	postsecondary institution
demographic profile	moderate	technology
liberal	postmodern family	traditional family
macrolevel		

Introduction

It has been said that one of the few constants is change. Clark (1994) notes that large trends in society are acting on the profession of health education as never before. Health seems to be the current watchword of populace in the United States. With increasing numbers of citizens interested in health information, a reliance on technology for information delivery and acquisition, rapidly changing demographic patterns, and a heightened skepticism of the medical establishment, the world that will confront health educators in the future is vastly different from that of only a decade ago. These changes present the health educator with enormous opportunities. The focus of this chapter will be to explore future developments in the discipline of health education/promotion and, hopefully, to create a sense of excitement and anticipation in the challenges that lie ahead.

Picture yourself as having just arrived to the United States from another planet. The year is 1970. Assume that the first thing you see is a one-hour television news program. Based solely on that program and the commercial messages during the station breaks, how would you describe the lives of people on the planet you are visiting? Now, transport yourself ahead to the year 1995, and repeat the same exercise. Although the purpose of this chapter is not to dwell on comparative history, it is noteworthy that, in a brief, twenty-five-year span, the United States and many other countries have changed so dramatically as to be almost unrecognizable. Certainly, some of the problems faced by individuals; communities; and local, state, and federal governments are the same and the dress styles and modes of transportation have not changed much, but demographic and societal changes, some subtle and others not so subtle, have altered the landscape forever. Several of these changes have profound implications for the way health education will be practiced in the next century.

The first chapter section will discuss changing demographic patterns. Societal trends that are predicted to play a role in the practice of health education into the next century will be featured. Issues related to credentialing and preparation will be covered next. Using this information as a foundation, the chapter will conclude by postulating about the impact of these changes for the health educator in the school, community/public health, worksite, and medical care settings. One caveat is in order prior to this discussion: obviously, no one knows exactly what the future will hold. The information presented is meant to stimulate thinking about the role health educators will play from now until the years 2020–2030.

Demographic Changes

Over the past thirty years, the population growth rate in the United States has increased at about 1 percent per year. While this stable growth pattern is probably manageable for the long term, a more in-depth study of the **demographic profile,** the breakdown of the United States population by age group, sex, race, and ethnicity, shows a dramatically altered picture from that of just ten years ago. It is this consistently changing demographic profile—specifically, a greater percentage of minority residents and an ever aging population—that has important implications for the future practice of health educators.

Minority Population Changes

Clark (1994) states, "We are undergoing a massive change in culture in our society. We are literally looking different as a nation and the conventional majority values and norms are being challenged as we become a more diverse, more ethnic, more integrated culture. Health educators have long prided themselves with working across cultures . . . . The cultural changes are . . . greater than we have experienced previously" (p. 137). Simons-Morton, Greene, and Gottlieb (1995) point out that the increasing racial and ethnic diversity in the United States results from the fact that many of the recent immigrants are from South America, Mexico, and Asia and not from western Europe, as was the case in the 1800s and early 1900s. In addition, they mention that in the United States minority groups often have higher birth rates than do whites. These two factors are largely responsible for driving the changes previously alluded to. Just what is the magnitude of the change?

Statistics from the U.S. Bureau of the Census (1993) indicate that in 1980 the U.S. minority population was 11.7 percent African American, 6.4 percent Hispanic, 1.5 percent Asian or Pacific Islander, and 0.6 percent Native American. Table 10.1 shows the projected percentage figures for each of these population groups for the years 2000, 2010, 2020, and 2030 (U.S. Bureau of the Census, 1996).

From Table 10.1 it is readily apparent that the greatest percentage increase over the next thirty years will come from the Hispanic and Asian/Pacific Islander groups. The percentage increase of Hispanics and Asians from 2000 until 2030 is 61.5 percent and 65 percent, respectively. During this same time period, the percentage of non-Hispanic whites in the population will fall from 71.4 percent in the year 2000 to about 60.5 percent in the year 2030, a decrease of about 15 percent.

Clark (1994) mentions that at least one ramification of these changes, increasing numbers of ethnic minority students in public school, is already being felt in the classrooms of our nation. By the year 2000, 35 percent of the children in public schools in the United States will be minorities. Additionally, in New York City in the next decade, 35 to 40 percent of the residents will be Hispanic, 25% African American, and 25 percent white. The escalating minority population makes an already diverse nation even more so and presents health educators with an ever widening array of opportunities and challenges as we race toward the twenty-first century.

TABLE 10.1 Projected U.S. Population Percentages of African Americans, Hispanics, Native Americans, and Asians or Pacific Islanders: 2000, 2010, 2020, and 2030

	Year			
Race	2000	2010	2020	2030
African American	13.0%	13.5%	14.0%	14.4%
Hispanic	11.7%	13.8%	16.3%	18.9%
Native American	0.9%	0.8%	0.8%	0.8%
Asian/Pacific Islander	4.0%	4.8%	5.7%	6.6%

Aging

Another demographic factor that will impact the practice of health education in the future is the aging population. The U.S. Bureau of the Census (1996) lists persons age sixty-five or older as representing 12.8 percent of the U.S. population. Between the years 2010 and 2030, the population over sixty-five is expected to grow by nearly 75 percent, while that of individuals under sixty-five will increase only 6.5 percent. To further illustrate this trend, the median age of the U.S. population in 1990 was 33.1 years. In the year 2000, it is predicted to be 35.9 years; in 2010, it will be 37.2; in 2020, it will be 37.6; in 2030, it will be 38.5.

One of the major reasons for the aging trend relates to the fact that older Americans are living longer than ever before. Other causative factors accentuating aging are that married couples in the United States are having fewer children, and the baby boomer cohort (those born between 1946 and 1964) is now reaching middle age. This group's massive size causes it to have a dominant effect on U.S. population statistics. "Clearly the aging of the American population creates an increased need for health-related programs for older adults" (Schuster, 1995, p. 338).

Societal Trends

There probably has not been a time when societal change has been as rapid as in the latter three or four decades of the twentieth century. For example, since 1960,

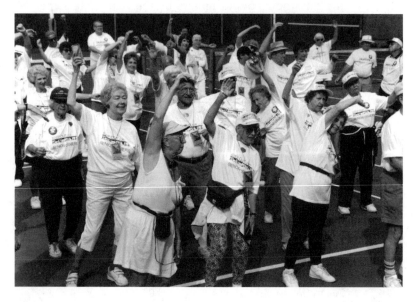

Health promotion for the elderly will be in increasing demand in the next century. (Spencer Grant/ Stock, Boston)

there have been changes in societal mores and practices, such as more openness to cohabitation, a greater tolerance for premarital sex, more vocal and open gay relationships, a greater number of single-parent households, an increase in child abuse, more violence, an increase in the amount and availability of pornographic materials, massive changes in the number of ethical issues related to medicine, alterations in the way the medical establishment is organized and medical care is delivered, a decreasing respect for authority of any kind, declining support for public schools, an infusion of and a reliance on technology, and a distrust of the political process in general. All of these factors play a big role in shaping the structure of society in the future. This section will discuss several of the major societal trends that experts agree will impact health education into the new millennium.

Technology

"Tool up, tool up, the 21st century is around the corner" (Clark, 1994, p. 141). This quote aptly sums up the charge to health educators in the area of technology. There have been great advances in technology in many areas—for instance, medicine, automobiles, and home appliances—over the past several decades. However, the **technology** we are referring to is in the use of educational technology.

One would be hard pressed to find a campus today that did not feature student computer labs in numerous locations. Access to a computer is almost a prerequisite for taking a class in any discipline. Many courses are conducted using fiber optics and satellites to beam "real time" lessons in a different part of campus or to remote locations. Students can acquire the information needed to complete assignments using technological advances such as the on-line search services on the Internet, computerized reference databases, CD-ROMs, and videodiscs. There are several electronic journals that are available only in electronic form; no printed hard copy is available. This knowledge explosion trend fueled by new innovations in educational technology shows no sign of diminishing.

What does this mean for health educators? Butler (1997) declares that future health educators must be able to access information, select and use the data obtained, make sound decisions about the appropriateness of the data, and create solutions that meet the needs of the audience with whom they are working. Clark (1994) believes that, while technology will be central to the future use of health education, the emphasis will need to be on user-friendly technology. In short, health educators will need to help others learn how to learn. This means that the health educator's role will not only include serving as a resource for health information but also helping the public develop skills in finding valid sources of health information and teaching them to evaluate the accuracy of that information.

Family Structure

The American family structure has changed dramatically since the 1960s. The **traditional family** (two parents and their children) is becoming less and less common because of factors such as high rates of divorce, smaller families, postponed marriage and childbearing, teenage and nonmarital childbearing, stepfamilies, homosexual couples, and dual-earner marriages (Acock & Demo, 1994). These changes have spawned a new sociological family descriptor, the **postmodern family** (Cheal, 1991; Stacy, 1991).

Acock and Demo (1994) state, "There is no doubt that the shape and composition of families have changed profoundly" (p. 11). In 1960, 87.7 percent of children under the age of eighteen lived with two parents, and only 9.1 percent with one parent. By 1992, this number had decreased to 70.7 percent living with two parents and 26.6 percent living with only one parent (U.S. Bureau of the Census, 1992). The quoted figures are for all races.

When comparing statistics for African American families with statistics for all races combined, the picture is even worse. In 1960, 67 percent of children under eighteen lived with both parents, and 19.9 percent lived with the mother only. In 1992, 35.6 percent lived with both parents and 53.8 percent lived with the mother only (U.S. Bureau of the Census, 1992).

The impact caused by these new structures is being felt throughout our society. Children are the most affected. Many parents today provide less guidance and support, and many seem to lack the commitment needed to be parents. Uhlenberg and Eggebeen (1986) write, "We suggest that it is an erosion of the bond between parent and child—one characterized by parental commitment and willingness to sacrifice self-interest—that is the significant cause of declining well-being of American adolescents after 1960" (p. 38).

Simons-Morton, Greene, and Gottlieb (1995) document other stressful changes in the family. They mention that the high costs of providing for a family today have almost necessitated that a family have two incomes. This places a strain even on nuclear families with two parents; affordable daycare services for the children must be obtained. For many low-income and single-parent families, the choice is no care or supervision at all—a situation that puts children at risk. In addition, fewer employers are offering health insurance, particularly in service-oriented positions that often pay minimum wage and are a major source of employment for many low-skilled workers. As a result, nearly 21 percent of children in the United States are living in poverty (*Kids Count Data Book*, 1995). The linkage between these factors may be a predisposing condition leading to an increased rate of child abuse (McKenzie & Pinger, 1995).

The changes previously noted have massive implications for health educators. Family structures look to remain diverse in the coming years and will probably operate on a new set of norms. Clark (1994) emphasizes that family structures of the future" will demand new laws, new policies, new procedures, and new health education in recognition of these new types of family" (p. 137). In other words, new methods of reaching individuals, families, and communities will need to be created in order to improve the health of all family members in accordance with their needs.

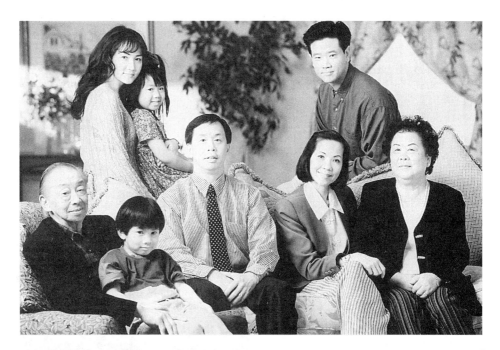

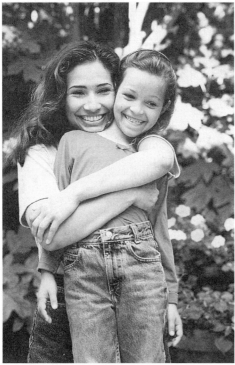

Health educators need to tailor their messages to many family types. (above—Bruce Ayres/Stock, Boston; left—Stewart Cohen/Stock, Boston)

Political Climate

As was mentioned earlier, there remains little doubt that today there is an increasing frustration with politics and politicians in general. Whether a person is a **conservative,** one who generally distrusts governmental regulations and tax-supported programs for addressing social or economic problems; a **moderate,** one who usually acts in a more situationally specific manner in regard to using tax-supported programs to solve societal problems; or a **liberal,** one who generally desires more government programs to attack social and economic problems, there seems to be no end to the bickering and infighting that goes on among members of various political parties. Many of the political issues considered in Congress relate to health. The landmark agreement between the tobacco industry and the states over the sale and marketing of tobacco products to minors, the repeal of a motorcycle helmet law in Texas, the passage of a physician-assisted suicide law in Oregon, and the settlement of a lawsuit related to the storage of nuclear waste in Idaho are examples of legislation that directly impacts the health of the populace.

A further example of the battle of political agendas as they relate to health follows. Sullum (1996) postulates that the public health establishment has assumed the role of protecting people from themselves by lobbying for seatbelt laws, fewer tobacco ads, restrictions on sales and advertising of alcoholic beverages, and gun control laws. In short, he believes that many of the public health programs today are an infringement on personal freedoms. Fineberg (1996) does not disagree with the fact that individuals are largely responsible for their own health. He advocates, however, that "public health must continue to recognize and to concern itself with the major threats to contemporary well-being" (p. 18).

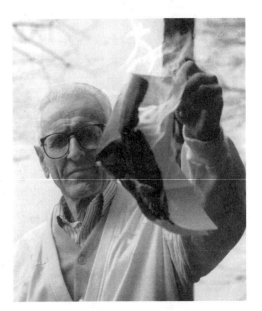

An awareness of political issues that affect health will be even more crucial in the future. (AP Photo/Carlos Osorio)

As citizens and professionals, the involvement of health educators in the political process is important. O'Rourke (1989) states, "Health education not only seeks to change lifestyles, but to create public understanding of the political issues involved in public health programs" (p. 9). He goes on to challenge all health educators to assume a **macrolevel view** of health problems. Using this approach, health educators move from a position of assisting behavior change one person at a time to community-based interventions. In implementing the community-based programs, success often depends on the health educator having a working knowledge of the political process and how it impacts every decision. Butler (1997) adds, "Forming coalitions, authoring legislation, writing letters, and lobbying by professional organizations are effective ways to affect public policy through the political system" (p. 344).

In the future it will be imperative for health educators to be politically active. To paraphrase Clark (1994), there is a great need for health educators to capture the energy and power of all in order that health promotion/education agendas are realized in the coming years. Clark goes on to say, "We need governments that are operating on the basis of healthful policies, regulations, and programs. We need organizations that enact healthful policies, maintain healthful facilities, implement healthful programs. We need individuals who are healthful in their behavior, and in the physical and psychological aspects of their life. All these levels must be involved to engender improved health status in society" (p. 140). In short, future health educators will need to sharpen their advocacy skills.

Medical Care Establishment

In her article on future directions in health education, Clark (1994) lists several societal trends that are powerful forces for change. One of these is the erosion of the powerbase of the medical care establishment. No longer are physicians' decisions going unquestioned by either patients or insurance providers. There is a strong desire on the part of citizens to be participants in their own care and to be provided with options. Clark (1994) also notes that the health goals of the public are slowly shifting from a "longevity mentality" to one focusing on quality of life.

Simons-Morton, Greene, and Gottlieb (1995) point out several reasons for this trend. While few would question the fact that our medical care system has been responsible for saving countless lives, it has become apparent to many that health is largely a reflection of personal lifestyle choices and living standards and not a medical care system. They further emphasize that medical care tends to concentrate on secondary and tertiary care and to ignore the value of primary prevention.

These points are substantiated in a landmark study done by McGinnis and Foege (1993), who changed the paradigm by analyzing the factors responsible for the leading causes of death. They concluded that the majority of the factors are lifestyle-related and not readily amenable to medical intervention.

The public is receptive to the notion that health education can make a difference in disease management (Butler, 1997; Clark, 1994). In addition to the reasons previously discussed, several other factors bode well for enhanced opportunities for health educators in future years—the advent of managed care, the fact that almost 37 million Americans have no health insurance, the restructuring of both the Medicare and Medicaid systems, and the growing influence of insurers. Given these circumstances, health educators can facilitate patient choice by helping patients understand their options regarding physician choice, health care insurance plan, type of care, and intensity of services. In addition, they can assist medical organizations by increasing patient satisfaction through contributing to more one-on-one contact, improving patterns of communication between patient and provider, and enhancing patient compliance with treatment regimens (Butler, 1997; Cree, 1997; Lorig, Manzonson, & Holman, 1993).

Professional Preparation and Credentialing

Although the issues of professional preparation and credentialing were extensively covered in Chapter 6, both have implications for the future practice of health education. Thus, spending a brief amount of time highlighting the reasons health education practice might be impacted by these issues is of some importance.

Professional Preparation

In this discussion, it is not our intent to provide a list of courses that must be taken to become a "better" health educator. Coursework is by nature specific to the institution you are attending. Course titles and descriptions vary widely from one program to another. As you are aware, the coursework you will take in your degree program is interdisciplinary. What we will attempt to accomplish is to provide some ideas, concepts, and objectives for you to consider as you enter your preparation program.

The social changes previously discussed in this chapter are the driving force behind challenging the health educator of the future to be proactive in meeting the demands placed on her. What tasks will a health educator need to be able to perform to be effective in the decades ahead? Clark (1994) helps answer this question by making several salient points in speaking about health education in the future:

1. The mission will be less providing factual information and more helping people become more analytical thinkers—thus, enabling them to deal better with complex issues and uncertainty.
2. There will be newer, stronger partnerships with the medical establishment. This collaboration will give a new power to health education and will capitalize on the idea that health education makes a difference in disease management.
3. Educators will need to analyze situations and examine past and future trends to see the threats to quality of life. Long-term, not short-term, thinking will be a must.

4. A greater emphasis will be placed on values clarification. Health educators must learn to account for the effects of culture and then find processes that reach people with different values.
5. Mechanisms need to be perfected for designing and delivering multilevel approaches to optimize health education in addressing priority health problems. Education at the community level will be the focus of the predominate number of health interventions.
6. There will be an enhanced need for quality research, so that the effectiveness of health education methodologies can be ascertained. The need for cost-effective, efficient strategies will remain.
7. Health educators must determine how to use technology to help people learn.
8. The need to integrate education, health, and social services within the schools will become more recognized. The gap between school and community services will close.
9. Environmental activism will continue to emerge, and health educators can play an important role in facilitating multidimensional programs that cross all socioeconomic and political boundaries.
10. In the final analysis, people will judge the success of health education by whether or not their quality of life has improved.

Several of Clark's thoughts are echoed by O'Rourke (1989), when he challenges health educators to be more macrolevel- oriented. In other words, there is an ever growing need to facilitate health education interventions at the community level (as opposed to the individual level, or **microlevel**). Inherent in this charge is that those who reside in the community where the intervention occurs will be totally involved in the planning from the outset. English and Videto (1997) affirm these observations when they state, "Regardless of our place of practice, our ability to identify and meet the needs of our local communities and neighborhoods is likely to be the measure that will determine our success as health educators . . . successful programs use community involvement" (p. 4).

Finally, it is apparent that tomorrow's health educators must be able to respond rapidly to changes in all avenues of society. When planning, implementing, and evaluating programs and working in multidimensional settings, they must enter into collaborative relationships with health care professionals from other disciplines in a spirit of cooperation. Health educators who are not afraid to be innovative; who respect but do not fear change; who are not just purveyors of information but community builders and facilitators of learning; who continue to be curious and learn themselves; who have a sense of adventure; and who seek the truth through thoughtful research, study, and dialogue—those are the individuals who will lead our profession into the next several decades.

Credentialing

The history of and reasons for credentialing were thoroughly covered in Chapter 6, yet there are several facets of credentialing that need reemphasis, as they have profound implications for the future practice of health education.

BOX **10.1**

Practitioner's Perspective

Name:	Joanne Mitten
Current Position/Title:	Chief, Bureau of Health Promotion
Employer:	Idaho Department of Health and Welfare
Major(s):	M.H.E.—Idaho State University
	B.S., Microbiology—Miami of Ohio
Minor(s):	None

Primary job responsibilities: My major responsibilities are budget management; personnel supervision; proposing and enforcing policies, procedures, and rules; quality assurance; evaluation; and communication coordination.

How I obtained my position: I obtained my position through experience in health education. I started by developing, implementing, and evaluating health promotion activities in community-based organizations such as the YMCA. I was then hired as a health education specialist for the state, and I earned my master's degree in health education from Idaho State University. Over a ten-year period, I wrote grants as a health education specialist and program supervisor. Eventually, the unit became so large it was classified as a bureau, and I was named the bureau chief.

What are future trends in health education/health promotion?

1. A return to population-based health promotion—a focus on community health and what it takes to be a healthy city or healthy community
2. A return of interest by employers to improved health as a means of cost savings. Health educators will be hired in managed care settings and other health care organizations to develop healthy work environments and plan health education for subscribers, so that healthy behaviors can be adopted or maintained. Prevention may not save money, but it is less costly than treatment by almost any measure.
3. More partnerships with social and behavioral sciences
4. More focus on evaluating policy changes and how they impact behavior
5. Health promotion strategies being used in more than chronic disease prevention and school health, health education empowering people to move off welfare and onto jobs, and health education assisting social services programs such as child protection and Medicaid
6. Health promotion specialists at more policy- and decision-making levels in federal, state, and local governments—advising and making health policy to change environments to be healthier for all with less cost

What I like most about my position: I have never been bored in my twelve years in health promotion. I like having a huge network of resources, being a partner with local groups, assuring quality health education and health promotion standards through evaluation, being on "the cutting edge" of what is happening nationally, evaluating programs, and grant writing.

What I like least about my position: I dislike administrative duties, because they leave me less time to participate in health promotion program development and evaluation.

Recommendations for health education students who want to have positions similar to mine:

1. Think big—step out of your box and see whom or what you can connect with. Look for the assets and how to bring them together to address problems. Don't concentrate only on "needs."

2. Develop solid writing skills and good verbal communication skills; be clear and concise.

3. Work on developing coalition-building and community empowerment skills.

4. Obtain experience in program evaluation; get some program planning experience.

5. Take a social marketing or marketing course.

6. Let research be your guide. Remember, however, that the research I am talking about needs to applied and usable in the field.

Finally, I see a health educator as being analogous to the conductor of an orchestra. The health educator must know who all the stakeholders and players must be and she/he gathers them together to work to achieve a similar goal or objective, just as the conductor gathers the necessary and appropriate musicians to play musical pieces. The health educator is not necessarily the expert at any one of the roles in solving the problem, just as the conductor is not fluent in playing each instrument. The conductor can read the music, and the health educator can "read" the community entities involved. Both create a plan and provide leadership to carry the plan to the finish.

The credentialing process as it now stands begins with the candidate's submitting a transcript of coursework in health education to the National Commission for Health Education Credentialing (NCHEC). On verification by NCHEC that the candidate has completed coursework leading to a degree in health education and the coursework has focused on the responsibilities and competencies of an entry-level health educator, the applicant is given permission to sit for the certification exam. Exam questions are based on the seven responsibilities and competencies for entry-level health educators. An individual who passes the exam is awarded a Certified Health Education Specialist (CHES) credential.

This process is not without its detractors. The major reason for disagreement stems from the fact that all individuals who are seeking a CHES certification must complete the same process. This tends to skew the credential in favor of creating a generic health educator. Many practicing health educators argue that the skills needed to teach health in a school setting differ from those needed to conduct a community program at a local American Cancer Society office or to direct health promotion programs at a worksite. For example, school health educators often see the need to be content specialists, while community health educators are more process- and skills-oriented.

Simons-Morton, Greene, and Gottlieb (1995) accurately mention that health education is a diverse profession. Health educators practice in a variety of settings (e.g., school, worksite, community, health care); they may work with different populations (e.g., adults, the aged, children, minorities); they may be process specialists (e.g., program planners, program implementers, program evaluators); or they may be content specialists (e.g., specialists in HIV/AIDS, chronic diseases, injury or violence prevention, nutrition). Should there be a generic credential? Perhaps in the future there will be "practice-specific" credentials. At any rate, it is important to be aware of this issue, as it probably will be debated for years to come.

An important consequence of having a CHES credential is that of eligibility for reimbursement for services rendered. As managed care sweeps the country, there is a growing tendency on the part of insurers to limit the types of providers eligible for reimbursement. Without some external credential or license, it is highly doubtful that any health education services rendered in a medical care setting will be reimbursed (personal conversation with Idaho Blue Shield Human Resources Dept. representative, 1997).

There is, however, an exciting development related to CHES credentialing that has implications for both increased recognition of the credential and the issue of reimbursement. On April 9, 1997, Governor Mike Huckabee of Arkansas signed into law the Health Educator Practice Act. This law establishes a board of health education to regulate the practice of persons who function as health educators in Arkansas. With few exceptions, the law requires that health educators hold the national credential CHES to be able to practice health education in the state (Hager, 1997, p. 23).

Another issue related to credentialing was raised by Butler (1997). He states, "The CHES credential places much more emphasis on the acquisition of skills than on health content. This concept is somewhat in conflict with many of the textbooks written for content areas such as human sexuality or substance abuse. . . It also conflicts with the philosophies of many institutions that continue to emphasize courses in health content" (p. 334). In this manner, professional preparation programs are affected by the credentialing process. There is little doubt that discussions related to this issue will continue into the next century.

Implications for Practice Settings

Chapter 7 detailed that there are a variety of settings in which health educators can choose to practice. the worksite, school, health care, or community/public health. Each setting has its own unique characteristics. The content areas covered, the population characteristics, and the competencies required differ, according to the organization's mission and structure (Simons-Morton, Greene, &

Gottlieb, 1995, p. 425). However, they are also similar in that the goal of health education is to create a climate that facilitates the improvement of health status for every member of the population served by the setting. The first part of this chapter described various influences destined to impact the health of the populace into the next century. This section briefly summarizes the future role of the health educator in each setting.

School Setting

"Children don't learn as well when they are not healthy" (Seffrin, 1994, p. 397). "Schools in the future will be a key in collaboration to serve kids' health and social service needs" (Clark, 1994, p. 140). These statements characterize the goal of school health education and provide a direction for the school health educator to follow. If children's well-being is to be maintained or enhanced, a comprehensive approach to providing health education is needed (Allensworth & Kolbe, 1987). The comprehensive approach referred to consists of eight components that are integrated to provide for all of the health needs of the children and adolescents attending the school: classroom school health education lessons, the school lunch program, health screenings, physical education, a healthy and safe school environment, the availability of trained school counselors, faculty and staff health promotion, and family and community support for education and health. Actually implementing this model is a tall order. In their discussion summarizing a study on school health policies and programs, Kolbe and colleagues (1995) said,

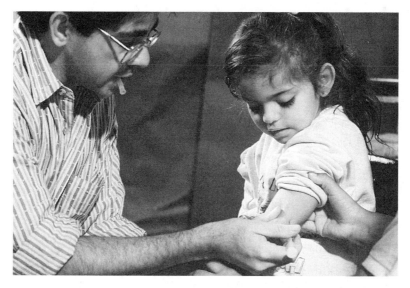

Schools can serve as sites for offering preventive health services and education. (Russell D. Curtis/Photo Researchers)

School health policies and programs, particularly at the school level, may not adequately address several of the most serious public health problems today such as violence, unintentional injuries such as motor vehicle crashes, and unintended pregnancies. School health services that do not respond to these problems, classroom instruction that is inadequate in scope and depth, and school health policies that only include punitive rather than remedial responses to violations must be replaced with more responsive programs. (p. 343)

Should you choose to practice health education in a school setting, what skills and abilities must you possess if schools are really going to incorporate a comprehensive health education program to address the health needs of children and adolescents, both now and in the future? Given the information on influences on health in this chapter and incorporating information from Chapter 7 on settings for health education, following is a list of skills that we think are imperative. You must be able to:

1. Create a logical scope and sequence to health content units that incorporate age-appropriate information
2. Prepare and deliver lessons that are participatory in nature, stress skill development, and foster attitudes necessary for problem solving and informed decision making
3. Use both qualitative and quantitative strategies to evaluate your lessons, your units, and the district health education program
4. Assess the health needs of the students, faculty, and staff
5. Assure that health and counseling services are provided for students
6. Create or coordinate a parent/community health education advisory council
7. Actively participate in local, state, regional, and national professional organizations
8. Use technology to assist in both updating your own skills and delivering health education messages to your school and community
9. Learn about, cultivate a sensitivity toward, and instill in your teaching an awareness of the influence of culture on health
10. Assist teachers at all grade levels in obtaining age-appropriate health education materials and help coordinate a classroom scope and sequence for all grade levels in your district
11. Serve as resource person and liaison between the school health setting and other settings in which health education might occur
12. Acquire sound oral and written communication techniques
13. Work both independently and as a member of a team
14. Apply behavior-change strategies and what is known about environmental influences on behavior to the classroom setting

School health educators who possess these skills will be well prepared to lead programs that enhance the health of the students and teachers in their schools.

Worksite Setting

It is no secret that the workplace of today bears little resemblance to that of only twenty years ago. Because many employers want to attract the top employees and because the employers realize that employee satisfaction is a key ingredient in productivity and retention, worksites have introduced an array of programs for employees and their families that provide continuing education, recreational opportunities, health promotion, and financial planning. In particular, worksites have become an increasingly important setting for health education/health promotion programs. The 1992 National Survey of Worksite Health Promotion Activities (USDHHS, 1993) found that 81 percent of worksites with fifty or more employees offered at least one health promotion activity, compared with 66 percent in 1985. Typically, the health promotion programs address injury prevention, exercise, the control of smoking, stress management, and alcohol and other drug abuse (Simons-Morton, Greene, & Gottlieb, 1995). An increasing number of sites are expanding their programs to include occupational safety and health issues such as the influences of physical, chemical, and psychosocial work exposures on employee health (Glasgow, McCaul, & Fisher, 1993).

Earlier in this chapter, the influence of changing demographic patterns on health education was discussed. However, there is another factor that must be taken into account when anticipating the future direction of worksite health promotion. According to the U.S. Bureau of Labor Statistics, between 1989 and the year 2000, 42.8 million people will join the U.S. workforce, but only 32 percent will be white males. The rest will be women and minorities (Motawani, Hodge, & Crampton, 1995).

The expansion of worksite health promotion programs bodes well for the future of health education and the concurrent need for an increasing number of trained health educators. Reasons for this growth have been chronicled by Green and Kreuter (1991), who state that the growth

> has been influenced by four phenomena: 1) changing demographic profiles in most workplaces, 2) growing concern for the burden on industry of medical care costs, health insurance premiums, the costs of lost productivity in unhealthy workers, 3) the recognition of the greater influence of behavior and environment on health, and 4) emerging evidence that health education and health promotion strategies have been effective in altering the behavioral and environmental precursors of health. (p. 308)

These trends have broad implications for the practice of worksite health education/promotion into the future. Keeping in mind the information presented both earlier in this chapter and in Chapter 7, the following competencies are baseline for the future practice of health education in worksite settings:

1. Recognize the importance of cultural and demographic influences on individual and group health behavioral choices

2. Coordinate needs assessments of worksite populace and conduct evaluations of program components
3. Identify and work with aspects of the corporate organizational climate that facilitate or impede participation
4. Prepare and conduct prevention presentations to worksite sub-groups
5. Conduct fitness assessments and participate in health screenings
6. Use up-to-date technology to market programs to worksite supervisors, employees, and their families through newsletters, brochures, Internet chat groups, and other media
7. Plan and manage a budget
8. Coordinate employee coalitions/steering committees to maximize employee input into program components
9. Function as a resource person for health information for employees and their families
10. Be able to apply behavior-change strategies and what is known about environmental influences on behavior to the worksite setting
11. Implement programs in a consistent manner with management philosophy
12. Attain a working knowledge of epidemiological and statistical principles and applications
13. Acquire sound oral and written communication techniques
14. Work both independently and as a member of a team

Incorporation of these competencies into the professional preparation program will help ensure the student is ready to begin practice as a worksite health educator.

Community/Public Health Setting

The community setting has the greatest variety of options for the practice of health education. For example, health educators are employed in many local, city, state, and federal health departments; in many federal agencies; in county extension agencies; in volunteer health organizations (e.g., American Cancer Society, American Heart Association, American Red Cross); in churches; in homeless shelters; in grassroots community organizations; and in prisons. One of the reasons for the diversity of opportunities is that the mission, goals, and objectives of one community agency may differ dramatically from those of another. Some of the agencies might have a health educator serving in the role of coordinator of services or as fund-raiser, while in another agency the educator plans, conducts, and evaluates programs. Another, more obvious reason for increased opportunity for employment is that almost every locale in the United States has one of the aforementioned groups.

The purpose of community health organizations is to both monitor and improve the health of the public they serve. Mullen and colleagues (1995) affirm the notion of the importance of community health promotion by making the point that the setting allows the educator to focus on reaching defined populations. Forming coalitions of key groups and community organizations has been shown to increase peoples' participation and mobilize residents to take action to enhance the health of all community members (Clark & McLeroy, 1995, p. 277). O'Rourke (1989) champions the philosophy that the only way to generate a measurable improvement in the health status of populations is through the use of community health population-level interventions. His remarks are based on the premise that individual-level interventions, which are often the most common, are less cost-effective. In this era of using health education/promotion to help reduce health care costs, and with an increasing need for community-level programs, community health educators are well positioned to take the lead in enhancing the health of citizens from all regions of the United States.

With employment opportunities for community health educators on the rise, what skills will the community health educator of the future need in order to function effectively? Following is a list of competencies or attributes that will be critical to the effective practice of community health education. They are not in any specific order of importance.

1. Recognize the importance of cultural and demographic influences on individual and group health behavioral choices
2. Maintain competence in the use of technology to access and deliver health-related information
3. Learn and use strategies to seek information, guidance, and support from community members regarding their health needs
4. Assess strengths of communities in building a plan to assist them in meeting their health needs
5. Be able to apply behavior-change strategies and what is known about environmental influences on behavior to the community setting
6. Learn coalition-building strategies
7. Actively participate in local, state, regional, and national professional organizations
8. Study and apply the fundamentals of obtaining extramural funding
9. Use a variety of marketing strategies to reach diverse community constituencies
10. Learn to be flexible, as the job probably will involve changing and varied responsibilities
11. Learn another language
12. Advocate policies that enhance the role of prevention and provide for universal access to health services when needed
13. Have the ability to work in teams
14. Attain a working knowledge of epidemiological and statistical principles and applications
15. Acquire excellent oral and written communication techniques
16. Work independently and as a member of a team

A well-trained community health educator will undoubtedly have an increased role in contributing to the health of populations. With the increasing health awareness of the American public and the multitude of cultural changes in society, community health educators have a bright and exciting future.

Health Care Setting

Health care settings employ health educators in a variety of institutions and in a multitude of ways. Health educators can be employed in for-profit and public hospitals, health maintenance organizations (HMOs), medical care clinics, and home health agencies. They might be involved in conducting one-on-one patient education; planning and implementing education programs for enrollees or other medical providers; coordinating community education programs on a variety of health topics; conducting program evaluations; marketing the health services available through the hospital, clinic, or HMO; conducting health promotion activities for the employees; or serving as a member of a community health promotion team.

Clark (1994) mentions that there is an ever increasing receptivity among medical providers, insurance companies, and the public to the idea that health education can make a positive contribution in the prevention and management of disease. Clark predicts that medicine will be a partner with health education, partly due to the erosion of influence among the medical establishment, the changes in the structure of the health care delivery system toward managed care, and the fact that prevention is more cost-effective than treatment.

Redman (1993) and Rankin and Stallings (1996) echo these thoughts. Both researchers note that in the past 20 years patient education in the health care setting has moved from an interesting innovation to a required service. This change has prompted a huge shift in practice norms by most clinical health care professionals, resulting in the need for trained personnel to assure that the education that occurs in the health care setting meets the needs of both the patient and the provider and motivates the patient to both adopt a healthier lifestyle and comply with any treatment regimen.

With the advent of medical acceptance of the value of health education in patient care, the outlook is positive for more employment opportunities in health care settings for health educators. What skills, competencies, and attributes will be absolutely necessary for the health educator of the future who seeks employment in a health care setting? Following is a list (not in any significant order):

1. Obtain a working knowledge of epidemiological and statistical principles and applications
2. Maintain competence in the use of technology to access and deliver health-related information
3. Be able to apply behavior-change strategies and what is known about environmental influences on behavior to the health care setting

4. Recognize the importance of cultural and demographic influences on individual and group health behavioral choices
5. Use up-to-date technology to market programs to patients, employees, and their families through newsletters, brochures, Internet chat groups, and other media
6. Provide training in health education theory to other members of the health care team
7. Become familiar with the clinical disease process
8. Advocate policies that enhance the role of prevention and provide for universal access to health services when needed
9. Prepare and deliver lessons that are participatory in nature, that stress skill development, and that foster attitudes necessary for problem solving and informed decision making
10. Coordinate interdisciplinary teams/steering committees to maximize input into program components
11. Learn to be flexible, as the job probably will involve changing and varied responsibilities
12. Serve as a liaison between the health care setting and other settings in which health education might occur
13. Function as a resource person for health information for patients and their families
14. Learn another language
15. Acquire sound oral and written communication techniques
16. Work independently and as a member of a team

With rapid changes occurring in medical care delivery today, there is much reason for health educators to be optimistic about employment opportunities. As the public demands health education/promotion and disease prevention as a part of their medical care treatment plan, health educators will increasingly be identified as the best prepared to assist individuals in adopting healthy lifestyles.

Alternative Settings

Besides the four traditional practice settings previously discussed, there are several other possibilities that look to be viable alternatives for the practice of health education into the next century. The purpose of this section is to very briefly introduce these choices, so that individuals who are interested can research these areas further.

The first alternative is to teach health education in a **postsecondary institution,** usually defined as an institution that educates people after they graduate from high school. There will continue to be a need for qualified instructors. Minimum standards for obtaining one of these positions is usually a master's degree in health education and two to five years of experience for a community college or vocational school position, and a doctorate and two to five years of experience for a college or university position.

For students who are interested in combining the fields of health education and journalism, positions can be found in both the print and TV media as reporters for newspapers, magazines, and TV stations, researching stories on health. A broad-based knowledge of health issues and a passion for writing and/or speaking are necessary qualifications.

Because of the increasing interdependence among nations and because there are many areas of the world in which health assistance is badly needed, there will continue to be health educator positions available in foreign countries. Examples include positions with organizations such as the Peace Corps, Project Hope, the United Nations, the Pan American Health Organization, and the World Health Organization. Many national church organizations also send interdisciplinary health teams to international locations to improve the health of the populace. Often, the health educator must have a college degree, some experience, and ability to speak a foreign language.

Medical supply companies, pharmaceutical companies, sports equipment manufacturers, health food stores, and textbook publishers often employ health educators in sales positions. A college degree is required. In addition, a willingness to travel, excellent oral and written communication skills, and an ability to work with all types of people are necessary prerequisites.

Because of the aging of the U.S. population, there is an escalating demand for health educators in long-term care institutions and retirement communities. Usually, a college degree is required. Excellent oral and written communication skills are essential, as is a desire to listen and learn from the wisdom of individuals residing in these communities.

There is an increasing number of opportunities for health educators in an entrepreneurial and consultant role. As self-employed persons, these individuals are free to set up their own practice, hiring out as consultants to organizations that need to temporarily hire someone with expertise in grant writing, program planning and evaluation, software development, professional speaking, or technical writing. Other possibilities include contracting with several small businesses to conduct worksite health promotion, freelancing with HMO's and other insurance providers to offer health education services (reimbursement will be an issue), serving as content specialist (e.g., stress management, eating disorders, substance abuse) to businesses and corporations, becoming a certified personal trainer, and teaching part-time in colleges, community colleges, or evening community education programs.

Now that the differences in the various practice settings have been explored, it is important to re-emphasize the fact that there are common tasks for health educators that transcend the individual practice setting. Dr. John Seffrin, director of the American Cancer Society, eloquently reminds us of the direction health education must take no matter where the practice setting, if it is to realize its potential. In his scholar's address, given to members of the American Association for Health Education (AAHE) in St. Louis in March 1997, he describes four actions for present and future health educators:

1. Look at ourselves as major players in keeping Americans healthy; to that end, work with policy makers to affect legislation that truly promotes health.
2. Collaborate with other health professionals in both the for-profit and the not-for-profit sectors.
3. Strive to exhibit greater professional solidarity; be an advocate for the profession of health education and the role-trained health educators can contribute as part of the health care team.
4. Advocate for those who do not have a voice; be a spokesperson in the political arena, and work to assure that health services and health education/promotion are available for all.

Summary

This chapter began with the notion of change as a constant. Although no one can actually "see" into the future, it is obvious that the need to be prepared to be flexible in order to adapt to ongoing change is imperative. This is an exciting time to become a health educator. Opportunities have never been greater and the future has never looked brighter. There is little doubt that health education will continue to expand in all of the more traditional as well as some of the nontraditional settings. Health educators have the training and expertise to make a positive difference in enhancing the quality of life for all people.

In conclusion, a quote from Dr. Bob Gold's (1997) address at the American Public Health Association meeting in Indianapolis so succinctly and eloquently sums up both the present and future roles of the health educator: "As for the future, your task is not to foresee, but to enable it." In many ways you have the opportunity to make the practice of health education have an ever-widening influence in enhancing the health of the populace. We wish you every success as you begin your journey.

REVIEW QUESTIONS

1. Identify three worksite settings in which health educators will practice to a greater degree than they do today.
2. How will each of the societal changes discussed in the chapter impact the practice of health education in the worksite setting? the medical care setting? the school setting? the community/public health setting?
3. What are the implications of CHES credentialing in each of the four major practice settings?
4. How will changing demographic patterns affect the practice of health education in nontraditional settings?
5. List three reasons health educators should be optimistic about the future and provide reasons for your choices.
6. What is meant by the statement "health educators need to become advocates for the profession"?

ACTIVITIES

1. Make a list of five of your strongest attributes. Make a second list of five tasks you most like to do. Using these lists and what you know about health education, write a paragraph description of the "perfect" health education job for you.

2. Construct and administer a short survey to the health education faculty at your institution on what they see as major influences on the future practice of health education. Compile your results and share them with the class.

3. Interview two graduates from the health education program in which you are studying who are now practicing in the field of health education. Make certain they are in different settings—for instance, one in a school, one in community/public health. Try to ascertain their feelings about their jobs and the influences they see impacting the way they practice, both now and in the future.

4. Assume the year is 2005. You are responsible for writing a job description that will be used to advertise for a new community/public health educator position. Write out the description, making sure to include the qualifications and duties the applicant will have to possess.

REFERENCES

Acock, A. C., & Demo, D. H. (1994). *Family diversity and well-being.* Thousand Oaks, CA: Sage.

Allensworth, D. D., & Kolbe, L. J. (1987). The comprehensive school health program: Exploring an expanded concept. *Journal of School Health, 57*(10), 409–412.

Butler, J. T. (1997). *Principles of health education and health promotion* (2nd ed.). Englewood, CO: Morton.

Cheal, D. (1991). *The family and the state of theory.* Toronto: University of Toronto Press.

Clark, N. M. (1994). Health educators and the future: Lead, follow, or get out of the way. *Journal of Health Education, 25*(3), 136–141.

Clark, N. M., & McLeroy, K. R. (1995). Creating capacity through health education: What we know and what we don't. *Health Education Quarterly, 22*(3), 273–289.

Cree, J. (1997, May). Personal conversation, Idaho State University Family Practice Residency.

English, G. M., & Videto, D. M. (1997). The future of health education: The knowledge to practice paradox. *Journal of Health Education, 28*(1), 4–8

Fineberg, H. V. (1996). Seeking equilibrium in a problem-driven field. *Priorities, 8*(2), 18.

Glasgow, R. E., McCaul, K. D., & Fisher, K. J. (1993). Participation in worksite health promotion: A critique of the literature and recommendations for future practice. *Health Education Quarterly, 20*(3), 391–408.

Gold, R. (1997, November). Address at the American Public Health Association Convention, Indianapolis, IN.

Green, L. W. & Kreuter, M. W. (1991). *Health promotion planning: an educational and environmental approach* (2nd ed.). Mountain View, CA: Mayfield.

Hager, B. L. (1997). The professionalization of health educators in Arkansas: The Health Educator Practice Act. *The CHES Bulletin, 8*(2), 23.

Idaho Blue Shield Human Resources Department. (1997, May). Personal conversation.

Kids Count Data Book. (1995). New York: Annie E. Casey Foundation.

Kolbe, L. J., et al. (1995). The School Health Policies and Programs Study (SHPPS): Context, methods, general findings, and future efforts. *Journal of School Health, 65*(8), 339–343.

Lorig, K. R., Manzonson, D. P., & Holman, H. R. (1993). Evidence suggesting that health education for self-management in patients with chronic arthritis has sustained benefits while reducing health care costs. *Arthritis and Rheumatism, 36*(4), 439–446.

McGinnis, J. M., & DeGraw, C. (1991). Healthy Schools 2000: Creating partnerships for the decade. *Journal of School Health, 61*(7), 292–296.

McGinnis, J. M., & Foege, W. H. (1993). Actual causes of death in the United States. *Journal of the American Medical Association, 270*(18), 2207–2212.

McKenzie, J. F., & Pinger, R. R. (1995). An introduction to community health. New York: HarperCollins.

Motawani, J., Hodge, J., & Crampton, S. (1995). Managing diversity in the health care industry: A conceptual model and an empirical investigation. *Health Care Supervisor, 13*(3), 16–23.

Mullen, P. D., et al. (1995). Settings as an important dimension in health education/promotion policy, programs, and research. *Health Education Quarterly, 22*(3), 329–345.

O'Rourke, T. (1989). Reflections on directions in health education: Implications for policy and practice. *Health Education, 20*(6), 4–14.

Rankin, S. H. & Stallings, K. D. (1996). Patient education issues, principles, and practices. New York: Lippincott.

Redman, B. K. (1993). *The process of patient education.* St Louis: Mosby.

Schuster, C. (1995). Have we forgotten the older adults? An argument in support of more health promotion programs for and research directed toward people 65 years and older. *Journal of Health Education, 26*(6), 338–344.

Seffrin, J. R. (1994). America's interest in comprehensive school health education. *Journal of School Health, 64*(10), 397–399.

Seffrin, J. R. (1997, March). *AAHE scholar's address.* St. Louis: American Alliance for Health, Physical Education, Recreation, and Dance Convention.

Simons-Morton, B. G., Greene, W. H., & Gottlieb, N. H. (1995). *Introduction to health education and health promotion* (2nd ed.). Prospect Heights, IL: Waveland Press.

Stacy, J. (1991). *Brave new families.* New York: Basic Books.

Sullum, J. (1996). What the doctor orders. *Priorities, 8*(2), 8–16.

Uhlenberg, P., & Eggebeen, D. (1986). The declining well-being of American adolescents. *The Public Interest, 82,* 25–38.

U.S. Bureau of the Census. (1992). *Statistical abstract of the United States* (112th ed.). Washington, DC: U.S. Department of Commerce.

U.S. Bureau of the Census. (1993). *Statistical abstract of the United States* (113th ed.). Washington, DC: U.S. Department of Commerce.

U.S. Bureau of the Census. (1996). *Statistical abstract of the United States* (116th ed.). Washington, DC: U.S. Department of Commerce.

U.S. Department of Health and Human Services (USDHHS). (1993). *1992 national survey of worksite health promotion activities summary report.* Washington, DC: Public Health Services.

APPENDIX A

Code of Ethics (Unabridged Version), Society for Public Health Education, Inc.

Society for Public Health Education Code of Ethics (1983)

Preamble

Health educators, in using educational processes to influence human well being, take on profound responsibilities. Their professional situation is varied and complex; they work with people of different backgrounds, in diverse settings, and have varying responsibilities in this country as well as overseas. Health educators are involved in their discipline, their colleagues, their employers, their constituents, their government's position, other interest groups, and process and issues affecting the general welfare of people, locally, nationally, and internationally.

In a field of complex involvements, value conflicts generate ethical dilemmas. It is a prime responsibility of health educators to anticipate and to resolve them in such a way as not to do damage either to the constituency with whom they work or their profession. Where these conditions cannot be met, the health educator would be well advised not to be involved.

The health educator must be committed to the principles of self-determination and liberty. Ethical precepts which guide the design of strategies and methods must ultimately reflect a respect for the right of individuals and communities to affirm their own ways of living.

The following principles are deemed fundamental to health educators' responsible ethical pursuit of their profession:

Article I: Relations with the Public

Health educators' ultimate responsibility is to the general public. When there is a conflict of interest among individuals, groups, agencies, or institutions, health educators must consider all issues and give priority to those whose goals are closest to the principles of self-determination and enhancement of freedom of choice.

Source: Reprinted with permission from the Society for Public Health Education, Washington, D.C.

Section 1
Health educators must protect the right of individuals to make their own decisions regarding health as long as such decisions pose no threat to the health of others.

Section 2
Health educators should be candid and truthful in their dealings with the public.

Section 3
Health educators should not exploit the public by misrepresenting or exaggerating the potential benefits of services or programs with which they are associated.

Section 4
As people who devote their professional lives to improving people's well being, health educators bear a responsibility to speak out on issues which would have a deleterious effect upon the public's health.

Section 5
In all dealings, health educators should be honest about their qualifications and the limitations of their expertise.

Section 6
In a world where privacy is frequently threatened, health educators should protect the physical, social, and psychological welfare of the public and ensure their privacy and dignity.

Section 7
Health educators should involve clients actively in the entire educational change process so that all aspects are clearly understood by clients.

Section 8
Health educators affirm an egalitarian ethic. Believing that health is a basic human right, they act to ensure that neither the benefits nor the quality of their professional services are denied or impaired to all people to whom they are responsible.

Article II: Responsibility to the Profession

Health educators are responsible for the good reputation of their discipline.

Section 1
They should maintain their competence at the highest level through continuing study and training for example:

1. Active membership in professional organizations.
2. Review of professional, technical, and lay journals.
3. Previewing of new products and media materials.
4. Creation and distribution of new programs and materials including the publication of professional and lay papers.
5. Involvement in economic and legislative issues related to public health.
6. Assumption of a leadership or participative role in cooperative endeavors.

Section 2

When they participate in actions related to hiring, promotion, or advancement, they should ensure that no exclusionary practices be enacted against individuals on the basis of sex, marital status, color, age, social class, religion, sexual preference, ethnic background, national origin, or other origin, or other non-professional attributes.

Section 3

Health educators should protect and enhance the integrity of the profession by responsible discussion and criticism of the profession.

Article IV: Responsibility in Employing Educational Strategies and Methods

In designing strategies and methods, health educators must not compromise their professional standards, nor reduce the trust in health education held by the general public. They should be sensitive to the prevailing community standard and existing cultural or social norms. Health educators should also be aware of the possible impact of their strategies and methods upon the community and other health professionals.

The strategies and methods must not place the burden of change solely on the targeted population but must involve other appropriate groups to bring about effective change.

In the design/implementation of strategies and methods, health educators have an obligation to two principles: First, the people have a right to make decisions affecting their lives. Second, there is a moral imperative to provide people with all relevant information and resources possible to make their choice freely and intelligently.

Section 1

To protect public confidence in the profession, health educators should avoid strategies and methods that are clearly in violation of accepted moral and legal standards.

Section 2

In conducting programs, the health educator's responsibility is not only to the participants, but also to the community at large.

Section 3
The selection of strategies and methods should include the active involvement of the people to be affected.

Section 4
The potential outcomes, both positive and negative, that can result from the proposed strategies should be communicated to all the appropriate individuals who will be affected.

Section 5
Health educators should implement strategies and methods which direct change whenever possible by choice, rather than by coercion. However, where a community is being harmed, or would be harmed by others, actions which limit the freedom of the harm-producing agents are justified. Where voluntary action has not succeeded in producing a desired outcome, coercive strategies and methods may be necessary but should be employed most cautiously.

Article V: Responsibilities to Employers

In their relations with employers, health educators should:

Section 1
Be honest about their qualifications (education, experience, training), capabilities, and aims.

Section 2
Reflect seriously upon the goals of the organization for which they are to work and consider with great care their employer's stated aims and their past behavior, prior to entering any commitment.

Section 3
Act within the boundaries of their professional competence.

Section 4
Accept responsibility and accountability for their areas of practice, including responsibility for maintenance of optimum standards.

Section 5
Exercise informed judgment and use professional standards and guidelines as criteria in seeking consultation, accepting responsibilities, and delegating health education activities to others.

Section 6
Maintain competence in their areas of professional practice.

Section 7
Be careful not to promise outcomes or to imply acceptance of conditions contrary to their professional ethics.

Section 8
Avoid competing commitments, conflict of interest situations, secret agreements, and endorsement of products.

Article VI: Responsibility to Students

The preparation and training of prospective health educators entails serious responsibilities affecting the well being of the profession, the public, and the students. All those involved in such preparation and training, including teachers, administrators, and practicum supervisors, have an obligation to accord students the same respect and treatment accorded all other client groups, and to provide the highest quality education possible.

Educators should be receptive and seriously responsive to students' interests, opinions, and desires in all aspects of their academic work and relationships. The principles and methods of health education that are taught should be practiced in the education of future professionals. Teachers and educators should share their passion, convictions, commitments, and visions as well as their knowledge and skills with their students. Personal and professional honesty and integrity are the essential qualities of a good teacher.

Section 1
Selection of students for professional preparation programs should preclude discrimination on any grounds other than ability and potential contribution to the profession and the public health.

Section 2
The ethical dimensions of the practice of health education should be stressed at all levels of professional preparation.

Section 3
The educational environment—physical, social and emotional—should, to the greatest degree possible, be conducive to the health of all involved.

Section 4
The responsibilities of all teachers to their students include careful preparation; presentation of material that is accurate, up-to-date, and timely; providing reasonable and timely feedback; having and stating clear and reasonable expectations; and fairness in grading and evaluation.

Section 5
Faculty owe students a reasonable degree of accessibility. Other demands such as research and administration must be kept in balance with responsibilities to students.

Section 6
Students should receive counseling regarding career opportunities and assistance in securing professional employment upon completion of their studies.

Section 7
Field word and internships should be based upon the professional interests and needs of the student and should provide meaningful opportunities to gain useful experience and adequate supervision.

Article VII: Responsibility in Research and Evaluation

The health educator engaged in research and evaluation studies should:

Section 1
Consider carefully its possible consequences for human beings.

Section 2
Ascertain that the consent of participants in research is voluntary and informed, without any implied deprivation or penalty for refusal to participate, and with due regard for participants' privacy and dignity.

Section 3
Protect participants from unwarranted physical or mental discomfort, distress, harm, danger, or deprivation.

Section 4
Treat all information secured from participants as confidential.

Section 5
Take credit only for work actually done and credit contributions made by others.

Section 6
Provide no reports to sponsors that are not also available to the general public and, where practicable, to the population studied.

Section 7
Discuss the results of evaluation of services only with persons directly and professionally concerned with them.

Code of Ethics (Abridged Version), Society for Public Health Education, Inc.

SOPHE Code of Ethics

Health educators take on profound responsibilities in using educational processes to promote health and influence well being. Ethical precepts which guide these processes must respect the right of individuals and communities to make the decisions affecting their lives.

Responsibilities to Society

Health Educators:
- Affirm an egalitarian ethic, believing that health is a basic human right for all.
- Provide people with all relevant and accurate information and resources to make their choices freely and intelligently.
- Support change by freedom of choice and self-determination, as long as these decisions pose no threat to the health of others.
- Advocate for healthful change and legislation, and speak out on issues deleterious to public health.
- Are candid and truthful in dealings with the public, never misrepresenting or exaggerating the potential benefits of services or programs.
- Avoid and take appropriate action against unethical practices and conflict of interest situations.
- Respect the privacy, dignity and culture of the individual and the community, and use skills consistent with these values.

Responsibilities to the Profession

Health Educators:
- Share their skills, experience and visions with their students and colleagues.
- Observe principles of informed consent and confidentiality of individuals.
- Maintain their highest levels of competence through continued study, training and research.

Source: Reprinted with permission from the Society for Public Health Education, Washington, D.C.

- Further the art and science of health education through applied research and report findings honestly and without distortion.
- Accurately represent their capabilities, education, training and experience, and act within the boundaries of their professional competence.
- Ensure that no exclusionary practices are enacted against individuals on the basis of gender, marital status, age, social class, religion, sexual preference, or ethnic or cultural background.

APPENDIX C

The Code of Ethics for Health Educators

Association for the Advancement of Health Education Code of Ethics for Health Educators

Preamble

Health education is a process concerned with designing, implementing, and evaluating educational programs that enable individuals, families, groups, organizations, and communities to play active roles in achieving, protecting, and sustaining health. Its purpose is to contribute to health and well-being by promoting lifestyles, community actions, and conditions that make it possible to live healthful lives. Health educators have professional responsibilities to the community and society in which they work and live. They apply and make public their knowledge of health with integrity and dedication to the truth. Health education is not the answer to every health problem and should not be positioned as a stand-alone, independent strategy. However, carefully planned and implemented programs are an essential component of effective health promotion, disease prevention, treatment, and care.

Health education is based on humanitarian and democratic ideals. Health educators are dedicated to improving the health of individuals and groups through educational interventions and other strategies that are characterized by respect for competing value systems, an overriding commitment to self-determination, justice, and the right of individuals to make informed choices. Health educators employ a recognized body of knowledge about human health and disease in order to promote well-being. They liberate people through the honest exchange of accurate and valid information, with appropriate consideration and respect for human diversity and the right of individuals and communities to determine their own ways of living.

Effective health education is planned with input from representatives of target populations and is influenced by the nature of the health problem and setting (e.g., school, community, workplace, or health care organizations). Health education methodologies and strategies are uniquely tailored to address the circumstances of a given population, person, or situation, and are consistent with empirically supported health education and learning theories.

Source: This article is reprinted with permission from the *Journal of Health Education,* July/August, 1994, Vol. 25, No. 4, pp. 197–200. The *Journal of Health Education* is a publication of the American Alliance for Health, Physical Education, Recreation and Dance, 1900 Association Drive, Reston, Virginia 20191.

Health educators have knowledge of scientific, behavioral, cultural, and philosophical foundations of health and health behavior. As a result of their professional preparation, health educators are able to apply this knowledge in planning, implementing, and evaluating health education programs.

This Code of Ethics provides a common set of values designed to guide health educators in resolving many of the ethical dilemmas experienced in professional life. These guidelines regarding professional conduct of health educators require a commitment to behave ethically and to encourage and support the ethical behavior of others.

Article I: Responsibility to the Public

Health educators' ultimate responsibility is to educate people about health in order to promote wellness and quality of life. Health educators recognize that decisions about health are made at individual, family, peer, community, societal, and global levels. When there is a conflict of interest among individuals, groups, agencies, or institutions, health educators consider all issues and given priority to the principles of responsibility and freedom of choice.

Section 1
Health educators support the right of individuals to make informed decisions regarding their own health.

Section 2
Health educators encourage actions and social policies which support the best balance of benefits over harm for all affected parties.

Section 3
Health educators accurately communicate the potential benefits and consequences of services.

Section 4
Health educators act on conditions that can adversely affect the health of individuals and communities.

Section 5
Health educators are truthful about their qualifications and the limitations of their expertise and provide services consistent with these qualifications and limitations.

Section 6
Health educators are committed to providing professional services equitably to all people.

Section 7
Health educators respect the rights of others to hold diverse values, attitudes, and opinions.

Section 8
Health educators protect individuals' privacy and dignity.

Article II: Responsibility to the Profession

Health educators are responsible for the reputation of their profession. Their professional behavior is consistent with the Code of Ethics. When appropriate, they consult with colleagues in order to promote ethical conduct.

Section 1
Health educators maintain their professional competence through continued study and education.

Section 2
Health educators treat all individuals equitably in professional actions (e.g., hiring, promotion, retention, work assignments, and admission policies) regardless of age, gender, race, ethnicity, national origin, religion, sexual orientation, disability, socioeconomic status, or any basis prescribed by law.

Section 3
Health educators encourage and accept critical discourse in order to improve the profession.

Section 4
Health educators contribute to the development of the profession by sharing program components they have found to be effective.

Section 5
Health educators do not manipulate or violate others' rights in sexual, emotional, financial, or other ways.

Section 6
Health educators are aware of possible conflicts of interest and exercise integrity in these situations.

Section 7
Health educators give appropriate recognition to students and colleagues for their professional contributions.

Article III: Responsibility to Employers

Health educators recognize the boundaries of their professional competence. They provide services and programs for which they are qualified by education and experience and they are accountable for their professional activities.

Section 1
Health educators accurately represent their own qualifications and the qualifications of others they recommend.

Section 2
Health educators use current professional standards, theory, and guidelines as criteria when accepting consultations, when delegating health education activities, and when making referrals.

Section 3
Health educators accurately represent potential program outcomes to employers.

Section 4
Health educators make known competing commitments, conflicts of interest, and endorsement of products when the quality of health education delivered could be adversely affected by these activities.

Section 5
Health educators openly communicate to employers when expectations or job-related assignments conflict with professional ethics.

Article IV: Responsibility in the Delivery of Health Education

Health educators promote integrity in the delivery of health education and respect the fundamental rights, dignity, confidentiality, and worth of all people by adapting strategies and methods to the needs of different populations.

Section 1
Health educators are sensitive to the variety of cultural and social norms.

Section 2
Health educators promote the right of individuals and groups to be actively involved in all aspects of the educational process.

Section 3
Health educators use educational strategies and methods that reflect the Code of Ethics and applicable laws. If neither law nor the Code of Ethics provides guidance in resolving an issue, health educators consider other professional standards

as well as their own personal standards of ethical behavior, and consult other health educators.

Section 4
Health educators implement strategies and methods that enable individuals to adopt health lifestyles through choice rather than by coercion.

Section 5
Health educators conduct regular evaluations of program effectiveness.

Section 6
Health educators provide educational interventions that are grounded in a theoretical framework and supported by empirical evidence.

Article V: Responsibility in Research and Evaluation

Health educators contribute to the health of the population and to the profession through research and evaluation activities. When planning and conducting research or evaluation, health educators do so in accordance with federal and state laws and regulations, organizational and institutional policies, and professional standards.

Section 1
Health educators conduct research in accordance with recognized scientific and ethical standards.

Section 2
Health educators ensure that the consent of participants in research is voluntary and informed.

Section 3
Health educators implements standards to protect the rights, health, safety, and welfare of human research participants.

Section 4
Health educators maintain confidentiality and protect the privacy of research participants in accordance with law and professional standards.

Section 5
Health educators take credit, including authorship, only for work they have actually performed and give credit to the contributions of others.

Section 6

Health educators who serve as research or evaluation consultants discuss their results only with those to whom they are providing service, unless maintaining such confidentiality would jeopardize the health or safety of others.

Section 7

Health educators honor commitments they have made to research participants.

Section 8

Health educators report the results of their research and evaluation accurately and in a timely fashion.

The AAHE Code of Ethics was developed over a two year period of time by a committee appointed by the AAHE president. Over 500 health educators working in a variety of settings participated in providing opinions on the various drafts of the document. Credit is given to SOPHE's Code of Ethics which served as a basis for the development of this document. The preface includes information adopted from the report of the 1990 Joint Committee on Health Education Terminology and a joint document of WHO and IUHE published in 1991, titled "Meeting Global Challenges: A Position Paper on Health Education."

> **Association for the Advancement**
> **of Health Education**
> **1900 Association Drive**
> **Reston, VA 22091**
> **703/476-3437**

APPENDIX D

Responsibilities and Competencies for Entry-Level Health Educators

Responsibility I—Assessing Individual and Community Needs for Health Education

Competency A
Obtain health-related data about social and cultural environments, growth and development factors, needs, and interests.

Sub-Competencies
1. Select valid sources of information about health needs and interests.
2. Utilize computerized sources of health-related information.
3. Employ or develop appropriate data-gathering instruments.
4. Apply survey techniques to acquire health data.

Competency B
Distinguish between behaviors that foster, and those that hinder, well-being.

Sub-Competencies
1. Investigate physical, social, emotional, and intellectual factors influencing health behaviors.
2. Identify behaviors that tend to promote or compromise health.
3. Recognize the role of learning and affective experience in shaping patterns of health behavior.

Competency C
Infer needs for health education on the basis of obtained data.

Sub-Competencies
1. Analyze needs assessment data.
2. Determine priority areas of need for health education.

Source: From *A Competency-Based Framework for Professional Development of Certified Health Education Specialists*, NCHEC, New York, 1996.

Responsibility II—Planning Effective Health Education Programs

Competency A
Recruit community organizations, resource people, and potential participants for support and assistance in program planning.

Sub-Competencies
1. Communicate need for the program to those who will be involved.
2. Obtain commitments from personnel and decision makers who will be involved in the program.
3. Seek ideas and opinions of those who will affect, or be affected by, the program.
4. Incorporate feasible ideas and recommendations into the planning process.

Competency B
Develop a logical scope and sequence plan for a health education program.

Sub-Competencies
1. Determine the range of health information requisite to a given program of instruction.
2. Organize the subject areas comprising the scope of a program in logical sequence.

Competency C
Formulate appropriate and measurable program objectives.

Sub-Competencies
1. Infer educational objectives facilitative of achievement of specified competencies.
2. Develop a framework of broadly stated, operational objectives relevant to a proposed health education program.

Competency D
Design educational programs consistent with specified program objectives.

Sub-Competencies
1. Match proposed learning activities with those implicit in the stated objectives.
2. Formulate a wide variety of alternative educational methods.
3. Select strategies best suited to implementation of educational objectives in a given setting.
4. Plan a sequence of learning opportunities building upon, and reinforcing mastery of, preceding objectives.

Responsibility III—Implementing Health Education Programs

Competency A
Exhibit competence in carrying out planned educational programs.

Sub-Competencies
1. Employ a wide range of educational methods and techniques.
2. Apply individual or group process methods as appropriate to given learning situations.
3. Utilize instructional equipment and other instructional media effectively.
4. Select methods that best facilitate practice of program objectives.

Competency B
Infer enabling objectives as needed to implement instructional programs in specified settings.

Sub-Competencies
1. Pretest learners to ascertain present abilities and knowledge relative to proposed program objectives.
2. Develop subordinate measurable objectives as needed for instruction.

Competency C
Select methods and media best suited to implement program plans for specific learners.

Sub-Competencies
1. Analyze learner characteristics, legal aspects, feasibility, and other considerations influencing choices among methods.
2. Evaluate the efficacy of alternative methods and techniques capable of facilitating program objectives.
3. Determine the availability of information, personnel, time, and equipment needed to implement the program for a given audience.

Competency D
Monitor educational programs, adjusting objectives and activities as necessary.

Sub-Competencies
1. Compare actual program activities with the stated objectives.
2. Assess the relevance of existing program objectives to current needs.
3. Revise program activities and objectives as necessitated by changes in learner needs.
4. Appraise applicability of resources and materials relative to given educational objectives.

Responsibility IV—Evaluating Effectiveness of Health Education Programs

Competency A
Develop plans to assess achievement of program objectives.

Sub-Competencies
1. Determine standards of performance to be applied as criteria of effectiveness.
2. Establish a realistic scope of evaluation efforts.
3. Develop an inventory of existing valid and reliable tests and survey instruments.
4. Select appropriate methods for evaluating program effectiveness.

Competency B
Carry out evaluation plans.

Sub-Competencies
1. Facilitate administration of the tests and activities specified in the plan.
2. Utilize data-collecting methods appropriate to the objectives.
3. Analyze resulting evaluation data.

Competency C
Interpret results of program evaluation.

Sub-Competencies
1. Apply criteria of effectiveness to obtained results of a program.
2. Translate evaluation results into terms easily understood by others.
3. Report effectiveness of educational programs in achieving proposed objectives.

Competency D
Infer implications from findings for future program planning.

Sub-Competencies
1. Explore possible explanations for important evaluation findings.
2. Recommend strategies for implementing results of evaluation.

Responsibility V—Coordinating Provision of Health Education Services

Competency A
Develop a plan for coordinating health education services.

Sub-Competencies
1. Determine the extent of available health education services.
2. Match health education services to proposed program activities.
3. Identify gaps and overlaps in the provision of collaborative health services.

Competency B
Facilitate cooperation between and among levels of program personnel.

Sub-Competencies
1. Promote cooperation and feedback among personnel related to the program.
2. Apply various methods of conflict reduction as needed.
3. Analyze the role of health educator as liaison between program staff and outside groups and organizations.

Competency C
Formulate practical modes of collaboration among health agencies and organizations.

Sub-Competencies
1. Stimulate development of cooperation among personnel responsible for community health education program.
2. Suggest approaches for integrating health education within existing health programs.
3. Develop plans for promoting collaborative efforts among health agencies and organizations with mutual interests.

Competency D
Organize in-service training programs for teachers, volunteers, and other interested personnel.

Sub-Competencies
1. Plan an operational, competency-oriented training program.
2. Utilize instructional resources that meet a variety of in-service training needs.
3. Demonstrate a wide range of strategies for conducting in-service training programs.

Responsibility VI—Acting as a Resource Person in Health Education

Competency A
Utilize computerized health information retrieval systems effectively.

Sub-Competencies
1. Match an information need with the appropriate retrieval system.
2. Access principal on-line and other database health information resources.

Competency B
Establish effective consultative relationships with those requesting assistance in solving health-related problems.

Sub-Competencies
1. Analyze parameters of effective consultative relationships.
2. Describe special skills and abilities needed by health educators for consultation activities.
3. Formulate a plan for providing consultation to other health professionals.
4. Explain the process of marketing health education consultative services.

Competency C
Interpret and respond to requests for health information.

Sub-Competencies
1. Analyze general processes for identifying the information needed to satisfy a request.
2. Employ a wide range of approaches in referring requesters to valid sources of health information.

Competency D
Select effective educational resource materials for dissemination.

Sub-Competencies
1. Assemble educational material of value to the health of individuals and community groups.
2. Evaluate the worth and applicability of resource materials for given audiences.
3. Apply various processes in the acquisition of resource materials.
4. Compare different methods for distributing educational materials.

Responsibility VII—Communicating Health and Health Education Needs, Concerns, and Resources

Competency A
Interpret concepts, purposes, and theories of health education.

Sub-Competencies

1. Evaluate the state of the art of health education.
2. Analyze the foundations of the discipline of health education.
3. Describe major responsibilities of the health educator in the practice of health education.

Competency B
Predict the impact of societal value systems on health education programs.

Sub-Competencies

1. Investigate social forces causing opposing viewpoints regarding health education needs and concerns.
2. Employ a wide range of strategies for dealing with controversial health issues.

Competency C
Select a variety of communication methods and techniques in providing health information.

Sub-Competencies

1. Utilize a wide range of techniques for communicating health and health education information.
2. Demonstrate proficiency in communicating health information and health education needs.

Competency D
Foster communication between health care providers and consumers.

Sub-Competencies

1. Interpret the significance and implications of health care providers' messages to consumers.
2. Act as liaison between consumer groups and individuals and health care provider organizations.

APPENDIX E

Eta Sigma Gamma Chapters: Locations and Dates of Installation

Chapter	Location	Date of Installation
Alpha	Ball State University, Muncie, IN	1968
Beta	Eastern Kentucky University, Richmond, KY	1969
Gamma	California State University, Long Beach, CA	1970
Delta	California State University, San Diego, CA	1970
Epsilon	University of Maryland, College Park, MD	1970
Zeta	Trenton State College, Trenton, NJ	1970
Eta	Central Michigan University, Mt. Pleasant, MI	1970
Theta	University of Nebraska, Lincoln, NE	1972
Iota	University of Toledo, Toledo, OH	1973
Kappa	SUNY College of Cortland, Cortland, NY	1973
Lambda	Indiana State University, Terre Haute, IN	1974
Mu	Western Kentucky University, Bowling Green, KY	1974
Nu	Indiana University, Bloomington, IN	1974
Xi	Purdue University, West Lafayette, IN	1974
Omicron	Slippery Rock University, Slippery Rock, PA	1974
Pi	Western Illinois University, Macomb, IL	1974
Rho	Kent State University, Kent, OH	1974
Sigma	James Madison University, Harrisonburg, VA	1974
Tau	University of Illinois, Champaign-Urbana, IL	1975
Upsilon	Russell Sage College, Albany, NY	1975
Phi	University of Northern Colorado, Greely, CO	1976
Chi	University of Utah, Salt Lake City, UT	1976
Psi	Brigham Young University, Provo, UT	1976
Omega	Illinois State University, Normal, IL	1976
Alpha Alpha	Southern Illinois University, Carbondale, IL	1976
Alpha Beta	Eastern Kentucky University, Richmond, KY	1976
Alpha Gamma	California State University, Long Beach, CA	1976
Alpha Delta	Florida State University, Tallahassee, FL	1976
Alpha Epsilon	University of New Mexico, Albuquerque, NM	1977
Alpha Zeta*	California State University, Northridge, CA	1977
Alpha Eta	Texas Tech University, Lubbock, TX	1977
Alpha Theta	Adelphi University, Garden City, NY	1977
Alpha Iota	University of Southern Mississippi, Hattiesburg, MS	1977
Alpha Kappa	University of Central Arkansas, Conway, AK	1977
Alpha Lambda	University of Florida, Gainesville, FL	1977
Alpha Mu	University of Tennessee, Knoxville, TN	1978

Alpha Nu	University of North Carolina, Greensboro, NC	1978
Alpha Xi	Penn State University, University Park, MD	1978
Alpha Omicron	Temple University, Philadelphia, PA	1978
Alpha Pi	Texas A & M University, College Station, TX	1978
Alpha Rho	Montclair State University, Montclair, NJ	1978
Alpha Sigma	Arizona State University, Tempe, AZ	1978
Alpha Tau	Oregon State University, Corvallis, OR	1979
Alpha Upsilon	Central Washington University, Ellensburg, WA	1979
Alpha Phi	Texas Women's University, Denton, TX	1979
Alpha Chi	St. Francis College, Brooklyn, NY	1979
Alpha Psi	The Ohio State University, Columbus, OH	1980
Alpha Omega	University of Nebraska, Omaha, NE	1980
Beta Alpha	University of Minnesota, Duluth, MN	1980
Beta Beta*	University of South Carolina, Columbia, SC	1980
Beta Gamma	Bowling Green State University, Bowling Green, OH	1980
Beta Delta	Eastern Michigan University, Ypsilanti, MI	1980
Beta Epsilon	University of Maine, Farmington, ME	1980
Beta Zeta	Towson State University, Towson, MD	1980
Beta Eta	Sam Houston State University, Huntsville, TX	1980
Beta Theta	Easter Carolina University, Greenville, NC	1980
Beta Iota	Eastern Tennessee State University, Johnson City, TN	1980
Beta Kappa	Mankato State University, Mankato, MN	1981
Beta Lambda*	University of Oregon, Eugene, OR	1981
Beta Mu*	Northeastern University, Boston, MA	1981
Beta Nu	Eastern Illinois University, Charleston, IL	1982
Beta Xi	West Chester University, West Chester, PA	1982
Beta Omicron	Worcester State College, Worcester, MA	1982
Beta Pi*	University of Georgia, Athens, GA	1983
Beta Rho*	Louisiana State University, Baton Rouge, LA	1983
Beta Sigma	Wayne State University, Detroit, MI	1983
Beta Tau	University of Arkansas, Fayetteville, AK	1983
Beta Upsilon*	Texas A & I University, Kingsville, TX	1983
Beta Phi	University of Wisconsin, La Crosse, WI	1983
Beta Chi	University of Alabama—Birmingham, Birmingham, AL	1984
Beta Psi	State University of New York, Brockport, NY	1984
Beta Omega	New Mexico State University, Las Cruces, NM	1984
Gamma Alpha	Western Washington University, Bellingham, WA	1984
Gamma Beta	University of Richmond, Richmond, VA	1984
Gamma Gamma	Virginia Tech, Blacksburg, VA	1986
Gamma Delta	Southern Illinois University, Edwardsville, IL	1987
Gamma Zeta	Plymouth State University, Plymouth, NH	1988
Gamma Eta	University of Cincinnati, Cincinnati, OH	1988
Gamma Theta	Youngstown State University, Youngstown, OH	1991
Gamma Iota	Georgia College, Milledgeville, GA	1991
Gamma Kappa	Liberty University, Lynchberg, VA	1992
Gamma Lambda	University of Texas—El Paso, El Paso, TX	1993
Gamma Mu	Western Michigan University, Kalamazoo, MI	1993
Gamma Nu	University of Nevado—Reno, Reno, NV	1993
Gamma Xi	East Stroudsburg University, East Stroudsburg, PA	1995

Gamma Omicron	Springfield College, Springfield, MA	1995
Gamma Pi	Hofstra University, Hempstead, NY	1995
Gamma Rho	Truman State University, Kirksville, MO	1996
Gamma Sigma	Appalachian State University, Boone, NC	1996
Gamma Tau	University of North Texas, Denton, TX	1996
Gamma Upsilon	Georgia Southern University, Statesboro, GA	1996
Gamma Phi	North Carolina Central University, Durham, NC	1998
Gamma Chi	Clemson University, Clemson, SC	1997
Gamma Psi	Western Oregon State University, Monmouth, OR	1997
Gamma Omega	William Paterson College, Wayne, NJ	1997
Delta Alpha	Iowa State University, Ames, IA	1997
Delta Beta	University of Montana, Missoula, MT	1998
Delta Gamma	Cleveland State University, Cleveland, OH	1998
Delta Delta	California State University, San Bernardino, CA	1998

Source: Reprinted by permission of the National Office of Eta Sigma Gamma.

*These chapters were inactive at the time of this writing.

GLOSSARY

A New Perspective on the Health of Canadians the Canadian publication that presented the epidemiological evidence supporting the importance of lifestyle and environmental factors on health and sickness and called for numerous national health promotion strategies to encourage Canadians to become more responsible for their own health.

abstracts short summaries of research studies that have appeared in selected journals.

accreditation "the process by which a recognized professional body evaluates an entire college or university professional preparation program" (Cleary, 1995, p. 39) (Chapter 6).

action stage a stage of the transtheoretical model in which a person is overtly making changes.

adjusted rate a rate that is statistically adjusted for a certain characteristic such as age, expressed for a total population.

administrative and policy diagnosis "an analysis of the policies, resources and circumstances prevailing in an organizational situation to facilitate or hinder the development of the health promotion program" (Green & Kreuter, 1991, p. 429) (Chapter 4).

American Alliance for Health, Physical Education, Recreation and Dance (AAHPERD) a professional alliance of six national associations (American Association for Active Lifestyles and Fitness, American Association for Health Education, American Association for Leisure and Recreation, National Association for Girls and Womens Sports, National Association for Sport and Physical Education, National Dance Association) and six district associations (Central, Eastern, Midwest, Northwest, Southern, and Southwest).

American Association for Health Education (AAHE) a professional association within AAHPERD.

American College Health Association (ACHA) a professional association comprised mostly of individuals who work in colleges and universities.

American Public Health Association (APHA) a professional association for those individuals working in the fields of public health.

American Red Cross (ARC) a quasi-governmental organization.

American School Health Association (ASHA) a professional association comprised of individuals interested in coordinated school health programs.

Asclepiads a brotherhood of men associated with the Asclepian temples who first began the practice of medicine based on a more rational basis.

Asclepios the Greek god of medicine, for whom many temples were built.

Association for Worksite Health Promotion (AWHP) a professional association for those individuals employed in worksite settings or providing services to worksite settings.

Association of State and Territorial Directors of Health Promotion and Public Health Education (ASTDHPPHE) a professional association comprised of individuals who, by position, head their state or territory public health education efforts.

atomic theory Hippocrates' theory of disease causation.

attitude toward the behavior an attitude about a certain behavior; a construct of the theory of planned behavior.

bacteriological period of public health the period of 1875 to 1900, during which great advancements in the study of bacteria occurred.

behavioral capability the knowledge and skills necessary to perform a behavior.

behavioral diagnosis "delineation of the specific health-related actions that most likely effect, or could effect, a health outcome" (Green & Kreuter, 1991, p. 429).

behavior change philosophy involves a health educator using behavioral contracts, goal setting, and self-monitoring to help foster and motivate the modification of an unhealthy habit in an individual with whom the health educator is working.

beneficence "simply doing good" (Balog et al., 1985, p. 91) (Chapter 4).

benevolence see beneficence.

browser a software package used for exploring the World Wide Web—Netscape®, for example.

caduceus the serpent and staff symbol of medicine, which was the symbol of the Asclepian Temples.

certification "a process by which a professional organization grants recognition to an individual who, upon completion of a competency-based curriculum, can demonstrate a predetermined standard of performance" (Cleary, 1995, p. 39) (Chapter 6).

Certified Health Education Specialist (CHES) a health educator who has met all necessary requirements and has been certified by the National Commission for Health Education Credentialing, Inc.

chain of infection a model used to help explain the spread of a communicable disease from one host to another.

change process theories theories that focus on behavior change.

Coalition of National Health Education Organizations, USA (CNHEO) a coalition made up of representatives from eight professional associations, of which health educators are members.

code of ethics a written system of norms (or professional moral consensus, as some refer to it).

Code of Hammurabi the earliest written record concerning public health.

cognitive-based philosophy a philosophy that focuses on the acquisition of content and factual information to increase knowledge so a person is better equipped to make health-related decisions.

communicable disease "an illness caused by some specific biological agent or its toxic products that can be transmitted from an infected person, animal, or inanimate reservoir to a susceptible host" (McKenzie & Pinger, 1997, p. 84) (Chapter 1).

communicable disease model a model used to help explain the spread of a communicable disease from one host to another via the elements of agent, host, and environment.

community health "both private and public efforts of individuals, groups, and organizations to promote, protect, and preserve the health of those in the community" (McKenzie & Pinger, 1997, p. 4) (Chapter 1).

community health education health education programs conducted in departments of health, voluntary agencies, hospitals, religious organizations, and so on.

competencies "reflects the ability of the student to understand, know, etc." (National Commission for Health Education Credentialing, Inc., 1996b, p. 12) (Chapter 6).

comprehensive school health instruction the development, delivery, and evaluation of a planned curriculum, preschool through 12, with goals, objectives, content sequence, and specific classroom lessons which include, but are not limited to the following major content areas: community health, consumer health, environmental health, family life, mental and emotional health, injury prevention and safety, nutrition, personal health, prevention and control of disease, and substance use and abuse (Joint Committee on Health Education Terminology, 1991a, p. 102)

computerized databases computerized storage disks containing a large compilation of references; each database is specific to a general subject area (e.g., education, medicine) and provides access to the cumulative information found in several index or abstract sources on that subject area.

conservative a person who generally distrusts governmental regulations and tax-supported programs for addressing social or economic problems.

concepts the primary elements, building blocks, or major components of theories.

consequentialism theories that evaluate the moral status of an act by looking at its consequences (White, 1988) (Chapter 5).

construct a concept that has been developed, created, or adopted for use with a specific theory.

contemplation stage a stage of the transtheoretical model in which a person is seriously thinking about change in the next six months.

coordinated school health program a coordinated and integrated school-based program to impact the health of students, faculty, staff, administration, and the community as a whole; this would include food services, nursing services, school counseling and psychology, health instruction, physical education, administration, school environment, community involvement, and faculty/staff wellness.

computerized databases computerized storage disks containing a large compilation of references; each database is specific to a general subject area (e.g., education, medicine) and provides access to the cumulative information found in several index or abstract sources on that subject area.

credentialing a process whereby an individual or a professional preparation program meets the specified standards established by the credentialing body and is thus recognized for having done so.

crude rate the rate expressed for a total population.

cue to action a construct of the health belief model that motivates a person to act.

cultural sensitivity having and showing respect for cultures other than one's own.

culturally competent having the knowledge and interpersonal skills to understand, appreciate, and work with individuals from cultures other than one's own; it involves an awareness and acceptance of cultural differences, self-awareness, knowledge of the culture of those in the target population, and the adaptation of professional skills to respond to the target population's cultural differences (McManus, 1988) (Chapter 1).

death rates the number of deaths per 100,000 resident population, sometimes referred to as mortality or fatality rates.

decision-making philosophy the belief that the use of scenarios, case studies, and simulated problems is the best method to motivate persons to adopt positive health behaviors.

demographic profile a statistical breakdown of the population of a country, region, state, or city by age group, sex, race, and ethnicity.

diffusion theory a theory that provides an explanation for the movement of an innovation through a population.

disability-adjusted life years (DALYs) a measure of health that takes into effect the severity of the health condition, age, and impact on the future.

discipline "a branch of knowledge or instruction" (Landau, 1979, p. 182) (Chapter 1).

early adopters a group of people who are very interested in innovation, but they do not want to be the first involved.

early majority a group of people who may be interested in an innovation but will need some external motivation to get involved.

eclectic health education philosophy a philosophical approach held by health educators that no one philosophy is "right" for all times and circumstances and that the best philosophy involves blending the various philosophical approaches or using different approaches depending on the setting (school, community, worksite).

ecological perspective a means of examining the influences on health-related behaviors and conditions via five levels: intrapersonal (individual) factors, interpersonal factors, institutional (organizational) factors, community factors, and public policy factors.

educational and organizational diagnosis the delineation of predisposing, reinforcing, and enabling factors.

emerging profession an occupation which does not rank so clearly high or so clearly low on the attributes that distinguish an occupation from a profession (Barber, 1988) (Chapter 1).

emotional-coping response to learn, a person must be able to deal with the sources of anxiety that surround a behavior.

EMPOWER an acronym for a computer program that stands for Expert Methods for Planning and Organization within Everyone's Reach.

empowerment "a social action process that promotes participation of people, organizations and communities in gaining control over their lives in their community and larger society. With this perspective, empowerment is not characterized as achieving power to dominate others, but rather power to act with others to affect change" (Wallerstein & Bernstein, 1988, p. 380) (Chapter 1).

enabling factor "any characteristic of the environment that facilitates action and any skill or resource required to attain a specific behavior" (Green & Kreuter, 1991, p. 431) (Chapter 4).

endemic occurs regularly in a population as a matter of course.

environment "all those matters related to health which are external to the human body and over which the individual has little or no control" (Lalonde, 1974, p. 32) (Chapter 1).

environmental diagnosis "a systematic assessment of factors in the social and physical environment that interact with behavior to produce health effects or quality-of-life outcomes" (Green & Kreuter, 1991, p. 432) (Chapter 4).

epidemic   an unexpectedly large number of cases of disease in a population.

epidemiological diagnosis   "the delineation of the extent, distribution, and causes of a health problem in a defined population" (Green & Kreuter, 1991, p. 431) (Chapter 4).

epidemiology   "the study of the distribution and determinants of diseases and injuries in human populations" (Mausner & Kramer, 1985, p. 1) (Chapter 1).

epistemology   the study of knowledge (Thiroux, 1995) (Chapter 1).

Eta Sigma Gamma (ESG)   the national health education honorary society.

ethical   good/bad, and right/wrong.

ethics   the study of morality, is one of the three major areas of philosophy, also referred to as moral philosophy, (Thiroux, 1995) (Chapter 5).

expectancies   values people place on expected outcomes.

expectations   beliefs about the likely outcomes of certain behaviors.

formalism (deontological or nonconsequential-ism)   "theories which look at the nature of the individual act and determine morality from whether that act is right or wrong in itself" (Mellert, 1995, p. 130) (Chapter 5).

freeing/functioning philosophy   proponents of this philosophy help the person make the best health choices possible for that person, based on the individual's needs and interests, not on societal expectations.

goodness (rightness)   a state or quality of being good; one of the five principles of common moral ground.

graduate teaching assistantship   an award given a graduate student who teaches for the program and in return is usually granted tuition assistance and a stipend.

graduate research assistantship   an award given a graduate student who works closely with one or more faculty members on a research project; the student is usually granted tuition assistance and a stipend in return for the work.

governmental health agencies   agencies designated as having authority for certain specific duties or tasks outlined by the governmental bodies that oversee them.

hard money   funds used to support health education positions and programs that are part of the regular budget of an employer.

health   "the state of complete mental, physical and social well being not merely the absence of disease or infirmity" (WHO, 1947) (Chapter 1).

health behavior   see lifestyle.

health belief model   an intrapersonal theory that "addresses a person's perceptions of the threat of a health problem and the accompanying appraisal of a recommended behavior for preventing or managing the problem" (Glanz & Rimer, 1995, p. 17).

health care organization   "consists of the quantity, quality, arrangement, nature and relationships of people and resources in the provision of health care" (Lalonde, 1974, p. 32), also referred to as the health care system.

health care settings   locations for health education programs, including public and for-profit hospitals, free-standing medical care clinics, home health agencies, and physician organizations such as health maintenance organizations (HMOs) and preferred provider organizations (PPOs).

health education   "any combination of learning experiences designed to facilitate voluntary adaptations of behavior conducive to health" (Green et al., 1980, p. 7) (Chapter 1).

health field   a term that includes all matters that affect health; far more encompassing than the health care system.

Health Field Concept   a framework that was developed in Canada to study health; it has four elements; human biology, environment, lifestyle, and health care organization.

health literacy   the capacity of individuals to access, interpret, and understand basic health information and services and the skills to use the information and services to promote health.

health promotion   "the combination of educational and environmental supports for actions and conditions of living conducive to health (Green & Kreuter, 1991, p. 4) (Chapter 1).

health promotion and disease prevention   "the aggregate of all purposeful activities designed to improve personal and public health through a combination of strategies, including the competent implementation of behavioral change strategies, health education, health protection measures, risk factor detection, health enhancement and health maintenance" (Joint Committee on Health Education Terminology, 1991a, p. 102) (Chapter 1).

Healthy People   the first major U.S. government document recognizing the importance of lifestyle in promoting health and well-being.

Healthy People 2000   a document that contains the health objectives for the United States during the 1990s.

Hippocrates   a Greek physician from the Asclepian tradition that eventually became known as the father of medicine.

holistic philosophy   the philosophy that the mind and body blend into a single unit; the person is a unified being.

home page   analogous to a combination of a cover and table of contents in a book, a home page names a specific web site and directs the user to options within that site.

human biology   "all those aspects of health, both physical and mental, which are developed within the human body as a consequence of the basic biology of man [sic] and the organic make-up of an individual" (Lalonde, 1974, p. 31) (Chapter 1).

humanism   a philosophy characterized by having a concern for humanity; it also promotes the basic premise of the worth of human life and that individuals can achieve self-fulfillment.

Hygeia   the daughter of Asclepios granted the power to prevent disease.

hypertext   a type of document that allows convenient links to other documents found on the World Wide Web; it is a simple way of cross-referencing words or phrases with additional information; words or symbols that appear in color are hypertext words, and clicking on them provides links to related documents in the field (Rivard & Olpin, 1998).

hypertext markup language   the programming language used on the Internet.

hypertext transfer protocol   the protocol for exchanging hypertext documents between sites on the web.

impact evaluation   "the assessment of program effects on intermediate objectives including changes in predisposing, enabling, and reinforcing factors, and behavioral and environmental changes" (Green & Kreuter, 1991, p. 432) (Chapter 4).

implementation   "the act of converting program objectives into actions through policy changes, regulation and organization" (Green & Kreuter, 1991, p. 432) (Chapter 4).

indexes   reference books that provide links to articles from many refereed journals, books, and selected reports; each index is written to target specific subject headings, so one index is not all-encompassing for all subjects.

individual freedom (equality principle, or principle of autonomy)   "people, being individuals with individual differences, must have the freedom to choose their own ways and means of being moral within the framework of the first four basic principles" (Thiroux, 1995, p. 187) (Chapter 5).

innovators   the first people to adopt an innovation.

International Union for Health Promotion and Education (IUHPE)   a professional association open to individuals who are interested in health education worldwide.

Internet   an integrated network of computers that spans the entire world; the computers can transfer data to one another via phone lines, microwaves, fiber optics, and satellites (Kittleson, 1997) (Chapter 9).

justice (fairness)   "human beings should treat other human beings fairly and justly in distributing goodness and badness among them" (Thiroux, 1995, p. 184) (Chapter 5); a basic principle of ethics.

laggards   the last group of people to get involved in an innovation, if they get involved at all.

late majority   a group of people who are skeptical and will not adopt an innovation until most people in the social system have done so.

liberal   generally, a person who favors governmental programs to address perceived social and economic inequities between segments of society.

licensure   "a process by which an agency or government (usually a state) grants permission to individuals to practice a given profession by certifying that those licensed have attained specific standards of competence" (Cleary, 1995, p. 39) (Chapter 6).

life expectancy   "the average number of years of life remaining to a person at a particular age and is based on a given set of age-specific death rates, generally the mortality conditions existing in the period mentioned. Life expectancy may be determined by race, sex, or other characteristics using age-specific death rates for the population with that characteristic" (NCHS, 1995, p. 287) (Chapter 1).

lifestyle "an aggregation of decisions by individuals which affect their health and over which they more or less have control" (Lalonde, 1974, p. 32) (Chapter 1).

likelihood of taking action chances that a person will behave in a particular way; a construct of the health belief model.

local health department a governmental organization that is located in a city or county.

locus of control one's perception of the center of control over reinforcement.

macrolevel having health education interventions targeted to the community as a whole, instead of to individuals.

maintenance the stage of the transtheoretical model in which a person is taking steps to sustain change and resist temptation to relapse.

Medicaid government health insurance for the poor.

Medicare government health insurance for the elderly and disabled.

mental health (termed *psychological health* by Goodstadt, Simpson, & Loranger, 1987) may include emotional health; may make explicit reference to intellectual capabilities; the subjective sense of well-being (Goodstadt, Simpson, & Loranger, 1987, p. 59) (Chapter 1).

metaphysics the study of the nature of reality (Thiroux, 1995) (Chapter 5).

miasmas theory a belief that vapors, or miasmas, rising from rotting refuse could travel through the air for great distances and result in disease when inhaled.

microlevel targeting health education interventions to individuals.

model a subclass of a theory.

moderate a person who acts in a more situationally specific manner in regard to using tax-supported programs to solve social problems.

modifiable risk factors changeable or controllable risk factors.

moral good/bad, and right/wrong.

moral philosophy see ethics.

M.P.H., M.Ed., M.S. degree designations available to master's-level health education students, depending on the institution they attend and their area of emphasis.

Multicausation disease model a model that explains the onset of disease caused by more than one factor.

National Commission for Health Education Credentialing, Inc. the organization that oversees the health education certification process.

National School Health Education Coalition (NaSHEC) a coalition of more than ninety associations and organizations that supports coordinated school health programs.

National Task Force on the Preparation and Practice of Health Educators the group that oversaw development of the roles and responsibilities of health educators and ultimately the CHES credentialing system.

networking establishing and maintaining a wide range of contacts in the field that may be of help when looking for a job and in carrying out one's job responsibilities once hired.

noncommunicable disease "disease that cannot be transmitted from infected host to susceptible host" (McKenzie & Pinger, 1997, p. 84) (Chapter 1).

nongovernmental health agencies agencies that "operate, for the most part, free from governmental interference as long as they meet Internal Revenue Service guidelines with regard to their tax status" (McKenzie & Pinger, 1997, p. 47) (Chapter 8).

nonmaleficence "the non-infliction of harm to others" (Balog et al., 1985, p. 91) (Chapter 5).

nonmodifiable risk factors nonchangeable or noncontrollable risk factors.

objective statement describing specific, measurable cognitive or affective changes in the learner. An objective establishes a performance standard for the learner.

outcome evaluation "assessment of the effects of the program on the ultimate objectives, including changes in health and social benefits or quality of life" (Green & Kreuter, 1991, p. 433) (Chapter 4).

ownership a feeling of responsibility for program outcomes.

Panacea the daughter of Asclepios granted the power to treat disease.

pandemic an outbreak of a disease over a wide geographical area, such as a continent.

participation the active involvement of those in the target population in helping identify, plan, and implement programs to address the health problems they face.

perceived barriers the cost of engaging in a health behavior; a construct of the health belief model.

perceived behavioral control a belief held by people that they have control over a behavior; a construct of the theory of planned behavior.

perceived benefits a belief that a particular health recommendation would be beneficial in reducing a perceived threat; a construct of the health belief model.

perceived seriousness/severity a belief that a health problem is serious; a construct of the health belief model.

perceived susceptibility a belief that one is vulnerable to a health problem; a construct of the health belief model.

perceived threat a belief that one is vulnerable to a serious health problem or to the sequelae of that illness or condition; a construct of the health belief model.

philanthropic foundations endowed institutions that donate money for the good of humankind (McKenzie & Pinger, 1998, p. 679) (Chapter 8).

philosophy a statement summarizing the attitudes, principles, beliefs, values, and concepts held by an individual or a group.

philosophy of symmetry a philosophy of health with physical, emotional, spiritual, and social components of health.

physical health the absence of disease and disability; functioning adequately from the perspective of physical and physiological abilities; the biological integrity of the individual (Goodstadt, Simpson, & Loranger, 1987, p. 59) (Chapter 1).

popular press publications publications ranging from weekly summary magazines (e.g., *Newsweek*) to monthly magazines (e.g., *Better Homes and Gardens*); often, articles include editorials; information from these sources should be heavily scrutinized before using.

postmodern family any family structure that differs from a family composed of two parents and their children.

postsecondary institution in the United States, an institution that provides further education after high school.

PRECEDE-PROCEED an acronym for a theory of implementation than stands for Predisposing, Reinforcing, and Enabling Constructs in Educational/Environmental Diagnosis and Evaluation and Policy, Regulatory, and Organizational Constructs in Educational and Environmental Development.

precontemplation stage the stage of the transtheoretical model in which a person is not thinking about change in the next six months.

predisposing factor "any characteristic of a person or population that motivates behavior prior to the occurrence of the behavior" (Green & Kreuter, 1991, p. 434) (Chapter 4).

preparation stage the stage of the transtheoretical model in which a person is actively planning change.

prevention the planning for and measures taken to forestall the onset of, limit the spread of, and rehabilitate after pathogenesis or other health problems.

primary data original data gathered by the health educator as part of a needs assessment; this includes data gathered from telephone surveys, focus groups, and interviews.

primary prevention preventive measures that forestall the onset of illness or injury during the prepathogenesis period.

primary sources published studies or eyewitness accounts written by the person(s) who actually conducted the study or observed the event.

process evaluation "the assessment of policies, materials, personnel, performance, quality of practice or services, and other inputs and implementation experiences" (Green & Kreuter, 1991, p. 434) (Chapter 4).

profession "the sociological construct for an occupation that has special status" (Livingood, 1996, p. 421) (Chapter 1).

professional health associations/organizations organizations that promote the high standards of professional practice for their respective professions, thereby improving the health of society by improving the people in the professions (McKenzie & Pinger, 1997) (Chapter 8).

Promoting Health/Preventing Disease: Objectives for the Nation a document containing 226 health objectives for the United States to be accomplished during the 1980s.

public health "the sum of all official (governmental) efforts to promote, protect, and preserve the people's health" (McKenzie & Pinger, 1997, p. 4) (Chapter 1).

public health agencies   also called "official governmental health agencies"; agencies usually financed through public tax monies and typically offering health promotion and education programs.

quasi-governmental health agencies   agencies that possess some of the characteristics of a governmental health agency but also possess some of the characteristics of nongovernmental agencies.

rate   "a measure of some event, disease, or condition in relation to a unit of population, along with some specification of time" (NCHS, 1995, p. 292) (Chapter 1).

reciprocal determinism   behavior changes result from an interaction between the person and the environment; change is bidirectional (Glanz & Rimer, 1995) (Chapter 4).

reduction of threat   a belief that a particular health recommendation would be beneficial in reducing a threat at a subjectively acceptable cost; a construct of the health belief model.

refereed journal   a journal that publishes original manuscripts only after they have been read and critiqued by a panel of experts in the field.

reinforcement   a response to behavior that increases the chance of recurrence.

reinforcing factor   "any reward or punishment following or anticipated as a consequence of a behavior, serving to strengthen the motivation for the behavior after it occurs" (Green & Kreuter, 1991, p. 434) (Chapter 4).

responsibilities   the seven major responsibilities of all entry-level health educators.

risk factors   inherited, environmental, and behavioral influences "capable of provoking ill health with or without previous disposition" (USDHEW, 1979, p. 13) (Chapter 1).

role delineation   the process of identifying the specific responsibilities, competencies, and sub-competencies associated with the practice of health education.

school health education   health education programs that instruct school-age children about health and health-related behaviors.

School Health Education Evaluation Study   a landmark study that examined the entire health program of selected schools in the Los Angeles area.

School Health Education Study   a nationwide study that examined the status of health education and resulted in the development of an important curriculum.

search engine   site on the World Wide Web specifically designed to search for all links associated with a word or phrase that the user wants information on; the search engines greatly decrease the time it takes to search for information on the web; examples are Yahoo®, Alta Vista®, and Hotbot®.

secondary data   pre-existing data used by a health educator in a needs assessment.

secondary prevention   preventive measures that lead to early diagnosis and prompt treatment of a disease or an injury to limit disability, impairment, or dependency and to prevent more severe pathogenesis.

secondary sources   articles that often provide an overview or a summary of several related studies or that chronicle the history of several related events, written by someone who did not conduct the study or observe first-hand the event that is written about.

self-control (self-regulation)   gaining control over one's own behavior by monitoring and adjusting it.

self-efficacy   people's confidence in their ability to perform a certain desired task or function.

social change philosophy   a philosophy emphasizing the role of health education in creating social, economic, and political change that benefits the health of individuals and groups.

social diagnosis   "the process of determining people's perceptions of their own needs or quality of life, and their aspirations for the common good, through broad participation and application of multiple information-gathering activities designed to expand understanding of the community" (Green & Kreuter, 1991, p. 45) (Chapter 4).

social ecology   an approach to health education that goes beyond individual behavior change to examine and modify the social, political, and economic factors impacting health behavior decisions.

social health   the ability to interact effectively with other people and the social environment; satisfying interpersonal relationships; role fulfillment.

Society for Public Health Education, Inc. (SOPHE)   a professional association for health educators.

Society of State Directors of Health, Physical Education, and Recreation (SSDHPER) a professional association comprised of individuals who, by position in a state/territorial department of education, represent their state/territory.

soft money funds to support health education positions and programs secured through grants or contracts, which may be discontinued at the end of a designated period.

Smith Papyri the oldest written document related to health, which describes various surgical techniques and dates back to 1600 B.C.

specific rate a rate for a particular population subgroup, such as for a particular disease (i.e., disease-specific) or for a particular age of people (i.e., age-specific) (Mausner & Kramer, 1985) (Chapter 1).

spiritual health a form of health associated with the concept of self-actualization; it sometimes reflects a concern for issues related to one's value system; alternatively, it may be concerned with a belief in a transcending unifying force (whether its basis is in nature, scientific law, or a godlike source) (Goodstadt, Simpson, & Loranger, 1987, p. 59) (Chapter 1).

sub-competencies "reflects the ability of the student to list, describe, etc." (National Commission for Health Education Credentialing, Inc. 1996b, p. 12) (Chapter 6).

subjective norm a belief held by people that others (individuals or groups) think they should do something and that they care about what others think; a construct of the theory of planned behavior.

technology any device used by society to increase access to or opportunity for people to be exposed to that device—for example, computers and television have increased educational access and opportunities for many people; thus, they are examples of technology.

tertiary prevention preventive measures aimed at rehabilitation following significant pathogenesis.

theories/models of implementation theories and models used in planning, implementing, and evaluating health education/promotion programs.

theory "a set of interrelated concepts, definitions, and propositions that presents a systematic view of events or situations by specifying relations among variables in order to explain and predict the events of the situations" (Glanz, Lewis, & Rimer, 1997, p. 21) (Chapter 4).

theory of planned behavior an intrapersonal theory that addresses individuals' intentions to perform a given behavior as a function of their attitude toward performing the behavior, their beliefs about what is relevant, what others think they should do, and their perception of the ease or difficulty in performing the behavior.

traditional family a family having two parents and their children.

transtheoretical model also known as the stages of change model, is an intrapersonal theory that addresses an "individual's readiness to change or attempt to change toward healthy behaviors" (Glanz & Rimer, 1995a, p. 17).

truth telling (honesty) to tell the truth; one of the five principles of common moral ground.

Uniform Resource Locators (URL) identifiers for each site on the World Wide Web; specify locations, or addresses.

value of life a basic principle of ethics: no life should be ended without very strong justification.

variable the operational (practical use) form of a construct.

voluntary health agencies "agencies that are created by concerned citizens to deal with health needs not met by governmental agencies" (McKenzie & Pinger, 1998, p. 684) (Chapters 7 and 8); these organizations rely heavily on volunteer help and donations to function.

wellness "an integrated method of functioning which is oriented toward maximizing the potential of which the individual is capable, within the environment where he [sic] is functioning" (Dunn, 1977, p. 9) (Chapter 1 and 3).

worksite health promotion health promotion and education programs offered by business and industry for their employees.

World Wide Web an interactive information delivery service that includes a repository of resources about most subjects; documents are related by subject area and linked together, thus creating a "web" (Larsson, 1996) (Chapter 9).

years of potential life lost (YPLL) a measure of premature mortality calculated by subtracting a person's age at death from seventy-five years.

CREDITS

Figure 1.1: From S.G. Deeds and M.J. Cleary, and B.L. Neiger (Eds.), *The Certified Health Education Specialist: A Self-Study Guide for Professional Competency,* 2nd ed., 1996. Copyright © The National Commission for Health Education Credentialing, Inc., Allentown, PA; **Figure 1.4:** From J.F. McKenzie and R.R. Pinger, *An Introduction to Community Health,* 1997. Sudbury, MA: Jones and Bartlett Publishers.www.jbpub. com. Reprinted with permission; **Figure 1.5:** From J.F. McKenzie and R.R. Pinger, *An Introduction to Community Health,* 1997. Sudbury, MA: Jones and Bartlett Publishers. www.jbpub.com. Reprinted with permission.

Quotes pp. 76, 78–79: From Eta Sigma Gamma Monograph Series, Volume 11(2) 1993. Copyright © Eta Sigma Gamma. Reprinted by permission. **Box 3.1:** Reprinted by permission of Kristy L. Jones, Health Education Specialist/Cancer Prevention and Control Supervisor, Idaho Department of Health and Welfare, Boise, ID.

Figure 4.1: From *Health Promotion Planning: An Educational and Environmental Approach,* Second Edition by L.W. Green & M.W. Kreuter. Copyright © 1991 by Mayfield Publishing Company. Reprinted by permission of the publisher; **Figure 4.2:** From *Introduction to Health Education,* by I.J. Bates and A.E. Winder. Copyright © 1984 by Mayfield Publishing Company. Reprinted by permission of the publisher; **Figure 4.4:** From E. Eng, "Room With a View for a Change." Keynote address to the 1997 Annual Meeting of the National Society of Public Health Education, Indianapolis, IN; **Figure 4.5:** From M. H. Becker, R.H. Drachman, & J.P. Kirscht, "A New Approach to Explaining Sick-role Behavior in Low Income Populations" in *American Journal of Public Health* 64, March, 1974. Copyright © 1974 American Public Health Association; **Figure 4.6:** From J. O. Prochaska, et al., "The Transtheoretical Model of Change and HIV Prevention: A Review" in *Health Education Quarterly,* 24(4), pp. 471–486. Copyright

© 1994 by Sage Publications. Reprinted by Permission of Sage Publications; **Figure 4.7:** From I. Ajzen, *Attitudes, Personality, and Behavior,* 1998, Dorsey Press. Copyright © 1988 Open University Press. Reprinted by permission; **Figure 4.8:** Adapted with the permission of The Free Press, a Division of Simon & Schuster from *Diffusion of Innovations,* Fourth Edition by Everett M. Rogers. Copyright © 1995 by Everettt M. Rogers. Copyright © 1962, 1971, 1983 by The Free Press.

Box 5.1: Reprinted by permission of John Jeffrey Barber, Health Educator, Indiana Dept. of Education, 251 E. Ohio St., State House, Rm. 229, Indianapolis, IN 46204-2798.

Box 6.1: Reprinted with permission from the Society for Public Health Education, Washington, DC; and American Association for Health Education.

Box 7.1: Reprinted by permission of Gretchen L. Anderson, Elementary Teacher, Pocatello, ID School District #25; **Box 7.2:** Reprinted by permission of Lisa Koslovsky, Youth Specialist, American Red Cross; **Box 7.3:** Reprinted by permission of Kimberly Jones, Health Education, Delaware County Health Department, Muncie, IN; **Box 7.4:** Reprinted by permission of Robert Pabst, Health/Fitness Technician, Tri-Health, Preventive Health Systems; **Box 7.5:** Reprinted by permission of Jill Sinclair Hopkins, Franciscan Health System of the Ohio Valley, Inc.

Box 8.1: Reprinted by permission of Cathy Nickels, Cancer Control Manager, Marion County (IN) Health Department; **Figure 8.1:** Reprinted by permission of the National Office of Eta Sigma Gamma.

Box 9.1: Reprinted by permission of Jenny J. Bair, Peer Education and Healthy Lifestyle Center Coordinator, Idaho State University, Department of Health & Nutrition Sciences; **Figure 9.2:** Text and artwork copyright © 1998 by Yahoo! Inc. All rights reserved. YAHOO! and the YAHOO! logo are trademarks of YAHOO! Inc; **Figure 9.3:** Text and artwork copyright © 1998 by Yahoo! Inc. All rights reserved. YAHOO! and the YAHOO! logo are trademarks of YAHOO! Inc.

Box 10.1: Reprinted by permission of Joanne Mitten, Chief, Bureau of Health Promotion, Idaho Department of Health and Welfare, Boise, ID.

Appendix A: Reprinted with permission from the Society for Public Health Education, Inc. Washington, DC.

Appendix B: Reprinted with permission from the Society for Public Health Education, Inc. Washington, DC.

Appendix C: This article is reprinted with permission from the *Journal of Health Education,* July/August, 1994, Vol. 25, No. 4, pp. 197–200. The *Journal of Health Education* is a publication of the American Alliance for Health, Physical Education, Recreation and Dance, 1900 Association Drive, Reston, Virginia 20191.

Appendix D: From *A Competency-Based Framework for Professional Development of Certified Health Education Specialists,* NCHEC, New York, 1996.

Appendix E: Reprinted by permission of the National Office of Eta Sigma Gamma.

INDEX

Page numbers followed by a *t* indicate tables;
italic page numbers indicate illustrations.

NCHEC. *See* National Commission for Health Education Credentialing
Neoplasms, malignant, 23
New Perspective on Health of Canadians, 56
NHANES. *See* National Health and Nutrition Examination Survey
Nineteenth century, health practices in, 48–49
Noncommunicable disease, 21
Nongovernmental health agencies, 192–213
Nonmaleficence, ethics and, 121
Nonmodifiable risk factors, 20
Nonresearch-based sources, accuracy of, evaluating, 222–223
Nontraditional health education positions, 185–186

On-line search services, 245

PAHO. *See* Pan American Health Organization
Pan American Health Organization, 192
Panacea, 37
Pandemic, public health and, 27
Pasteur, Louis, contribution of, 49
Philanthropic foundations, 194
Philanthropy, defined, 194
Philosophy
benefit of, 73–75
defined, 71–73
in health education, 82–85
moral, 118
Physical Education Index, 226
Physical health, defined, 7
Placement centers, use of, 187
Plague
bubonic. *See* Black Death
cause of, 44–45
health boards, 47

Planned behavior, theory of, 107, *108*
Planning models, 92–100
Pneumonia, as public health issue, 23
Political activity, of health educators, 249
Political climate, change in, 248–249
Postmodern family, 246
Practicums, planning, 187
PRECEDE-PROCEED model, 94–95
Precontemplation stage of change, 105
Preparation stage of change, 106
Priesthood, role in healing arts, in Greece, 37
Primary data, in assessment procedure, 148
Primary prevention, 18
Primary sources of data, 218
Profession
defined, 3
obligations to, ethics and, 129
Professional associations, joining, 187
Professional health associations, 194–213, 200–201t
joining, 213–214
Professional preparation, changes in, 250–254
Professionals
clients, obligations between, ethics and, 128
employers, obligations between, ethics and, 129
Program accreditation, 145–146
Program planning, model for, generalized, 98–100, *100*
Promoting Health/Preventing Disease: Objectives for Nation, 5, 57
Promotion and Education, 225
Psychological Abstracts, 227, 229

Psychological health, defined, 7
Public health
defined, 9
in United States, 50–59
Public health agencies, 167
Public health education, 165–170
advantages, disadvantages of working in, 171
sources of employment, 168
Public Health Reports, 225

Quarantine, to control disease, 50
Quasi-governmental health agencies, 191–192

Ransdell Act, 55–56
Religious groups, impact of, 194
Renaissance, health practices in, 45–48
Report of Sanitary Commission of Massachusetts, 51–53
Report on Inquiry into Sanitary Conditions of Labouring Population of Great Britain, 49
Report on Sanitary Commission of Massachusetts, 60
Research article
components of, identifying, 220
reading of, 221–222
Research assistantship, graduate school, 156
Resource in Education, 227
Resource persons, in health education, 150–151
Responsibilities, of health educators, 146–152
Risk factors, 20–21
modifiable, 20
Role delineation, 140
history of, 139–142
Romans, health practices, 41–42
Royalty, hygiene among, during Renaissance, 46